Psychiatric Primary Care

Psychiatric Primary Care

Linda Denise Oakley, RN, PhD, CS
Assistant Professor
School of Nursing
University of Wisconsin—Madison
Madison, Wisconsin

Claudette Potter, RN, MS, CS
Clinical Nurse Specialist
St. Mary's Hospital and Medical Center
Madison, Wisconsin

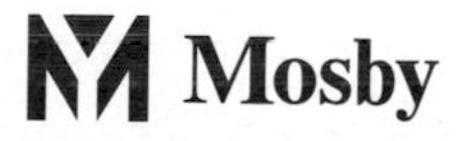

St. Louis Baltimore Boston Carlsbad Chicago Naples New York
Philadelphia Portland London Madrid Mexico City Singapore
Sydney Tokyo Toronto Wiesbaden

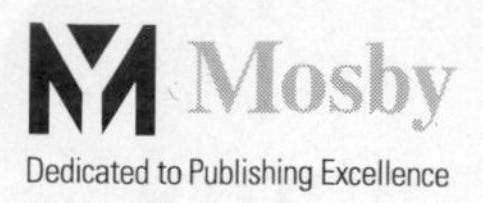

A Times Mirror
Company

Vice President and Publisher: Nancy L. Coon
Editor: Jeff Burnham
Developmental Editor: Linda Caldwell
Project Manager: Gayle Morris
Designer: Dave Zielinski
Manufacturing Manager: Karen Boehme

A NOTE TO THE READER:
The author and publisher have made every attempt to check dosages and nursing content for accuracy. Because the science of pharmacology is continually advancing, our knowledge base continues to expand. Therefore we recommend that the reader always check product information for changes in dosage or administration before administering any medication. This is particularly important with new or rarely used drugs.

Printed in the United States of America

Mosby-Year Book, Inc.
11830 Westline Industrial Drive, St. Louis, Missouri 63146

International Standard Book Number: 0-8151-7310-5

97 98 99 00 01 / 9 8 7 6 5 4 3 2 1

Reviewers

Frances Jane Lingenfelter Smith, MSN, RN, CSN
Clinical Nurse Specialist
Assistant Professor of Nursing
Psychiatric Mental Health Nursing
Department of Nursing
Lamar University
Beaumont, Texas

Jane L. Hill Burson, MS, MSN, CNS, RNC
Assistant Professor
School of Nursing
Northeast Louisana University
Monroe, Louisana

Preface

Why ***psychiatric*** primary care?

Psychiatric primary care is the assessment and management of common, mental disorders and psychosocial problems that may not require specialized psychiatric care. At a time when there is a growing public need and demand for accessible, skilled, mental health care (Arean and Miranda, 1996), hard hitting health care reforms and managed care strategies have effectively decreased access to specialized psychiatric care services. Under these "do more with less" health care objectives there can be no doubt that only those individuals who require specialized psychiatric care will be referred by a practitioner to a specialist. Most people will receive mental health care as a routine component of their primary care or, as defined here, psychiatric primary care.

Today, over half of the people who seek health care for mental disorders are treated by primary care practitioners (Gonzales, Magruder, and Keith, 1994). In order to effectively meet the mental health care needs of primary care patients, practitioners must be well grounded in basic mental health concepts, mental health care skills, and the application of interpersonal communication skills. Effective psychiatric primary care practice requires that practitioners have skills in interpersonal assessment, focused interviewing, and counseling.

With these practice needs in mind, we have developed a book for primary care practitioners that presents everything from basic mental concepts and terms to clinical examples of psychiatric primary care. *Part I, Mental Health Basics*, covers basic mental health concepts and mental health care skills, in a concise and informative manner. The last chapter of this section covers conditions of severe mental illness (SMI) that require specialized psychiatric care because of the potential risk of long-term disability. *Part II, Common Mental Disorders*, covers depression, stress, anxiety, substance abuse, and eating disorders—the mental disorders that practitioners are most likely to encounter in primary care settings. Each chapter in this section presents what we hope will be helpful information in terms of the assessment, counsel ing, prescribing, consultation, and referral aspects of each disorder.

In *Part III, Psychosocial Problems*, a range of psychosocial problems that practitioners routinely encounter are presented. Although these problems are common, effective intervention requires a clear understanding of how individuals may experience such problems. When faced with these problems, no two people will experience or express their distress in the same way. Therefore this section offers a focused discussion of common psychosocial problems and related needs. The section begins with an overview of the basics of psychosocial functioning and includes chapters on psychosocial problems related to sexuality, death and divorce, pain, and spiritual distress.

Because of their unique needs, children, adolescents, elders, survivors of trauma, individuals who may be suicidal, and those who experience partner violence are covered as special populations in *Part IV, Special Populations and Problems*. These populations are unique in that although they are vulnerable to the common mental disorders and psychosocial problems covered in the previous sections the disorders and problems are more likely to be experienced in ways that may require unique treatment approaches.

Part V, Practice Notes, covers two critical aspects of practice, mental health care laws and patient rights, and three of the most serious problems encountered in practice. The final chapter is a series of clinical examples intended to highlight important characteristics and symptoms of SMI and common mental disorders.

Although this book is intended to be helpful to primary care practitioners who may be less experienced in the assessment and management of common mental disorders and psychosocial problems, clinical specialists, physicians, midwives, social workers, nursing students, medical students, and physician assistants may also find this book to be a useful reference. As the reader will observe, our fundamental assumption is that the practice of psychiatric primary care requires the same purposeful attention to detail that is required in the practice of physical primary care. With this goal in mind we hope practitioners will find this book to be user-friendly, jargon-free, and informative.

Linda Denise Oakley
Claudette Potter

References

Arean PA, Miranda J: Do primary care patients accept psychological treatments? *Gen Hosp Psychiatry 16(1):22, 1996.*

Gonzales JJ, Magruder KM, Keith SJ. Mental disorders in primary care services: an update, *Public Health Reports* 109(2):251, 1994.

Brief Contents

Detailed Contents

Psychiatric Primary Care

Part I

Mental Health Basics

Mental Health Concepts 1

This chapter presents a brief overview of six basic concepts that are referred to throughout this book: mental health promotion, mental illness prevention, severe mental illness, mental disorders, psychosocial problems, and coping. Psychiatric primary care is, in large part, the practice of mental health promotion and mental illness prevention with primary care patient populations. Practitioners can expect to assess, diagnosis, and treat a range of mental disorders and psychosocial problems, which are defined in this chapter, but they should also have a clear understanding of severe mental illness and its effect on functioning and well-being. Coping is defined and presented with examples that clarify this common but often misunderstood concept.

Mental Health Promotion

Mental health cannot be defined in absolute terms. Generally, mental health is characterized by positive evidence of progressive, biopsychosocial development and adaptive biopsychosocial functioning. Clinical assessment findings demonstrate that the person has learned to effectively handle everyday biological, psychological, and social demands and is able to interact with other individuals and various physical environments in ways that support and strengthen the person.

Mental health promotion is defined simply as actions taken that maintain or improve mental health. Improvement, as it relates to mental health promotion, varies from person to person and is subject to developmental and situational factors. Given these variations, improvement is most reliably indicated by evidence of significant and positive changes in self-concept, self-esteem, day-to-day functioning, and the ability to effectively use support resources.

Keeping these clinical indicators of mental health and improvement in mind, practitioners must also consider each patient's less tangible, but sometimes more reliable, personal definitions. For many, mental health means achieved personal satisfaction and personal security. In effect, achievement acts as a precursor to the experience of feelings of satisfaction or security. When clinical and personal definitions of mental health are identified, the practitioner and patient have a basis for working together to reach shared goals.

Mental Illness Prevention

Mental illness prevention is the process of defining the mental disorders or psychosocial problems to which a person is susceptible, determining the basis of that susceptibility, and then taking action to decrease the person's susceptibility. Susceptibility to mental disorders and psychosocial problems is related to each individual's unique set of personal, situational, and developmental risk factors. Once identified, these risk factors become the target of actions aimed at preventing or minimizing the experience of mental disorders or psychosocial problems. As conceptualized here, risk assessment is the key to prevention.

Personal risk factors are specific characteristics, states, or traits that increase the probability that a person will experience a mental disorder or psychosocial problem. ***Situational risk factors*** are specific characteristics of a situation or circumstances the person is currently experiencing or has experienced. ***Developmental risk factors*** are specific, age-related characteristics. A range of personal, situational, and developmental risk factors are identified for each of the mental disorders and psychosocial problems reviewed in this book.

Risk factors are not generic predictors of mental disorders or psychosocial problems. Two people with identical risk factors may not have the identical risk level. Risk factors are contextual and at best indicate the probability of a mental disorder or psychosocial problem within a limited time period or set of circumstances. Changes in time and circumstances can significantly alter probability. Thus, risk factors used as generic predictors become meaningless stereotypes rather than important personal, situational, and developmental characteristics. Poverty, for example, is a strong situational and developmental risk factor, yet all impoverished people do not have the same probability of developing the same mental disorders or psychosocial problems within a given period of time.

The goal of mental illness prevention is to determine what risk factors are important for a particular person at a particular time, what specific mental disorder or psychosocial problem is related to those factors, and what actions can be taken to decrease the probability that this person will experience the specified disorder or problem. Despite the importance of risk-factor assessment and mental illness prevention, practitioners ***must remember*** that although mental disorders and psychosocial problems may be anticipated, this does not mean that disorders can be predicted or prevented. Survivors of trauma, abuse, violence, and disaster, for example, are at risk for experiencing multiple mental disorders and psychosocial problems. Yet some people are able to survive traumatic experiences intact and, once their safety is reestablished, are able to continue their lives with good mental health; many others are not so fortunate. The serious effects of trauma should not be confused with the failure of mental illness prevention measures. With trauma, the goal of prevention is to decrease the probability that the traumatic experience will generate chronic or long-term disorders or problems (Sartorius, 1993).

Severe Mental Illness

Severe mental illness (SMI) is the appropriate term for diseases that have a primary and profound effect on brain structure and function. The effect of SMI is manifested in high numbers of symptoms, prolonged symptom duration, and extreme symptom intensity. SMIs such as schizophrenia and bipolar disorder strike entire families, but currently it is impossible to predict who in the family will or will not develop the illness. Despite many advances in the science of observing and measuring human brain functions, we remain far from being able to map or predict SMI. Until then the thinking, feeling, behaving mind is a useful construct for understanding severe mental illness.

Changes in brain structure and function caused by SMI produce devastating transformations in a person's thoughts, feelings, and behaviors. For periods of time ranging from minutes to years, the person with SMI may experience the inability to distinguish the real from the unreal; his or her feelings can become vacant, overwhelming, or disembodied; behavior can become odd, absent, or excessive. For the affected person, SMI feels like a cold, lonely journey to a strange place. To significant others, SMI takes away the person's identity.

SMI is a diminishing and demoralizing experience. Without specialized psychiatric care, long-term biopsychosocial deterioration can occur. In the past, patients with SMI, particularly schizophrenia, were removed from society and required to live out their lives in secluded state hospitals. Now, with improved diagnosis and treatment, many people with SMI live and work in their communities. The requisite treatment goals for SMI are to produce symptom remission as quickly as possible, prevent chronic distress and disability, and promote and maintain the highest possible level of functioning. If there has been an extended period of stable functioning and symptom remission, some people may require only basic mental health care. Primary health care and basic mental health care needs can be met in primary care settings but resources should always be available for an unexpected or acute need for specialized psychiatric care.

Mental Disorders

The *Diagnostic and Statistical Manual of Mental Disorders, fourth edition* (DSM-IV) (American Psychiatric Association, 1994) defines mental disorders according to ***symptom criteria***. Symptom assessment criteria are the nature of each symptom and the total number, intensity, and duration of those symptoms. Based on symptom criteria, the person's symptoms either meet or fail to meet the criteria for a DSM-IV diagnosis. DSM-IV mental disorders may also be assessed in terms of the person's actual ***condition*** relative to the symptoms. Condition is expressed in a general statement of mild, moderate, or severe. When a person who has been diagnosed as having a DSM-IV diagnosis no longer meets the DSM-IV criteria for the diagnosis, the person's condition is subclinical and is specified as ***partial remission***, ***full remission***, or ***prior history***.

Full remission may or may not indicate that treatment is no longer required. For some people, full remission is contingent upon long-term or maintenance treatment. With some mental disorders, such as depression or substance abuse, residual symptoms, symptom recurrence, and full clinical relapse following full remission are common, and preventive treatment may be required. Practitioners should refer to DSM-IV guidelines for the recommended use of the term "full remission," with and without maintenance treatment. Practitioners should use the term "prior history" when symptoms no longer meet DSM-IV diagnostic criteria without maintenance or prevention therapy.

In primary care, there is always the potential of overmedicating when treating mental disorders, but undertreatment continues to be more common. Undertreatment typically takes one of two forms: inadequate medication (dose and duration) or the attempt to confirm a person's need for medication by "waiting to see" if it is needed. A cautious response is appropriate if symptoms are vague or confusing; however, the DSM-IV does not allow for a great deal of symptom ambiguity. Additional symptom information may be necessary, but more ***information*** should not be defined as more ***time***. The time criteria for DSM-IV disorders are clearly stated. Often more time only produces more symptoms or worse symptoms, not more information.

Practitioners should not overlook emotional pain when reviewing symptoms. Even mild symptoms can cause severe emotional pain. Practitioners should rely on DSM-IV symptom criteria to diagnose DSM-IV mental disorders but also take into account the experience of related emotional pain.

Psychosocial Problems

Compared to SMIs and mental disorders, psychosocial problems are common. A DSM-IV diagnosis of a psychosocial problem should be made when a person has experienced a stressor (demand or need) that cannot be ignored and his or her response to that stressor is maladaptive or ineffective. Stressors may be internal (e.g., negative thoughts) or external (e.g., discrimination). A complete DSM-IV diagnosis of a psychosocial problem should include both the stressor (e.g., partner conflict) that precipitated the person's response and the person's response to the stressor (e.g., anxiety).

Unlike SMIs or mental disorders, there are no specific types of DSM-IV psychosocial problems or diagnostic criteria. Psychosocial problems are stated in terms of the most relevant psychosocial context for the stressor and the response. The DSM-IV defines the following contexts for psychosocial problems: relational, academic, occupational, identity, religious/spiritual, acculturation, and phase of life. Once the problem is diagnosed, improvement should be defined as significant and positive change in both the stressor and the person's response to it. Both sides of the psychosocial-problem equation should be addressed.

The fact that a psychosocial problem can be diagnosed does not automatically mean that practitioners can, or are expected to, resolve it. The goal must always be improvement. The practice of primary care is sufficiently challenging without adding psychosocial problem resolution as an expected outcome. Still, practitioners should not view psychosocial problems as unimportant or unrelated to health and well-being. The practitioner may not only be an appropriate source of help for the patient, but the ***only*** source of help. Psychosocial problems that can be improved with basic mental health care are reviewed in Part III.

Coping

Understanding the concept of coping is fundamental to the practice of basic and specialized mental health care. Of the many theoretical and investigational definitions of coping the classic definition offered by Lazarus, Averill, and Opton (1974) is noted here. *Coping is a continuous process of appraisal and mastery that is influenced by personal and situational factors.* Appraisal predicts coping. People routinely take an accounting of their lived experiences. This accounting involves two or three steps that occur almost simultaneously. The first, ***primary appraisal***, is the determination of whether an experience is harmful, beneficial, irrelevant, or some combination thereof. The second appraisal is the ***determination of options***. Thus, coping is the process of defining an experience and the necessary response.

In basic mental health care a third step, ***reappraisal***, is also important. Reappraisal is reconsideration of the experience. For example, a harmful experience can be reappraised as a beneficial experience. Coping is the ultimate outcome of the entire process: it is everything that makes up the response from the primary appraisal to the reappraisal and can be simplified as actions (external) and thoughts (internal). People develop a pattern or style of coping because this allows for predictable responses. In addition to style, coping is significantly influenced by biochemical responses. For example, a person may at first appraise an experience as nonthreatening, but after developing gastric symptoms may reappraise it as very threatening. Overall, coping is viewed on a scale of effectiveness.

Practitioners will also encounter coping in the form of defense mechanisms. ***Defense mechanisms*** are powerful, unconscious psychological maneuvers that protect against anxiety caused by direct or indirect threats to the self, especially threats to self-concept and self-esteem. Defense mechanisms are unconscious but individuals can be highly aware, somewhat aware, or unaware of their patterns or ***defense style***. Analysis of defense style is not a basic mental health care skill, and it is not recommended that practitioners attempt to diagnosis or intervene at this level. This brief review of selected defense mechanisms and the three most common defense styles is presented to help practitioners recognize defense styles and to remind practitioners of the function of defenses and the hazards of mistaking defense style for deliberate conduct.

The three most common defense styles are referred to as ***mature***, ***neurotic***, and ***immature*** (Vaillant, Bond, and Vaillant, 1986). In theory, as people mature, their defense style matures. Mature defense styles are more effective in protecting self-concept and self-esteem than neurotic or immature defense styles. However, a person's normal defense style may be mature, but circumstances can affect one's normal coping responses. Thus, defense styles are both developmental and situational. Defense style is one of many ways people cope with threatening experiences. If a person's defense style unduly affects the health care process, practitioners may be able to decrease this by taking steps to support and protect the person's self-concept and self-esteem.

Immature defenses include denial, splitting, projection, acting out, and passive-aggressive behavior. ***Denial*** is the refusal to recognize reality. For example, Joe refuses to acknowledge that drinking 12 to 18 cans of beer every day is a symptom of alcohol abuse disorder. ***Splitting*** is the repeated division of the universe into "all good" or "all bad." For example, Joe insists that his former practitioner was good but "none of you new people are any good at anything." ***Projection*** is the attribution of one's own thoughts, feelings, or wishes to others. Joe may say to his practitioner, "You don't want to help me because you think I'm a loser." In fact, these are Joe's fears about seeking health care for alcohol abuse. ***Acting out*** is impulsive behavior and ***passive-aggression*** is the indirect expression of aggressive feelings. Joe may repeatedly ask the practitioner to explain why he should believe he has an alcohol abuse disorder but ignore the practitioner's answers. He only appears to cooperate and accept the practitioner's answer. By repeating the same question and making the practitioner repeat the answer Joe indirectly conveys his aggressive feelings.

Neurotic defenses include controlling, intellectualizing, and isolating. ***Controlling*** is the attempt to govern people, places, and events. Joe may insist that he is the head of his household and all decisions must be made or approved by him. ***Intellectualizing*** is the use of thoughts to avoid feelings. When asked how he feels about his drinking behavior, Joe responds, "I think a man that does a man's job likes to relax and drink a beer." Neurotic defenses contain circular thinking and immature defenses contain self-focused thinking. ***Isolating*** is the inability to experience thoughts and feelings about an experience because feelings are kept unconscious. Joe may insist he has no feelings about his drinking, positive or negative.

Mature defenses include humor, sublimation, and suppression. ***Humor*** is the ability to express thoughts and feelings without experiencing or inflicting discomfort. When asked if his drinking has been a problem for him, Joe says, "Only when I drink alcohol." ***Sublimation*** is the ability to redirect, without blocking or giving up, strong drives. Joe may feel angry about discussing his use of alcohol but rather than direct his anger at himself or the practitioner he loudly slaps his knee, states "I really hate this," and continues with the assessment. ***Suppression*** is resistance to acting on impulse. Joe may feel an intense desire to leave the clinic, but he does not act on this desire; instead, he completes the assessment.

As presented in this chapter, mental health promotion and mental illness prevention are universal health goals that should be addressed in primary care. All individuals face coping challenges that can be difficult, but how an individual copes with a given experience will determine the psychological impact of that experience.

References

American Psychiatric Association. *Diagnostic and statistical manual of mental disorders*, ed 4,. Washington, DC, 1994, The Association.

Lazarus RS, Averill JR, and Upton EM: The psychology of coping: issues of research and assessment. In Coelho G, Hamburg D and Adams J: *Coping and adaptation*, New York, 1974, Basic Books, Inc.

Sartorius N, Girolamp G, Gavin A, Geman G, and Eisenberg L: *Treatment of mental disorders*, Washington, 1993, American Psychiatric Press.

Vaillant GE, Bond M Vaillant CO: An empirically validated hierarchy of defense mechanisms, *Arch Gen Psychiatry* 43:786, 1986.

Mental Health Care Skills 2

The practice of psychiatric primary care requires working knowledge of basic therapy methods and mental health care skills. In this chapter, three basic therapy methods suitable to primary care are reviewed: interpersonal therapy, cognitive-behavioral therapy, and brief therapy. The basic mental health care skills described here are necessary tools for the practice of psychiatric primary care. Practitioners can expect to routinely use the basic psychosocial interview and the American Psychiatric Association's *Diagnostic and Statistical Manual of Mental Disorders, fourth edition* (DSM-IV), as well as the practice fundamentals of mental health assessment, counseling, case management, prescribing medication, consultations, and referrals. With experience, practitioners will identify the therapy methods and basic skills that are most effective for them, given their professional interaction style and patient population.

Therapy Methods

Interpersonal Therapy

In 1952, Hildegard E. Peplau, a pioneer in the development of interpersonal theory and practice, stated that the principal element of interpersonal practice is the beneficial human relationship. Modern interpersonal theorists and practitioners continue to apply this principle. Klerman, Weissman, Rounsaville, and Chevron (1984) identified primary or significant relationships as the focus of interpersonal therapy. They recommend that past and current significant interpersonal relationships be addressed in the assessment and treatment of mental disorders and psychosocial problems. These relationships should be assessed in terms of the quality and pattern of interpersonal interactions regarding such issues as authority, intimacy, trust, division of labor, and reciprocity. The goal of interpersonal therapy is to view personal experiences within the context of important relationships rather than as disconnected, individual phenomenon.

Interpersonal therapy acknowledges that interactions with others affect the onset, course, and remission of mental disorders and psychosocial problems. Few if any disorders or problems are without interpersonal antecedents or consequences (Klerman et al, 1984). The goal of interpersonal therapy in primary care is to take into account relevant interpersonal factors. For example, childhood, family relationships, and adult partner relationships are now standards of assessment and treatment for alcohol abuse disorders. Historically, the focus of assessment and treatment was limited to personal characteristics of the individual who abused alcohol (Weissman and Markowitz, 1994).

Cognitive-Behavioral Therapy

Cognitive-behavioral therapy is a method of producing change in distressing thought and behavior patterns. The goal of cognitive-behavioral therapy is to target the thoughts that support problem behaviors. Beck, Rush, Shaw, and Emery (1979) described basic negative thought patterns that contribute to maladaptive behaviors as well as the development of mood disorders such as depression. These thought patterns are negative views of self, negative interpretation of experiences, negative views of the future, selective attention or screening out information that does not support negative views, overgeneralization, magnifying or minimizing the significance of events, personalizing events that are not personal, and all-or-nothing thinking.

These negative thought patterns support problem behaviors, increase the risk of mood disorders, and cause significant psychological pain. Negative thoughts can be triggered or automatic. The person who has negative thoughts may or may not question their validity thereby effectively decreasing the probability of alternative or positive thoughts. One may become so accustomed to negative thoughts that one has little awareness of them despite their effect. Like listening to music that is unpleasant, if you hear it long enough, you may stop reacting to it and gradually come to accept the presence of the sound. Cognitive-behavioral therapy can be used to increase awareness of the sound and its unpleasant nature, and encourage actions aimed at stopping or changing the music. The goal of cognitive-behavioral therapy is to discover negative thought patterns and recognize their impact on behavior and mood.

Practitioners will find that people vary in their tolerance for this sort of self-scrutiny. Some enjoy self-awareness and are able to recognize their patterns and act to change them. Others may recognize their patterns but reject the idea that their thinking is related to their problems. There can be good reason for the latter reaction. To some, the implication of cognitive-behavioral therapy may be that "people are as happy as they make up their mind to be." No one in distress would welcome even the suggestion of such a cavalier attitude. To avoid implying such an attitude, practitioners can explicitly state the intended benefit of cognitive-behavioral therapy. In summary, the process of cognitive-behavioral therapy calls for developing answers to four questions: (1) what are the negative thoughts, (2) what are the behaviors based on those thoughts, (3) what is the level of self-awareness regarding the thoughts and behaviors, and (4) what is the tolerance for self-awareness and cognitive-behavioral change?

Brief Therapy

Brief therapy is a single-appointment method of identifying a target problem and discovering effective solutions. In order to be effective, target problems selected for brief therapy should represent "here and now" concerns. Brief therapy (Budman & Gurman, 1988), draws on six assumptions of psychological distress:

1. Children adopt faulty information or beliefs that can continue into adulthood.
2. Individuals are in constant interaction with their environments, and this interaction shapes both the individual and the environment.
3. Interpersonal relationships can moderate or exacerbate individual stress.
4. An individual's personality or character can be influenced by an interpersonal interaction of any duration (brief encounters to lifelong relationships).

5. The meaning of a life experience for an individual is largely determined by one's stage of development at the time of the experience.
6. Therapy requires significant personal change.

The goal of brief therapy is to motivate and mobilize the patient to continue to make identifiable positive changes. The immediate effectiveness of brief therapy is measured in the patient's satisfaction with being heard, understood, and helped. The amount of positive change accomplished at any given point is less important than the patient's level of motivation to create positive change. The key to the practice of brief therapy is ***careful identification of target problems***. Poorly defined problems hinder the patient's ability to discover solutions and also undermine motivation and mobilization. Brief therapy is not effective with chronic problems unless they can be redefined into "here and now" target problems, in which case a series of brief therapies can be employed, addressing one problem at a time.

Psychosocial Interview

The psychosocial interview is the process of obtaining accurate information about a patient's thoughts, feelings, and behaviors. Many interview formats have been developed. Depending on the practitioner's experience, the type and amount of information needed, and the patient's level of self-awareness, a psychosocial interview can last a few minutes or an hour. Practitioners have legitimate concerns about the effectiveness of psychosocial interviewing in primary care. It is not always possible to know how long an interview will take or, more importantly, to distinguish between relevant and irrelevant psychosocial information. There is also the potential of overlooking or misinterpreting subtle information. In addition, despite being called an interview, the psychosocial interview is much more than a series of questions and answers. It is also a powerful interpersonal interaction. For example, a practitioner who is interpersonally remote, preferring emotional distance to closeness, may obtain different if not less information than a more sociable practitioner.

Sensitive information can be a major pitfall of the psychosocial interview. Practitioners deal with highly sensitive information all the time, but there is a great deal of stigma attached to information that could be considered a symptom of a mental disorder or psychosocial problems. Practitioners can be prepared to state exactly what will and will not be done with sensitive information. Practitioners can start a psychosocial interview with a simple statement of intent, such as "I need to ask you several questions about...for the purpose of...." Starting the interview with a statement of intent makes the interview easier and more productive.

Using the DSM-IV

The DSM-IV (APA, 1994) is designed to generate comprehensive diagnoses of mental disorders and psychosocial problems, allow for calculation of diagnostic incidence and prevalence rates, and provide for effective communication of patient information. The DSM-IV was never intended to be an absolute or exhaustive mental health catalog. Practitioners will routinely encounter conditions not included in the DSM-IV, but the diagnoses that are included are presented in detail, with specific diagnostic criteria. A complete DSM-IV diagnosis includes the following five separate diagnoses:

- Axis I: Clinical condition
- Axis II: Personality or developmentally related conditions
- Axis III: Physical health status
- Axis IV: Psychosocial stressors
- Axis V: Global assessment of functioning

Specific symptom criteria are defined for the Axis I and II diagnoses: nature, number, intensity, and duration of symptoms. Symptom ***nature*** is the type or kind of symptom being experienced, ***number*** refers to the total number of symptoms, ***intensity*** is symptom severity, and ***duration*** is the total number of symptomatic days, weeks, months, or years.

Psychosocial problems may be listed as an Axis I or IV diagnosis. Axis III, physical condition, is a general statement of health or specific medical diagnosis such as hypertension. An Axis IV diagnosis, psychosocial stressor, is intended to be a list of specific negative life events and their severity. An example of an Axis IV diagnosis would be: Unexpected loss of employment (severe). Axis V, global assessment of functioning (GAF) is assessed on a 0 to 100-point scale, with 100 as the highest level of occupational/academic, social, and interpersonal functioning. GAF scores are current and for the previous year. Practitioners should become comfortable with DSM-IV language and the five-axis diagnostic system.

Assessment

Sociocultural Assessment

Sociocultural assessment (Alarcon, 1995) is the identification and evaluation of relevant sociocultural experiences, including social stigma, stereotyping, prejudice, and discrimination. A brief sociocultural assessment is recommended for two reasons. First, this assessment makes it possible for practitioners to provide culturally sensitive and culturally competent health care for patients as unique individuals. Second, negative sociocultural experiences such as prejudice are extremely stressful and therefore can be significant factors in understanding stress-related mental disorders and psychosocial problems. A sociocultural assessment should include but not be limited to the patient's social and cultural experiences with personal characteristics such as age, sex, education, income, ethnicity, religion, sexual orientation, and physical ability. Negative experiences with these personal characteristics can have significant effects on global functioning, including occupational and academic functioning.

Practitioners may question the need for a specific sociocultural assessment with the implication being that they treat all patients with respect. However, individuals who have experienced stigma, stereotyping, prejudice, or discrimination require more than generic respect. Effective mental health promotion and mental illness prevention require accurate assessment of stressful life experiences, including negative sociocultural experiences and stressors. At the same time practitioners cannot assume that stress-related mental disorders, psychosocial problems, or impaired functioning are automatic results of stressful sociocultural experiences. The actual effect of these experiences is determined by the person affected and the circumstances of the experience.

Symptom Assessment

Symptom assessment is a prerequisite skill for using the DSM-IV diagnostic system. In primary care settings some symptoms, such as crying or insomnia, are more likely to be assessed than other symptoms, such as worry or social withdrawal, because assessment is heavily influenced by individual variations in the symptom experience. For some, crying is significantly different behavior, but for others, it is not. Mental health symptom assessment is as much an art as a science. Florid symptoms can be just as confusing as invisible symptoms. A body temperature of 42 °C. would have little or no individual difference in experience or expression, but a mental health symptom can have significant differences. Crying can be a symptom of any number of experiences such as stress, alcohol withdrawal, anxiety, depression, fear, pain, confusion, or anger. Only by applying DSM-IV criteria is it possible to measure, rather than assume, the actual diagnostic significance of symptoms. A comprehensive symptom assessment reduces the risk of attributing too little or too much diagnostic significance to any single symptom.

Symptoms related to mental disorders or psychosocial problems rarely develop overnight; practitioners can therefore anticipate symptom history as being a significant part of symptom assessment. Symptom history should include the development of the symptom as well as its impact on functioning. Many patients become concerned by significant alterations in their thoughts, feelings, or behaviors. Absence of this reaction should be noted and evaluated. Usually there is little concern if the symptoms have been present for an extended period of time. In conclusion, symptom assessment must be comprehensive, accurate, complete, and current. Reassessment should be performed routinely or when a change in symptom profile occurs.

Intervention Assessment

Intervention assessment determines appropriate treatment and management. Unlike conditions that produce symptoms with little individual variation, mental disorders and psychosocial problems do create significant variations in individual experience, expression, and response. In part this variation can be attributed to individual differences in energy level, motivation, resources, and coping style. Personal characteristics such as these partially define the experience of symptoms as well as the efforts needed to increase the probability of symptom remission and full recovery. For example, emotional support as an intervention requires less patient energy and effort than cognitive-behavioral therapy. Similarly, a patient with a highly interpersonal coping style may respond better to interpersonal therapy than to cognitive-behavioral therapy. Patients who are not psychologically minded may be less tolerant of the interactions that define interpersonal therapy. An intervention assessment is an opportunity to evaluate the patient's psychosocial strengths and weaknesses as integral elements of treatment. Optimum intervention effectiveness requires that treatment and management plans be appropriate for both the individual and the mental disorder or psychosocial problem.

Counseling

Family Counseling

Family counseling is the process of bringing together the right people at the right time to address a stated problem. Family counseling is most effective when a specific problem with short-term goals can be identified. The structure and the process of family counseling depends on available physical space, relationships among the participating family members, and anticipated counseling outcomes. ***Structure*** includes the location of family counseling, the number of people who attend, their relationships with each other, and their roles within the family. ***Process*** refers to how the family operates as a unit, especially in communication, decision making, and resource allocation.

Family counseling is not family therapy. Family counseling assists a group of related people in their efforts to unite and accomplish shared goals. Family therapy, on the other hand, is a sustained effort toward accomplishing major changes in family structure and process. Family therapy can require months or years and usually at least two health care providers. Family counseling is often limited to one to three brief meetings.

The first step of family counseling is to identify and assemble the participating family members. The meeting should begin with each participant presenting his or her concerns about the stated problem. The practitioner draws on this information to identify shared views and applies this consensus to help the family develop a plan of action. The family may want the practitioner to give them a plan of action. The outcome of complying with this wish is often less, rather than more, family participation. When families develop their own plans of action, they become activated, invested in the process, and able to claim responsibility for their success. Practitioners can actively help the family to recognize their problem and goals, but should allow the family to develop their own plan of action as much as possible. Some family members will be more helpful than others. Practitioners should focus on the problem at hand and the helpful family members.

The goal of family counseling is active problem solving with some level of participation by most of the family members. When family counseling is not effective, usually the family process rather than the problem itself has become the focus. Family members may debate ***how*** things are going to be done and avoid dealing with ***what*** will be done and ***who*** will do it. Once practitioners determine who will participate in a family counseling meeting, they have the opportunity to influence the counseling process. Although all participants should be willing and able to contribute, powerful family members should never be excluded. Ideally, participants should have daily contact with each other and firsthand knowledge of the circumstances that require family counseling. Each family member will make a unique contribution to the effectiveness of the counseling.

Individual Counseling

Individual counseling is actually a set of mental health skills (Jarrett and Rush 1994). Basic mental health counseling skills include providing emotional support (validation), advising (alternatives), coaching (reinforcement), teaching (information), reorganizing (structure), grounding (reality check), and owning (accountability). Just as family counseling differs from family therapy, individual counseling is not the equivalent of individual therapy. Individual therapy requires more time than individual counseling and, unlike counseling, therapy is intended to produce major changes in thought, feeling, and behavior patterns. Counseling can be limited to general promotion (improvement) and prevention (risk reduction) goals or can include treatment for symptoms related to mental disorders and psychosocial problems. The magnitude of hoped-for changes and improvements distinguish counseling from therapy. The following descriptions of seven basic counseling skills are presented as a brief review.

Providing emotional support is perhaps the most common counseling skill. Friends, partners, family members, and co-workers, as well as health care professionals, provide effective emotional support. The essential process of emotional support is for one person to validate the feelings of another; that is, to value another's experience and expression of feelings without analysis, interpretation, or judgment. Because it can be very draining for the person who is providing emotional support and because emotional support may have few actual effects, it should be combined with other forms of counseling. Emotional support is essentially an analgesic: the main effect is short-term emotional relief; people feel better. For the same reason, emotional support can be very effective when the problem is overwhelming feelings, such as grief, and emotional relief is the primary need.

Advising is also a common type of counseling, but when provided by health care professionals it should generate realistic alternatives. When friends advise each other, it is often in the form of recommendations or narrative descriptions of how they each might handle a particular problem. Developing realistic alternatives is a more deliberate process, requiring the active participation of the person being advised. The golden rule of advice counseling is that alternatives must be real. Consideration of unrealistic options serves no purpose other than to frustrate the person who needs to make a decision. The goal of advice counseling is developing alternatives so that people feel more in control, more hopeful, better able to make effective decisions, and are more willing to act on those decisions.

Coaching is the process in which a more experienced person supplements the efforts of a less experienced person who may require extra skills to perform a function, complete a task, or accomplish a goal. For example, new members of twelve-step recovery programs are encouraged to work with a sponsor as soon as they join the program. A sponsor is someone in the program who has accomplished program goals. In primary care, coaching supports the patient's efforts in ways that increase the probability of success. For example, Debbie, 43, complains that for the past 6 months, she has been trying to lose 20 pounds by limiting herself to 1000 calories per day, but she has not lost weight. Debbie feels extremely discouraged and angry with herself. Having worked with women in their 40s who want to lose weight, the practitioner offers to coach Debbie. She starts by developing with Debbie a 6-month weight-loss plan with equal emphasis on motivation, nutrition, fun, support, exercise, and calories. Because Debbie's plan only focused on calories, this new plan appeals to her.

Teaching is an extremely important part of counseling. For many patients, health care professionals are the only reliable source of accurate health information. Most primary care settings make a great deal of information available in the form of pamphlets, videos, posters, and community lectures. This generic information, on topics ranging from healthy hearts to family violence, is vital, but personal health teaching is also essential. Patients need specific information about their personal mental health and mental health care. Misinformation and inaccurate beliefs about mental disorders and psychosocial problems should be identified and revised at every opportunity. Unfortunately, practitioners and patients do not always agree on what is misinformation or inaccurate beliefs. For example, Ed believes that depression is caused by negative events, such as the death of a loved one or a disaster. He has had severe symptoms of major depression for the last 6 weeks but insists that he is suffering from a virus that must be treated with antibiotics. He states he is not depressed because nothing bad has happened to him. Ed needs accurate information about depression in general, and more information about his own experience of and response to symptoms of depression. Without this teaching, it is not likely that Ed will accept or fully participate in treatment.

Reorganizing is the process of helping a person to build structure out of chaos. This form of counseling is particularly helpful when patients seem unable to sort through or absorb information or focus their efforts, and subsequently become immobilized. Immobilization is often described as being stuck or spinning one's wheels, becoming exhausted, and accomplishing little. Reorganizing is appropriate when the solution to a problem is a plan of action. If the patient's disorganization is due to mental confusion or disorientation, the cause rather than the effects of the confusion or disorientation must be treated. Reorganizing is most effective when a patient is trying to accomplish a goal or perform a task but is unable to get started or keep going. This goal or task should be clear and the patient should not be operating under a great deal of ambivalence toward accomplishment. Reorganizing is the development of a "first things first" plan of action, identifying for today what must and can be done. The goal of reorganizing is to support mobilization by identifying a specific, realistic starting point. For example, Chip has been informed by his employer that unless his work performance improves, including coming to work on time, he will be fired. This is the third job Chip has had in the last 18 months and he is worried that he would not be able to find another job if he is fired again. He states that if he got help for his severe insomnia he would be able to work better and would not have to worry about losing his job. Chip's anxiety keeps him awake at night and makes it difficult for him to complete his work during the day. The practitioner learns that Chip's wife filed for divorce last week. Rather than trying to cope with the job and the divorce at the same time, Chip is advised to take a 1-week medical leave of absence to get settled in a new apartment and then meet with his employer the following week to establish a specific list of work-performance expectations.

Grounding is a reality check. It is similar to reorganizing but instead of helping patients get started again it helps them to "face facts." Grounding is not always a welcomed experience, so patience and a matter-of-fact approach is recommended, particularly when it appears that the patient equates facing facts with giving up or admitting defeat. Hopes, by definition, exceed reality and therefore are more comforting. Grounding is not confrontation, dashing hopes, or slapping someone in the face with reality. The purpose of providing patients with a reality check is to support the patient's effort to cope with, rather than avoid, unpleasant facts.

Owning is accountability. The goal is to support patients' efforts to accept responsibility for their choices. Practitioners often hear patients describe their choices as though they had no control over them and the choice "just happened." Disowning one's choices can provide immediate relief from negative feelings, but the long-term effect is increased feelings of personal incompetence. Regardless of life circumstances, people make choices every day and every choice has an effect. In working with patients to improve their ability to evaluate their choices and accept accountability, practitioners must ensure that the patient is not blamed or shamed. Blaming and shaming negate the promised benefit of owning, that by accepting the importance of their choices patients can improve their skills in making choices.

Case Management

Case management is the fundamental process of organizing and dealing with multiple components of a patient's health and health care. Case management, in the practice of psychiatric primary care, requires ongoing, easy access to skilled and reliable practice partners. This should include, at the minimum, close working relationships with peer practitioners in your setting, a psychiatric specialist, a pharmacist, and a community practice specialist. When case management is effective, patient information and the required health care services and resources are available and accessible. Practitioners should develop practice partnerships as one of the first steps in developing a primary care practice, for two reasons. First, practitioners who develop practice partnerships are more likely to use them and thus better able to meet the mental health care needs of their patients. Second, having developed these resources, practitioners are able to focus on providing, rather than finding, mental health care. In most primary care settings, fundamental case management resources include expert skills in severe mental illness (SMI), drug/alcohol dependence disorders, psychiatric medications, and access to community resources (Hromco, Lyons, Nikkel 1995).

Prescribing Psychiatric Medications

Most psychiatric medications are prescribed for symptoms of thought disorder, mood disorder, and related behaviors (Preskorn, Burke, Fast, 1993). Specific information is presented in the prescribing sections of the chapters on mental disorders in Part II.

Neuroleptic Medications

Neuroleptic medications (antipsychotic) are prescribed for thought disorders such as schizophrenia and for any disorder that produces psychotic symptoms, such as hallucinations or delirium. Neuroleptic medications may be prescribed as treatment for a disorder, to relieve psychotic symptoms, or to prevent the recurrence or relapse of acute symptoms (thought disorder or psychosis). Neuroleptic medications do not produce physical addiction or emotional dependence. Abrupt rather than tapered withdrawal of these medications, however, will produce significant negative effects, such as anxiety or nausea.

The exact mechanism of action of neuroleptic medications has not been identified. Researchers have shown that neuroleptics block the transmission or reception of specific types of neurotransmitters associated with specific thought and mood experiences. The clinical effectiveness of these medications supports the widely accepted hypothesis that thought disorder symptoms are related to excessive or altered effects of serotonin and dopamine in specific parts of the brain. Many patients who are prescribed neuroleptic medication for the treatment of a thought disorder also require medication to treat neuroleptic side-effect symptoms and may require medication for treatment of depression, anxiety, or mania symptoms.

Intramuscular (IM) forms of neuroleptic medications are available with single doses that are effective for approximately two weeks. These neuroleptics provide more consistent doses and fewer missed doses, which in turn provides better symptom control and in some cases fewer side effects. These benefits are particularly helpful when a patient is not able to reliably take oral neuroleptic medication. Commonly prescribed neuroleptic medications include fluphenazine (Prolixin), thiothixene (Navane), haloperidol (Haldol), clozapine (Clozaril), and risperidone (Risperdol). Eight general categories of neuroleptic medication side effects have been recognized and are listed below.

1. Central nervous system (sedation, drowsiness, insomnia, agitation)

2. Extrapyramidal (parkinsonism, akathisia, dystonic reaction)
3. Cardiovascular (orthostatic hypotension, tachycardia, cardiac arrhythmias)
4. Anticholinergic (dry mouth, constipation)
5. Endocrine (weight gain, ejaculation inhibition)
6. Skin reactions (rashes, pigmentation, photosensitivity)
7. Ocular (lenticular pigmentation, pigmentary retinopathy)
8. Blood dyscrasias, hepatic disorder, and seizures

Antidepressant, Antianxiety, and Antimanic Medications

Antidepressant, antianxiety, and antimanic medications are prescribed for symptoms of mood disorders. Antidepressants are widely prescribed and offer numerous benefits for many mood disorders. All antidepressants are thought to be equally effective, but each class of antidepressant has a somewhat unique side effect profile. Many antidepressants require 7 to 21 days to reach clinically effective plasma levels, which can be a significant problem because many patients have difficulty waiting for symptom relief. First-generation antidepressants (heterocyclics, e.g., imipramine) are highly anticholinergic. These medications should not be prescribed when the health history and physical exam reveals evidence of asthma, closed-angle glaucoma, cardiac arrhythmias, or congestive heart failure. These antidepressants must be started at low doses and gradually increased to therapeutic dose levels. The risk of lethal overdose is significant.

Second-generation antidepressants (tricyclics, e.g., nortriptyline) have fewer anticholinergic side effects than the first generation. Third-generation antidepressants (selective serotonin reuptake inhibitors [SSRIs], e.g., sertraline) have improved on the previous generations by having a more selective effect on cerebral neurotransmitters. Third-generation antidepressants selectively increase the level or effects of specific types of serotonin neurotransmitters. Based on the clinical effectiveness of antidepressants, the hypothesized cause of mood disorder symptoms is low or ineffective serotonin levels in specific areas of the brain.

Third-generation antidepressants have very little anticholinergic or central nervous system side effects. The side effects associated with these medications are anxiety and hyperactivity or "serotonin syndrome," which is palpitation, agitation, muscle twitching and, in rare cases, delirium. Compared to first- and second-generation antidepressants, SSRI medications can be expensive. Lethal overdose is rare (Preskorn, 1995).

The commonly prescribed antimanic or mood stabilizing medications are lithium, carbamazepine, and valproic acid. These medications are simple in their chemistry but require complex assessment and monitoring when prescribed. Anxiolytic or antianxiety medications are benzodiazepines, barbiturates, beta-blockers, antihistamines, and buspirones. Unlike other classes of psychiatric medications, these may produce symptom relief without treating the neurodysregulation causing the symptoms. Excluding the buspirones, these medications can produce significant physical or emotional dependence and the risk of lethal overdose is significant.

Patient Attitudes toward Psychiatric Medications

When prescribing psychiatric medications, the goals are to: (1) provide the right medication to the right person at the right dose and (2) establish an open channel of communication between the prescribing practitioner and patient. Practitioners ***prescribe*** psychiatric medications, but patients ***take*** medications. Practitioners should spend as much time as needed to ensure that the patient's definition of "taking" medication is based on factual and helpful information. For example, for some patients, psychiatric medications are never the solution; for others, psychiatric medication is the only solution. Similarly, some patients "take" psychiatric medication the way they take over-the-counter analgesics: they take a smaller-than-prescribed dose on "good days" and a larger-than-prescribed dose on "bad days." Patient attitudes can significantly affect patient behavior and, subsequently, medication effectiveness.

Taking medication for a mental disorder or psychosocial diagnosis is acceptable to some patients and unacceptable to others. Practitioners should determine each patient's attitude toward taking medications that are intended to produce significant changes in thoughts, feelings, or behaviors, in order to identify problems that may occur after the patient has started taking the medication. In assessing patient attitudes toward psychiatric medication, practitioners should note the patient's general resilience and reliability, the patient's attitude toward psychiatric medication in general, and the patient's attitude toward the specific medications being considered. Practitioners can count on little or no disclosure when patients believe they have to say the right thing to receive a prescription. The intent is not to challenge or question the patient's attitude but to use the prescribing process to help the patient define "taking" prescribed psychiatric medication in a useful and factual manner.

General resilience and reliability can be useful indicators of medication-taking behavior. ***Resilience*** is indicated by tolerance, patience, and stamina. ***Reliability*** refers to honesty, decision making, and predictability. The best-case scenario for prescribing psychiatric medication is a person who, based on the psychosocial interview and assessment findings, is not likely to give up or become disturbed by the absence of instant improvement or the presence of minor side effects, and who gives the practitioner truthful information, works with the practitioner in developing acceptable choices, and follows through. If the patient does not have acceptable levels of personal resilience or reliability, often there is a significant other who does and who is willing to be involved in the prescribing process.

Most psychiatric medications produce mild side effects before they produce symptom remission and general clinical improvement may not be noticeable for weeks. Under these conditions, it is not uncommon for patients to take a newly prescribed medication, such as antidepressant or antianxiety medications, for 5 to 6 days, then stop taking it or insist on trying a different one. Patients may complain that a psychiatric medication is ineffective because when they take it they feel no effects, too many effects, or even feel worse. In the absence of severe side effects or other prohibiting factors (e.g., cost), the practitioner's first response can be to reassess the patient's attitude toward taking the prescribed medication. Psychiatric medications are similar to other medications: teaching and counseling are critical elements of prescribing.

In some states informed consent is required when psychiatric medications are prescribed. Practitioners may be required to obtain written informed consent, indicating that the patient understands why the medication is being prescribed, what benefits are anticipated, and what the potential risks and side effects are. In some settings, patients with active suicidal thoughts or recent suicidal behavior may only be prescribed psychiatric medications by a specialist. Informed consent with psychiatric medications need not be more or less complicated than with any other health care procedure. The consent process can actually support the prescribing process by helping patients to understand and participate in their mental health care.

Additional critical issues to take into consideration when prescribing psychiatric medications are cost, combination medications, long-acting IM medications, and benefits versus risk analysis. These issues are discussed in the prescribing sections of the chapters in Part III.

☎ Consultation and Referral

Consultation differs from case management in that consultation is not an ongoing arrangement but is usually very brief. The goal of consulting is to obtain expert information to support the practitioner's assessment, diagnosis, and treatment planning. Most primary care settings have detailed consultation protocols for working with experts. In addition to those protocols, practitioners should consult with a psychiatric specialist when, during the course of providing basic mental health care, transference, countertransference, or boundary violations are noted.

Transference is the patient's transferral of positive or negative feelings from an original relationship onto the relationship with the practitioner. The patient's feelings are not the result of actual experiences with the practitioner. ***Countertransference*** occurs when a practitioner transfers feelings from another relationship onto the relationship with the patient. ***Boundary violations*** are behaviors that violate the practitioner's or patient's personal space (physical or psychological). A violation means that a line of respect has been crossed. The person who is violated typically feels anger and shame and may act out these emotions. Practitioners who encounter or are concerned about transference, countertransference, or boundary violations will benefit from consulting with a specialist to either resolve the situation or make alternative treatment arrangements for the patient.

Referral differs from case management (which is continual) and consultation (which is brief) in that practitioners refer patients to a specialist. When specialized care is no longer needed, the specialist discharges the patient to primary care. Rather than seeing a team of providers who work together, the patient sees a series of individual providers but primary care practitioners often do not discharge a referred patient.

References

Alarcon RD, editor: Cultural psychiatry. *Psych Clin North Am* 18:3, 1995.

Beck AT, Rush JA, Shaw BF, Emery G: *Cognitive therapy of depression*, New York, 1979, Guilford Press.

Budman SH, Gurman AS: *Theory and practice of brief therapy*, New York, 1988, Guilford Press.

American Psychiatric Association: *Diagnostic and statistical manual of mental disorders,* ed 4, Washington, DC, 1994, The Association.

Hromco JG, Lyons JS, Nikkel RE: Mental health case management: characteristics, job function, and occupational stress, *Comm Mental Health* J, 31(2):111, 1995.

Jarrett RB, Rush AJ: Shorterm psychotherapy of depressive disorders: current status and future directions, *Psychiatry* 57(2):115,1994.

Klerman G, Weissman M, Rounsaville B, and Chevron E: *Interpersonal psychotherapy of depression*, New York, 1984, Basic Books, Inc.

Peplau HE: *Interpersonal relations in nursing*, New York, 1952, GP Putnam's Sons.

Preskorn SH, Burke MJ, Fast G: Therapeutic drug monitoring: principles and practice, *Psych Clinic North Am* 16(3):611, 1993.

Preskorn S: Comparison of the tolerability of bupropion, imipramine, nefazodone, paroxetine, sertraline, and venlafaxine, *Journal of Clinical Psychiatry* 56(Suppl 6):12, 1995.

Weissman MM, Markowitz JC: Interpersonal psychotherapy: current status, *Arch Gen Psychiatry* 51(8):559,1994.

Review of Severe Mental Illness 3

This chapter presents a comprehensive review of schizophrenia and schizoaffective disorder along with brief overviews of bipolar disorders, personality disorders, paraphilias, and dissociative disorders. These disorders typically cause severe short-term impairment of psychosocial functioning and, in some cases, long-term psychiatric disability and therefore are classified as severe mental illness (SMI). Because of the risk of psychiatric disability, individuals with SMI should receive specialized psychiatric care but practitioners should have a fundamental understanding of the complex and extraordinary human experience of SMI.

Schizophrenia and Schizoaffective Disorder

Schizophrenia is a thought disorder that appears to affect the cerebral frontal lobes, limbic system, and basal ganglia, but the exact nature of the changes in brain structure and function that cause schizophrenia is unknown (Buckley, Buchanan, Schulz, Tamminga 1996). The primary effect of the cerebral changes associated with schizophrenia is a neurochemical dysregulation. Schizophrenia strikes families. One percent (1%) of the general population is diagnosed with schizophrenia; 8% of the siblings of individuals with schizophrenia will develop schizophrenia; 12% of those who have one parent with schizophrenia will develop schizophrenia; and 47% of those who have an identical twin with schizophrenia will develop schizophrenia (Africia and Schwartz, 1995). The first episode severe enough to be diagnosed as schizophrenia usually occurs in the late teens to late 20s. However, it may be diagnosed much earlier or later in life because the illness is correlated with other factors: prenatal insult (e.g., maternal substance abuse) developmental insult (e.g., neglect) schizotypal personality disorder, and toxic response to stimulants, opiates, and hallucinogens,

There are several types of schizophrenia, many of which are just beginning to be recognized, but the typical course of illness is years of persistent symptomatology punctuated by recurrent acute episodes, often without complete remission between episodes. This pattern quickly erodes psychosocial functioning and can completely demoralize the individual, to the point where coping consists of giving up one's identity, becoming a schizophrenic rather than a person with schizophrenia. With time and specialized psychiatric care, about half of the people with schizophrenia improve and regain their identity and ability to function. There is no way of knowing for sure who will and will not recover from schizophrenia, but healthy premorbid functioning appears to be related to recovery. This observation may indicate that those individuals without a significant history of healthy functioning may have a more severe form of schizophrenia (International Symposium, 1995).

The American Psychiatric Association's *Diagnostic and Statistical Manual of Mental Disorders, fourth edition,* (DSM-IV) defines four types of schizophrenia: ***paranoid***, ***disorganized***, ***catatonic***, and ***undifferentiated***. The type of schizophrenia is defined by the individual's predominant symptoms. In paranoid schizophrenia, the predominant symptom is ***suspicion***. In disorganized schizophrenia it is ***incoherence***; in catatonic schizophrenia it is ***withdrawal***, and undifferentiated schizophrenia has no predominate symptom.

Symptoms are classified as residual or acute, positive or negative. ***Residual symptoms*** are less intense but more persistent than acute symptoms. ***Acute symptoms*** can be severe enough to produce psychosis, a partial or complete break with reality. ***Positive symptoms*** are external (e.g., odd behavior and speech), making the individual aware of and responsive to interactions with others. ***Negative symptoms*** are internal (e.g., silent rocking), removing the individual from interaction with others and environments (Vazquez-Barquero, 1996). The predominant negative symptoms are withdrawal, apathy, and isolation. Long-term use of neuroleptic medications can induce pseudoparkinsonism, sedation, and dysphoria side effects that mimic negative symptoms (VanPutten, 1974).

The major symptoms of schizophrenia are hallucinations, incoherence, fear, poor grooming, withdrawal, suspicion, apathy, loss of energy, delusions, odd affect, and impaired occupational, academic, social, and interpersonal functioning (Harvey, Curson, Pantelis, Taylor, and Barnes, 1996). These symptoms can produce troubling secondary reactions, especially fear, anger, and sadness.

Hallucinations are altered sensory perceptions (vision, hearing, smell, touch, taste) that do not reflect reality. Hallucinations can be made worse by stress. ***Auditory hallucinations*** (Carter, Mackinnon, Copolov 1996) are the most common and can range from a small sound to the conversations of groups of people. Individuals can react to hallucinations in many ways, including fear, anger, and pleasure. Individuals may recognize the sounds or voices they hear and refer to them by name. Individuals may also experience auditory hallucinations as being in control or as commands that they must obey. ***Command hallucinations*** are potentially dangerous. They can be as simple as a command to "touch your arm" or as dangerous as a command to step in front of a car or harm someone. Early warning signs of command auditory hallucinations include a sudden increase in agitation or in behaviors intended to silence the commands. Accusing and blaming auditory hallucinations are more common than command hallucinations but equally upsetting.

Visual hallucinations can be sustained or fleeting and contain full or partial imagery. Individuals report seeing things as complex as insects or as simple as a door opening and closing. Smell, touch, and taste hallucinations may be unrecognized until the individual engages in compensatory behavior. For example, a patient who smells or tastes poison in food may refuse to eat. ***Touch hallucinations*** are somewhat more rare than the others but with an equal range of symptom types, from feeling insects crawling on one's skin to feeling violated. Hallucinations are assessed in terms of their content and process and whether or not they are triggered by internal (e.g., anxiety) or external (e.g., crowds) factors.

Schizophrenic symptoms include sweeping and unpredictable mood changes. Individuals can also appear to be totally lacking in mood or somehow vacant. Of the many moods and feelings associated with schizophrenia, fear and anger are among the most important. ***Fear*** can take the form of anything from social withdrawal to social aggression. For many, the worst fear is that of never recovering. From 25% to 50% of individuals with schizophrenia attempt suicide and 10% succeed (Africia, 1995). ***Poor grooming*** is a common symptom of schizophrenia usually due to the high level of organization and motivation needed to bathe and dress according to social standards. Poor grooming can also be the result of other symptoms, such as insomnia or confusion.

Delusion differs from hallucination in that it is a fixed false belief, whereas a hallucination is a false sensory perception. Delusional thoughts are not factual but, unlike hallucinations, they can be nearly impossible for others to invalidate by pointing out reality. Individuals who are delusional do not recognize or accept information that contradicts their beliefs. Delusional thinking generally is experienced as a fixed (unchanging) or loose (frequently changing) system of connected ideas. An example of a ***fixed delusional system*** is a man who believes the government has made arrangements to have him murdered. His system of beliefs contains ideas about himself, the government, and murder that are connected to form a murder conspiracy. The system is fixed because the ideas and connections do not change: new ones are not added, established ones are not subtracted, and the delusional system does not invade other areas of the man's thinking. A ***loose delusional system*** is just the opposite. Ideas and their connections change frequently, significantly, and unpredictably. If the government delusional system were loose instead of fixed, yesterday this man may have believed that he worked for the government or that a totally different group of people was pursuing him for totally different reasons. Tomorrow his delusional system may contain new ideas; for example, he may believe that he alone has some vital information. Loose delusional systems are unique in that real people and events can become incorporated. The man may begin to believe, for instance, that health care staff or family members are working for the government and plan to harm him.

Thought broadcasting and thought insertion are two extremely frightening symptoms of schizophrenia that are delusional in nature but may not occur as systems. ***Thought broadcasting*** is the belief that others can hear one's thoughts, either directly or via electronic or communication devices. ***Thought insertion*** is the belief that others are placing thoughts into one's mind. Individuals experiencing either symptoms may engage in bizarre or dangerous efforts to protect their thoughts. The symptoms presented here are characteristic of schizophrenia but are also classic symptoms of psychosis associated with any number of conditions, such as head injury or toxic reaction to street drugs. These symptoms cause the individual and significant others a great deal of distress and can severely impair functioning, but for many individuals these symptoms can be improved or completely remitted with antipsychotic medication.

Schizoaffective disorder is a thought disorder with significant mood symptomatology. The major symptoms of schizoaffective disorder include all the symptoms of schizophrenia, but the predominant symptom is dysphoria, elation, or both.

Neuroleptic Medications

When medication is effective, individuals with schizophrenia function well and live normal lives. Those who do not have a good response to medication or cannot tolerate it may endure years of poorly controlled symptoms and severe psychiatric disability (Szymanski et al 1996). One of the results of effective medication treatment for schizophrenia is that more and more individuals are able to obtain management care from practitioners as a component of their overall health care. Maintenance medication treatment for schizophrenia, according to Csernansky and Newcomer (1995), involves three treatment goals: relapse prevention, mental health promotion, and minimization of medication side effects. Of these three, the biggest challenge for practitioners is relapse prevention. Relapse occurs even with extremely effective neuroleptic treatment. All neuroleptic medications can also produce upsetting side effects, however, so practitioners who prescribe neuroleptic medications should develop a treatment plan that allows for early recognition of both symptom relapse and medication side effects.

The most common side effects of neuroleptic medications are referred to as ***extrapyramidal symptoms***. The following extrapyramidal symptoms (EPS) should be carefully distinguished from acute or persistent symptoms of schizophrenia (Neuchterlein, Gitlin, and Subotnik, 1995).

- Akathisia, or severe restlessness, causes pacing, fidgeting, and a range of odd gestures and body movements. Approximately 20% of those taking antipsychotic medication will experience this side effect.

- Pseudoparkinsonism, or muscle stiffness, affects muscles in the face, arms, and legs. Drooling and fine hand tremors can also occur.
- Dystonia, unlike akathisia or pseudoparkinsonism, has a sudden onset as an acute reaction to neuroleptic medication. Dystonia symptoms are painful muscle cramps in the face, tongue, jaw, and neck that twist and contort the face, head, and neck. Up to 5% of those taking neuroleptic medications will have a dystonic reaction within hours or days after starting medication.
- Tardive dyskinesia (TD) is irreversible and disabling. This devastating side effect is thought to be the result of cerebral synapse hypersensitivity caused by prolonged exposure to neuroleptic drugs. Approximately 20% of the people who take neuroleptic medications for longer than 2 years will develop TD, and it is more common in women then men. TD symptoms include bizarre lip movements such as smacking and puckering, chewing movements, wormlike movements of the tongue in and out of the mouth, extreme side-to-side jaw movements, and rhythmic or discoordinated sweeping movements of the arms and legs. These symptoms usually disappear during sleep and are increased by anxiety or stress.

There are basically two types of neuroleptic medications: low potency (high dose) and high potency (low dose). Low-potency medications tend to produce more side effects than high-potency medications, and both low-dose and high-dose medications are more effective with positive symptoms than negative symptoms. The atypical neuroleptics, such as resperidone and clozaril, have been developed to be high potency, low EPS, effective with negative symptoms, and safe for long-term use. Standard EPS treatment lowers the dose of antipsychotic medication or starts anti-EPS medication such as trihexyphenidyl (Artane), benztropine mesylate (Cogentin), diphenhydramine hydrochloride (Benadryl), and amantadine hydrochloride (Symmetrel). Anti-EPS medications can effectively reduce EPS symptoms but they can intensify the anticholinergic side effects of most neuroleptics. In most cases, people gradually adapt to the neurohormonal changes produced by neuroleptic medications and no longer experience EPS.

Bipolar Disorder

Bipolar disorder is a severe mood disorder defined by episodes of elation (mania/hypomania) and dysphoria (depression). Patients describe it as an emotional roller coaster ride of unpredictable highs and lows. Bipolar disorder, formerly known as manic depressive illness, is similar to schizophrenia in that the first acute episode typically occurs in the early or late 20s, the disorder strikes families, and there is significant alteration in brain structure and function that can be relieved with medication. The DSM-IV describes two types of bipolar disorder. Type I is single or recurrent episodes of mania, hypomania, or both. Type II is single or recurrent episodes of depression with at least one episode of hypomania, no episodes of mania, and no episodes of mixed mania and depression. The essential difference between the two types is that the predominant symptom of Type II is depression.

The symptoms of bipolar disorder, the course of illness, and the severity of episodes can range from mild to extreme. Acute episodes can last for days or months. When symptoms are severe, a manic episode, which is essentially a psychotic episode, is often mistaken for schizophrenia. Hypomania is less intense than mania and can even be experienced as a pleasurable high. Depressive episodes often last longer than manic or hypomanic episodes.

Individuals alternate between moods at different rates, with periods of days, weeks, months, or years between acute episodes. The amount of symptom-free time between acute episodes also varies for each individual. Symptoms of mania and hypomania are so individualized that it is difficult to present a standard symptom profile. When manic, a person can be sweet, fun loving, and sociable, or hostile, irritable, and aggressive. Thinking may or may not be impaired. But symptoms of psychosis, such as delusions, hallucinations, and paranoia, do occur. When manic, people often act on drives (e.g., having sex, spending money, stealing) that they normally would inhibit. The most unique symptoms of mania are rapid thoughts and rapid speech. The person feels intense pressure to talk. Speech is typically explosive and often words do not keep up with or follow the thoughts that preceded them.

When a person is manic, there is an intense need to keep busy. If the person has an activity they can do for hours, this symptom is less obvious. But if the person has nothing to do, substitute behaviors such as collecting small items and changing clothing may occur. Whether pleasant or aggressive, manic people are in effect driving 100 mph without brakes, and thus are literally unable to control their thoughts, speech, or behavior. There can be little or no need for sleep or food. Depending on how long the episode continues, significant weight loss and exhaustion can occur.

Depression involves the usual symptoms of dysphoria, negative thinking, and fatigue. This experience is more difficult because some people come to believe that depression is the price they must pay for the pleasures of mania and hypomania. This is not only untrue but also it is an unnecessary burden and probably more a symptom of depression than a reasoned belief. The most difficult aspect of bipolar disorder is that people may deny the diagnosis because they experience the mania or hypomania as pleasurable and have long symptom-free periods between episodes. The main effect of denial is failure to take the needed medication. The almost-universal early warning sign of a new manic episode is refusal to take one's medication. The distressing effects of acting on this impulse are obvious (Soloman et al 1995).

Personality Disorders

The core symptoms of personality disorders are atypical thought and behavior patterns, unstable mood, interpersonal conflict, recurrent crisis, and hypersensitivity to stress (Paris, 1994; Paris, Zweig-Frank, Bond, Guzder 1996). Similar to those with bipolar disorder, patients with personality disorder often reject the diagnosis, preferring to explain unusual experiences as unique rather than as symptoms. The etiology of personality disorders is incomplete personality development. Many experiences can interfere with personality development such as abuse or other trauma, that interrupts, distorts, or redirects the evolving personality. For this reason, a diagnosis of personality disorder requires evidence of symptoms beginning in early adolescence or early adulthood.

Personality is represented by recurrent patterns of thoughts, feelings, and behaviors that in effect define the individual. Personality affects all areas of psychosocial functioning and shapes the individual's view of the world. Personality is also a conduit for interpersonal interactions and relationships, serving the individual's needs for satisfaction, security, and status. With personality disorders, the treatment goal is to improve functioning and stabilize mood and behavior. However, because of the nature of personality disorders, particularly the hypersensitivity to stress, patients with personality disorders frequently experience and require treatment for other mental disorders and psychosocial problems, such as depression, anxiety, substance abuse, and interpersonal conflict. The DSM-IV categorizes 10 specific personality disorders into one of three clusters. Cluster A disorders (paranoid, schizoid, schizotypal) are individuals who appear to be odd or eccentric. Cluster B disorders (antisocial, borderline, histrionic, narcissistic) are individuals who appear dramatic, emotional, or erratic. Cluster C disorders (avoidant, dependent, obsessive-compulsive) are individuals who appear anxious or fearful. DSM-IV symptom criteria restrict the use of these diagnoses to individuals who have inflexible and maladaptive patterns that cause marked functioning impairment, distress, or poor impulse control, and these patterns are evident in a range of personal and social situations.

Paranoid personality disorder, characterized by suspicion, is expressed as a belief that others wish to exploit, harm, or deceive the individual. The loyalty or trustworthiness of others is questioned and tested repeatedly, and insults or perceived injuries are not forgiven or forgotten. This includes recurrent suspicion and loyalty-testing of spouses or sexual partners.

Schizoid personality disorder, characterized by detachment, is manifested by a lack of desire for participation in close relationships or pleasurable activities. There is little experience or expression of emotion or affect.

Schizotypal personality disorder, characterized by social and interpersonal deficits, is indicated by discomfort with and limited ability to participate in close relationships, cognitive-perceptual distortions, and odd behavior. Symptoms may include delusions, odd beliefs, unusual perceptions, unusual thoughts or speech, suspicion, and inappropriate affect or mood. This disorder is related to schizophrenia in that it can serve as a premorbid condition.

Antisocial personality disorder, characterized by disregard for others, is most notable for rejection of rules and laws, and responsibility, exploitation, impulsivity, irritable aggression, recklessness, predatory or opportunistic behavior, and lack of remorse. There also appears to be a relentless drive for satisfaction.

Borderline personality disorder, characterized by instability and impulsivity, is indicated by abandonment anxiety, unstable relationships defined as love or hate, unstable self-concept, impulsive risky behavior, recurrent suicidal behavior, gestures or threats of self-mutilation, unstable mood, chronic emptiness, anger, and stress-related paranoia or dissociative reaction. The individual may be highly demanding of others and experience intense episodes of uncontrolled rage. This disorder is distinctive in the intensity of and recurrence of self-harm (intent and behavior) and the significant rate of individuals with this diagnosis who have a history of childhood sexual abuse.

Histrionic personality disorder, characterized by emotional attention-seeking, is manifested by an excessive need to be the center of attention and by sexually seductive behavior. Moods and emotions appear superficial and there is significant emphasis placed on physical appearance. Language is excessive and is used to create an impression rather than for expression. For example, a report of an ordinary work meeting becomes, "Everybody in the room said my idea was the best they had ever heard." This disorder is also associated with self-dramatizing, suggestibility, and a pattern of assigning more intimacy to relationships than actually exists.

Narcissistic personality disorder, characterized by a grandiose sense of self, differs from histrionic in that, along with the feeling that one is special, the individual requires admiration, has a strong sense of entitlement, and exploits others to achieve personal gain. Symptoms may also include arrogance and a lack of empathy for others.

Avoidant personality disorder, characterized by social inhibition, feelings of inadequacy, and hypersensitivity to disapproval, involves a marked unwillingness to be in a position that requires significant interpersonal contact or intimacy. The individual experiences an intense need to avoid criticism and rejection and strong feelings of inadequacy or inferiority.

Dependent personality disorder, characterized by clinging and subordination, causes the individual to seek advice and reassurance and to have others assume responsibility for major areas of his or her life. The individual fears loss of support, lacks the confidence to initiate, and goes to extraordinary lengths to obtain nurturance. There are significant feelings of helplessness when alone, so the person repeatedly seeks relationships as a source of nurturance and as a way to decrease the fear of not having someone to take care of them (Overholster, 1996).

Obsessive-compulsive personality disorder, characterized by a preoccupation with control, limits the individual's ability to be flexible, open, or efficient. There is a marked preoccupation with details, order, and organization. Completing a project is difficult because the person cannot meet excessively high performance expectations. Work and productivity are valued over relaxation and friendship. With this disorder, there may be an insistence on absolutes where there are none, such as with personal values or some standards of morality. The individual may keep objects of no apparent importance or value simply to avoid throwing them away. He or she works with others reluctantly, unless they submit to the same excessive expectations. Stubbornness and penny-pinching are also characteristic of this disorder.

According to the DSM-IV, a diagnosis of personality disorder is appropriate when multiple areas of the individual's life are affected by symptoms of the disorder. Having one or two traits is not sufficient for a diagnosis. Personality disorders are extremely complicated and require long-term specialized care. However, many people with personality disorders are never diagnosed and never receive treatment because they are able to express their symptoms without experiencing or inflicting overwhelming distress; thus they are able to contain their symptoms within their life-style. When they seek mental health care, often it is for other conditions, such as depression, substance dependence, or suicidal behavior. Unless they can be convinced that the secondary disorder is related to a personality disorder, they may have little motivation to continue with therapy.

Of the disorders reviewed here, those most likely to be treated, because life-style alone is not enough to contain the symptoms, are the borderline, antisocial, and obsessive-compulsive personality disorders: borderline, because of recurrent self-harm and mutilation; antisocial, because of harm to others; and obsessive-compulsive, because of irrational demands on others.

Paraphilias

Para means "going beyond", "to exceed or deviate", and ***philia*** means "a tendency toward; an attraction." The term paraphilia is used to describe strong sexual attraction and arousal that is excessive, abnormal, or unacceptable. This definition is difficult to use in clinical practice because people often deny that their sexual attraction and arousal is excessive, abnormal, or unacceptable. Therefore legal standards have been developed. Paraphilias involve pattern of attraction and arousal involving nonhuman objects, children, or nonconsenting adults, and suffering or humiliation (of self or others). The attraction, arousal and related behavior must be persistent for at least 6 months. The attraction and arousal experience can be constant or episodic, and may or may not be acted upon. This attraction and arousal may be the core of the individual's life, a substitute behavior to alleviate frustration, anxiety, or anger, or a nominal element of the person's life.

As with all DSM-IV disorders, each specific type of paraphilia is defined by the predominant symptom. ***Exhibitionism*** is attraction to and arousal by exposure. ***Fetishism*** is attraction to and arousal by objects such as shoes. ***Frotteurism*** is contact, usually rubbing or bumping, with a person who has not consented or who may be unaware of the contact. ***Pedophilia*** is attraction to and arousal by prepubescent children. ***Masochism*** is attraction to and arousal by humiliation and ***sadism*** is attraction to and arousal by the suffering of others. ***Voyerism*** is sexual arousal by observing an unsuspecting person nude or engaged in sexual activity.

Dissociative Disorder

Dissociative disorder is essentially a psychological escape when physical escape is impossible. According to the DSM-IV, the dissociative process is the separation of perceptions, identity, memory, and consciousness. This separation can occur in real time and be acute or chronic. Dissociative experiences range from ordinary brief episodes to severe disorders. An ordinary dissociative experience is, for example, "tuning out" while driving to work. Rather than paying attention to the drive, you let your mind attend to something more interesting and the drive to work is accomplished with automatic behaviors. The DSM-IV defines four types of dissociative disorders according to the nature, duration, and intensity of the "separation." These disorders can develop suddenly or follow a gradual, episodic, or chronic course. Dissociative disorders severely damage self-concept and interpersonal attachments, interactions, and relationships (Kluft & Fine, 1993).

Dissociative amnesia is characterized by one or more episodes of lost recall. The individual is unable to recall significant personal information, usually related to an intense trauma. This experience causes significant distress or psychosocial functioning impairment. The individual has gaps in his or her report of life events. For example, a woman in her early 40s is unable to recall her childhood before age 10. During those years she lived with her mother and father. Both parents were violent and abused alcohol. This disorder is also referred to as localized or selective amnesia. With ***localized amnesia*** there is no recall of a specific period of time. ***Selective amnesia*** means that only parts of a time period or event are recalled. ***Generalized amnesia*** is the lost recall of one's entire life, ***continuous amnesia*** is lost recall following an event or period of time until the current time, and ***systematized amnesia*** is lost recall of a specific type of information, such as events related to one specific person or place.

Dissociative fugue is characterized by a sudden loss of recall and finding oneself in a strange or unfamiliar place. An individual suddenly appears in a place that is strange or unfamiliar and does not know who or where he or she is. In extremely rare cases individuals have adopted a new identity and started a new life.

This disorder does not have significant symptomatology, so the individual, though distressed, could go unnoticed. This disorder is also related to the experience of overwhelming trauma or stress. An episode of dissociative fugue can last from hours to months.

Dissociative identity disorder is characterized by the experience of at least two whole and distinct personalities, each with the ability to control behavior. There is also lost recall of personal information and the experience cannot be attributed to blackouts associated with substance abuse and dependence. According to the DSM-IV there can be a period of 6 to 7 years between the first symptoms of the disorder and the diagnosis; therefore the awareness or evidence of different personalities tends to be gradual. Stress is a factor because it can cause symptoms to become acute. The multiple personalities may or may not have awareness, or co-consciousness, of each other's existence. When there is evidence of potential personal benefit, especially financial or legal, the absence of malingering or a factitious disorder must be confirmed.

Depersonalization, as a dissociative disorder, is characterized by persistent or recurrent episodes of detachment from one's self. The experience of depersonalization is to perceive oneself as the uninvolved observer of a stranger. Individuals observe, rather than experience, their emotions and their bodies. They may be unable to speak and there is a perception of being out of control or not able to command one's thoughts, feelings, or behavior. Depersonalization occurs as a secondary experience of other severe disorders, such as schizophrenia, but can be diagnosed as a separate disorder. As a separate disorder, depersonalization is often triggered by a life-threatening danger. Depersonalization does not impair one's sense of reality, but there is significant distress. For example, victims of violent crime may carefully report their experience in detail but repeatedly state, "I just don't believe this happened to me."

References

Africia B, Schwartz SR: Schizophrenia disorders. In Goldman H: *Review of general psychiatry* (ed 4). Norwalk, CT, 1995, Appleton & Lange.

Buckley PF, Buchanan RW, Schulz SC, Tamminga CA: Catching up on schizophrenia, *Arch Gen Psych* 53(5):546, 1996.

Carter DM, Mackinnon A, Copolon DL: Patient's strategies for coping with auditory hallucinations, *J of Nervous and Mental Disease*, 194(3):159, 1996.

Csernansky JG, Newcomer JG: Maintenance drug treatment for schizophrenia. In Bloom FE, Jupfer DJ (eds): *Psychopharmacology: the fourth generation of progress*, New York, 1995, Raven Press.

Harvey CA, Curson DA, Pantelis C, Taylor J, Barnes T: Four behavioral syndromes of schiziphrenia, *British J of Psych*, 168(5):562, 1996.

International Symposia Report: Current concepts in schizophrenia: new standards for assessment and treatment, *J Clin Psych*, 56:5, 1995.

Kluft R, Fine C: *Clinical perspectives on multiple personality disorder*, Washington, DC, 1993, American Psychiatric Assocation.

Neuchterlein, K, Gitlin M, Subotnik K: The early course of schizophrenia and long-term maintenance neuroleptic therapy, *Arch Gen Psych*, 52:3, 1995.

Overholser JC: The dependent personality and interpersonal problems, *J of Nervous and Mental Disease*, 184(1):8, 1996.

Paris J: The etiology of boderline personality disorders: a biopsychosocial approach, *Psychiatry*, 57(4):316, 1994.

Paris J, Zweig-Frank H, Bond M, Guzder J: Defense styles, hostility, and psychological risk factors in male patients with personality disorders, *J of Nervous and Mental Disease*, 184(3):453, 1996.

Reus VI: Mood disorder. In Goldman H: *Review of general psychiatry*, ed.4, Norwalk, CT,1995, Appleton & Lange.

Solomon P, Keltner G, Miller J, Shea MT, Keller M: Course of illness and maintenance treatment for patients with bipolar disorder, *J Clin Psych*, 56:1, 1995.

Szymanski SR, Cannon TD, Gallacher F, Erwin RJ, Gur RE: Course of treatment response in first-episode and chronic schizophrenia, *Am J Psych* 153(4):549, 1996.

Van Putten T: Why do schizophrenic patients refuse to take their drugs? *Arch Gen Psych*, 31:67, 1974.

Vaxquez-Barquero JL, Lastra I, Nunez MJ, Castanedo SH, Dunn G: *British J Psych* 168(6):693, 1996.
Ziedonis DM, Fisher W: Assessment and treatment of comorbid substance abuse in individuals with schizophrenia, *Psych Ann* 24:477, 1994.

Part II

Common Mental Disorders

Depression Disorders 4

This chapter reviews the assessment and management of three depression disorders: major depression, dysthymia, and adjustment disorder depression. Depression disorders are painful and debilitating conditions that can impair psychosocial functioning and cause significant psychosocial disability. Depression disorder is a total experience far more intense and complex than brief feelings of sadness. It is the experience of meaningful negative changes in thoughts, feelings, and behaviors that can affect any area of psychosocial functioning, but interpersonal interactions and relationships are particularly sensitive.

➲ Who Is at Risk

Because depression disorders are common in many groups, significant risk factors have been identified. Risk factors significantly increase the probability of depression disorder onset. According to the Agency for Health Care Policy and Research (AHCPR) 1993, the most important depression risk factors are: personal history of depression disorder, family history of depression disorder, history of suicide behavior, female gender, youth (under 40), postpartum, physical illness, inadequate social support, and substance abuse. Because risk-factor assessment makes early diagnosis possible and early diagnosis improves the probability of full recovery, these risk factors are reviewed in detail.

Gender

Women are more likely to be diagnosed with depression for two reasons. First, women are socialized to experience and express distress with the types of thoughts, feelings, and behaviors that are used to define clinical depression. Second, women are exposed to chronic gender-specific stressors in their female social roles. As a result of traditional masculine socialization, distressed males are more likely to abuse alcohol, withdraw, and become irritable, whereas distressed females are more likely to cry, seek support from others, or become sad. When gender differences in the expression of distress are taken into account the rate of depression for women and men is not so different.

Personal History Of Depression

The best criterion for full recovery following treatment for depression is a minimum of 1 year of symptom remission and effective psychosocial functioning. This criterion is important because the rate of relapse during the first 6 to 18 months following treatment is approximately 50%. The high risk of relapse following treatment for depression has been attributed to two common treatment complications: persistent mild symptoms and inadequate treatment. Research suggests that persistent mild symptoms of depression may be a manifestation of persistent neurotransmitter dysregulation; that is, mild symptoms may persist because the biological or psychological basis of the symptoms persists. Inadequate treatment addresses the symptoms of depression without dealing with depression-related changes in functioning. Partial symptom remission, short-duration symptom remission, and untreated psychosocial functioning impairments are significant depression risk factors. Individuals with a history of long-duration depression or multiple episodes have a greater risk of developing chronic depression with significant psychosocial disability (Keller, 1994).

Family History Of Depression

As a depression risk factor, family history can be thought of in the same terms as a personal history of depression. A family history of depression does not predict depression but it represents significant biological, psychological, and psychosocial functioning risk factors. Biological risk of depression based on family history is believed to have a genetic basis, whereas risk based on psychological and functioning factors is related to the highly stressful coping and interpersonal patterns that develop when members of one's family have a depression disorder. There are numerous specific biological models of family susceptibility to depression, ranging from theories of inherited biopsychosocial susceptibility to stress to theories of inherited chronic neurotransmitter dysregulation. Psychological and functioning theories focus on the stress of interacting with relatives who are depressed and the faulty learning experiences of children of depressed parents (Hagerty, 1995).

Physical Illness

Numerous physical conditions and disorders can be depression risk factors. Life-threatening illness, chronic illness, or unexpected illness can induce significant feelings and thoughts of helplessness and hopelessness, exposing the individual to multiple stressors. Physical illness that causes pain, fear, or unwanted changes can increase the risk of depression by undermining the individual's ability to cope with the illness effectively. Negative changes related to physical illness can also cause negative changes in self-concept and body image, two components of personal identity that are critically related to effective coping.

The American Psychiatric Association's *Diagnostic and Statistical Manual of Mental Disorders, fourth edition*, (DSM-IV) provides a comprehensive list of mental disorders, including depression, that are directly caused by physical illnesses such as thyroid disease, cancer, and bronchitis. Physical illness is an indirect cause of depression when the individual's otherwise highly effective coping skills are no longer available due to the illness. Lastly, physical illness is related to depression in that many people have somatic rather than psychological symptoms of depression. Rather than feeling sad or irritable, they may have headaches, backaches, and stomach aches, but physical causes for physical symptoms must be ruled out before a diagnosis of somatic depression can be considered. One of the most important and often overlooked physical conditions related to depression is physical fatigue. Effective psychosocial coping with everyday life requires physical stamina. When fatigued, people can become extremely susceptible to negative thoughts and thus susceptible to depression (Beck, Rush, Shaw and Emery, 1979).

Ineffective Psychosocial Functioning

Ineffective psychosocial functioning is one of the most difficult depression risk factors to generalize. It increases one's exposure to and experience of stressors, and stress is a major risk factor for depression. Effective psychosocial functioning can be defined as the ***performance of valued social roles*** and the ***use of effective***

coping skills. Individuals who do not have valued social roles can be at risk for depression when without such roles they develop a negative self-concept and low self-esteem. Poor coping skills can increase the risk of depression through an inability to protect the self-concept and self-esteem from threats as well as an inability to solve stressful problems. By making bad problems worse, ineffective coping skills can compound the negative impact of stressful problems. For example, Ed, a 45-year-old male, has been married for 3 months. To him, finally being able to say he is someone's husband means he is not a loser. Last night the couple had an unexpected, intense argument (stressor) about their money problems (stressor). Ed instantly blamed (immature defense) his wife for their money problems and their argument, but blaming did not protect Ed's self-concept or self-esteem from the stressors. Therefore he perceived the conflict with his wife as extremely threatening to him. He has returned to thinking of himself as a loser and has become silent and withdrawn.

Nonsupportive Environments

Both physical and interpersonal nonsupportive environments are important depression risk factors. Individuals are dependent on their physical and interpersonal environments for necessary resources, such as physical safety and emotional support. The two basic types of nonsupportive environment are those that lack or restrict access to needed resources and those that place excessive demands on the individual's resources. Individuals typically move among a variety of environments, supportive and some nonsupportive. Common nonsupportive environments include impoverished communities and highly stressful work environments.

Substance Abuse

Substance abuse directly and indirectly increases the risk of depression. The direct effects of substance abuse are chemical. Substances that produce dramatic CNS effects, psychosis, debilitating withdrawal symptoms, hangovers, or cravings significantly and directly increase the risk of depression. ***Abuse*** is defined as impaired functioning due to the large amounts of time spent seeking, using, and recovering from substance intoxication. Substance abuse also increases the risk of depression due to the related experience of important social losses. Substance abuse almost always causes lost relationships, lost income, lost identity, or lost hopes. Regardless of the source or nature of the loss, it is a major depression risk factor. The DSM-IV distinguishes depression disorders related to substance abuse from those that are not, and the term ***dual diagnosis*** is used when an individual has a substance abuse disorder along with other mental disorders.

* Common Symptom Onset Patterns

Depression symptom onset may occur gradually or suddenly, but regardless of the pattern, individuals vary in their awareness of and response to their symptoms. Individual awareness can range from full consciousness of the smallest changes in one's thoughts, feelings, and behaviors to a complete lack of consciousness of dramatic changes. Individuals who are psychologically attentive are more likely to be aware of symptoms than those who are not; there is no other meaningful explanation for these individual variations. ***Gradual symptom onset*** allows individuals to doubt and even invalidate their experience of symptoms. If one is unable to identify important problems or events that might account for negative changes in thoughts, feelings, and behavior, one may just assume that the problem is not serious and one will feel better tomorrow. Individuals are more likely to notice and respond to sudden symptoms. ***Sudden symptom onset*** is often described as waking up prepared to start the day only to find that one is unable to do so. In many cases the individual has had vague symptoms for some time but did not become concerned or fully aware of them until these symptoms began to impair functioning. Few people seek professional health care when they first begin to feel depressed since few are able to recognize their symptoms as symptoms.

❑ Common Assessment Problems

The assessment of depression disorders can be significantly complicated by negative reactions and by individual variations in the experience and expression of symptoms. Depressed individuals often complain that people who are not depressed fail to understand depression and therefore place unrealistic expectations on them to pull themselves together or accuse them of intentionally making things difficult for others. Negative reactions are unkind but they highlight the fact that depressed people can be depressing to be around (Coyne, 1976). Negative reaction is included here as an assessment problem because practitioners themselves are not immune to it. Interacting with depressed patients can be trying. Rather than ignoring this potential problem, practitioners should be aware of their reactions and ensure that they do not influence the assessment.

Individual variations in depression symptomatology can also present significant assessment problems. The assessment of depression is least complicated when the individual's symptoms conform to accepted norms. Traditional symptoms of depression in Western cultures are sadness, apathy, tears, and listlessness. Depressed individuals who are irritable, refuse to bathe, or complain a lot may not be recognized as depressed. How individuals experience and express depression is in part determined by their social learning. Different cultures, communities, social groups, and families have different accepted norms for depression. Depression may therefore be experienced and expressed as sadness, headache, sarcasm, aggression, silence, or anger. Depression can be most difficult to assess when the individual's expression conforms with non-Western norms or is highly individualized.

Depression Disorders

Major Depression

DSM-IV criteria for major depression requires five of the following eight symptoms for at least 2 weeks. Symptoms are assessed in terms of frequency, intensity, and duration (APA, 1994).

1. Dysphoria or apathy
2. Weight loss or significant change in appetite
3. Insomnia or hypersomnia
4. Physical restlessness or slowness
5. Fatigue
6. Feelings of worthlessness or guilt

7. Decreased concentration and inability to make decisions
8. Thoughts of death and suicide

Either dysphoria (sadness) or apathy (loss of interest) and impaired psychosocial functioning should be evident. Major depression is not the appropriate diagnosis for bereavement, depression related to substance abuse, or depression related to a medical condition.

Dysphoria or apathy

Depending on the individual, dysphoria or apathy can be very obvious or difficult to assess. Dysphoria generally appears as a slowed-down, dragged-out sadness. Apathy can be less apparent but typically is a lack of interest or boredom in an area where the person normally feels interest. Rather than saying they are no longer interested, some people may say that something that was of interest " doesn't matter" anymore or they may question a former interest with statements such as "what's the point?" Dysphoria or apathy can be expressed with irritability, anger, sarcasm, silence, hostility, arrogance, complaints of physical pain, or uncharacteristic changes in appearance. Depressed individuals may not shower or maintain their appearance because these things do not seem important.

Weight loss or significant change in appetite

Depressed individuals may report an increase or decrease in appetite, and weight loss is an important symptom of depression. Eating is a basic coping behavior, especially in response to stress. Increased eating as a coping behavior is not particularly effective, but at least the individual is trying to cope. Individuals may eat more as a way to distract themselves, avoid problems, or inflict self-punishment. Weight loss of 10 to 20 pounds indicates a vegetative state in which hunger is either not experienced or not acted on for an extended period of time.

Insomnia or hypersomnia

Sleeping more and sleeping less are both symptoms of depression. Why do some depressed individuals sleep all day and others can't sleep at all? One possible explanation is that serotonin, the neurotransmitter most strongly related to depression, is also related to sleep. Serotonin changes can therefore produce a range of sleep and mood changes. Sleep is also affected by stress; when distressed, some people sleep more, some cannot sleep at all and some cannot stop thinking about their concerns to allow for enough sleep. Because sleep changes are so varied as a symptom of depression, a good assessment standard for practitioners is whether or not the individual feels rested after a period of sleep. Research suggests that depression decreases the duration of deep sleep so that, regardless of the amount of time involved, the individual does not feel rested upon waking.

Physical restlessness or slowness

When depressed, some people feel hyperactive and restless while others feel robotic and slowed down. In either case the individual feels out of sync. Both restless and robotic psychomotor changes related to depression can be very apparent to the depressed individual as well as to significant others. Normal activities may take much longer to perform and complete. The restless depressed individual can take longer due to increased aimlessness and undirected activity; the robotic individual takes longer because of slow starts and frequent stops.

Fatigue

As a symptom of depression, fatigue differs from being slowed down or physically exhausted. Rather, it is experienced as a loss of will. Most people who feel this way are able to clearly articulate it. Activities such as watching TV, reading a book, or calling a friend seem to require excessive amounts of effort. Fatigue is an empty weariness not relieved by sleep or rest. Fatigue is an alarming symptom of depression especially after the depressed individual has unsuccessfully tried to remedy the problem with rest and relaxation.

Feelings of worthlessness or guilt

Depressed individuals may state that they feel worthless, guilty, or inadequate. Modern work and home environments that endlessly demand unrealistic levels of individual performance have made feelings of inadequacy more common and thus easier to overlook as a symptom of depression. Although common, feelings of inadequacy are nevertheless serious because they can lead to significant feelings of self-hate. Self-hate is a potentially dangerous level of feeling worthless because individuals can feel compelled to act out their self-hate in order to obtain some measure of relief. Feelings of worthlessness and self-hate are embraced because they create the illusion of control over painful feelings without actually having to confront those feelings.

Decreased concentration

Most individuals who experience a significant decrease in their ability to concentrate are alarmed by the experience. They may report being less able than usual to concentrate in performance situations, such as work or school, or in pleasurable activities, such as seeing a movie or reading a novel. In both performance and pleasure activities, individuals with decreased concentration report that they cannot put their mind on something and keep it there. In some cases, individuals may report that, rather than being unable to focus their attention, they have difficulty absorbing an experience. Decreased concentration can also be an inability to put thoughts together or the loss of one's train of thought in midsentence. Depending on the individual's routine needs for concentration, a decrease in it may not immediately be noticed as troubling. For example, a university student may be troubled sooner by this symptom. Confused or altered thinking are not symptoms of decreased concentration, but are serious cognitive symptoms that may be related to serious mental illness (SMI).

Thoughts of death and suicide

Thoughts of death and suicide are expected symptoms of major depression and reflect the negative thinking associated with it (Beck, 1979). Assessment of thoughts of death and suicide includes the content and process of those thoughts. An individual may need to be reassured that thoughts of death or suicide are symptoms of depression and, with treatment, will decrease along with other symptoms. This validation can make it somewhat easier to disclose what may be very disturbing thoughts. Practitioners should avoid giving the impression that a person's thoughts about death or suicide are either appropriate or inappropriate.

The assessment should also distinguish between thoughts of death and thoughts of suicide. ***Thoughts of death*** tend to be passive; their content is death, with little or no content regarding the cause. Examples of these would be thoughts of going to sleep without waking up or not waking up until a stressful situation has improved. ***Thoughts of suicide*** include the cause of death. A person who has thoughts of death might say "I would rather be dead than live like this," whereas a person with thoughts of suicide might say "I'd rather end my life than live like this." Some individuals may be more forthcoming with their thoughts about death than their thoughts about causing their death. Thoughts of death and suicide cannot be ranked in seriousness since neither in itself predicts behavior. Suicidal thoughts do not always lead to suicidal behavior, but this is always a possibility and should therefore be assessed.

Dysthymia

In comparison to major depression, DSM-IV symptoms of dysthymia are fewer and less intense but of greater duration. Dysthymia is essentially chronic mild depression. Symptoms should be evident for at least 2 years and should cause distress or impaired functioning. Overall the number of symptomatic days should exceed the number of symptom-free days. There may or may not be a prior history of major depression, but individuals with dysthymia may report having always been depressed and are learning to live with it. Individuals with dysthymia can develop major depression as a separate disorder. DSM-IV criteria for dysthymia are (APA, 1994):

1. Depressed mood on a regular basis for at least 2 years
2. During depression, 2 or more of the following are evident: poor appetite or overeating, insomnia or hypersomnia, low energy or fatigue, low self-esteem, poor concentration or difficulty making decisions, and feelings of hopelessness

3. Symptom-free periods no longer than 2 months
4. No episode of major depression during the first 2 years of dysthymia

Adjustment Disorder-Depression

Adjustment disorder-depression refers to the onset of depression symptoms in response to an identifiable negative event. With this disorder, individuals have experienced an event to which they cannot easily adjust. According to the DSM-IV, this event must have occurred within 3 months of symptom onset. The predominant symptoms of adjustment disorder-depression are depressed mood, tearfulness, or hopelessness. Symptoms may be emotional or behavioral in nature and should produce significant distress or functioning impairment. This diagnosis should not be used for cases of bereavement or post-traumatic stress disorder. The name of this diagnosis implies that it is a brief cause-and-effect disorder only, but adjustment disorders can be diagnosed as acute (within 6 months after the event) or chronic (more than 6 months after the event). Events related to adjustment disorders may be sudden, chronic, recurrent, single, or multiple. Adjustment disorder-depression differs from major depression in that the symptoms are fewer and milder; it differs from dysthymia in that the symptoms are moderate rather than mild and symptom duration is less than 1 year.

Management of Depression Disorders

➤ Counseling

When the depressed individual's level of distress and functioning impairment is not severe, brief therapy is usually effective in mobilizing positive thinking and effective coping (Jarrett and Rush, 1994). Counseling should focus on current rather than long-standing concerns. The most important skills here are listening and talking. Practitioners may be reluctant to counsel depressed individuals based on the incorrect assumptions that counseling will take too much time, and accomplish too little, that depressed patients are difficult and demanding, and that counseling is not necessary. Counseling is actually an effective use of the time spent with patients as well as an effective strategy for working with difficult individuals. The depressed primary care patient can benefit from emotional support, education, structure, and mobilization.

Depressed patients may have experienced negative action from their friends, family, co-workers, and partner, making positive emotional support an important patient need. Emotional support begins with the positive message that the individual is different from and more than one's symptoms of depression. This positive message can be very helpful to the depressed individual, who may overidentify with one's symptoms and lose one's identity as a person without depression. Explicit statements that symptoms do not define a person are particularly helpful for patients who may have forgotten what it was like when they were not depressed.

In order to be most effective, emotional support should be offered within the context of the interpersonal relationship of practitioner and patient. Even sincere emotional support can appear to be phony when it does not acknowledge the individual. Patients should be encouraged to express their experience of depression without fear of being judged or invalidated. Emotional support can address the negative thinking and hopelessness associated with depression.

Teaching is also an important early intervention in counseling depressed patients. Information about depression should for the most part be specific to the individual. Until they have significant symptom relief, few people are very interested in learning general information about depression. Most want to understand what is happening to them and what they can expect. Teaching should address the effect of the patient's symptoms on day-to-day functioning and the effort needed to improve. Teaching should help the patient to identify those factors that make symptoms or functioning worse and those that bring about improvement. This information is the basis for personalized mental health promotion and mental illness prevention. Of all the information that patients need to know, perhaps the most important is that depression can be an aggressive and invasive disorder that if left untreated can affect all areas of the patient's life.

Mobilizing is the process of helping the patient develop a plan of action to follow, starting with the first visit. Patients frequently ask practitioners to tell them what they could and should be doing for themselves. With depression, the answer should always be to take action and to do anything and everything that actively decreases the immobilizing effects of depression. Patients should identify personal goals related to their psychosocial functioning and the efforts needed to achieve them. Ideally this counseling produces a daily plan that provides structure, which is usually lacking for people with depression. The plan should include a daily measure of progress toward recovery. Patients should continually evaluate their activities by asking themselves, "Am I moving toward or away from recovery?" and then making every effort to follow their daily plan. Even simple plans, such as being out of bed and dressed by a certain time, meeting three obligations, going for a walk, and calling a friend, can be effective. A minimal plan for mobilizing depressed individuals should include interaction with supportive others, sleep and rest, restorative recreation, exercise, work, and doing something for someone else. The plan should severely limit the amount of time the individual spends alone. Patients may insist that they don't feel like doing anything, but practitioners can teach them to recognize this thinking as a symptom that can impair functioning if it is not addressed. The point is not to tax the depressed individual with meaningless performance expectations but to support recovery. Efforts to develop and follow a plan of action also support the patient's self-concept and self-esteem. Practitioners should tell patients that the expectation is that they will try.

℞ Prescribing

Many excellent psychotropic medication references are available and practitioners should refer to them when prescribing antidepressants (Friedman and Kocsis 1996; Richelson, 1993). A review is provided here of the prescription process in terms of safety issues, patient expectations, medication effectiveness, substance use and abuse, and cost. Selective serotonin reuptake inhibitors (SSRI) are effective and safer than earlier antidepressants due to a very low risk of lethal overdose. Prescriptions need not be limited to 7- to 10-day supplies. However, patient reliability and impulsivity should still be considered. Although the risk of lethal overdose with SSRI has been diminished, intentional or unintentional overdose, misuse, misplacement, and distribution of prescribed medications should be discussed. When the potential danger of a medication is not spelled out to patients, they may be less likely to take necessary precautions. Always remind patients to keep their antidepressants in a safe place. Medications left in pockets, purses, and backpacks and on tables and counters can be a hazard to curious children, impulsive adolescents, disoriented elders, or hungry pets.

Patient expectations

Practitioners should review the patient's positive and negative expectations about the potential effects of antidepressant medications. The appropriate patient expectation is symptom relief and remission over a period of 2 to 6 weeks. From 50% to 75% of depressed patients treated with anti-depressant medication will improve, but the rest experience little or no benefit. Practitioners should review why an antidepressant medication is being prescribed, what positive and negative effects can be anticipated, and the expected length of treatment. Unrealistic expectations of patients should be addressed but practitioners should keep in mind that it is difficult to keep one's expectations realistic when one's needs are high.

Effectiveness

Practitioners should identify specific target symptoms, including sadness or apathy, to be used as indicators of effective relief and remission. Symptom relief and remission should be defined individually. Patients should be reminded that effective treatment does not preclude experiencing normal changes in mood. According to the DSM-IV an episode of major depression can be considered remitted when there have been at least 2 months of subclinical symptoms or no symptoms. Problems (e.g., conflict with partner) usually improve with symptom relief but cannot be used as target symptoms. Two or three of the patient's predominant symptoms can be effective target symptoms. Practitioners should not imply or allow patients to infer that taking antidepressant medications will make them "feel better" in the usual sense of the term. Many people may not have noticeable effects from SSRIs.

Substance abuse

SSRIs do not produce pleasurable changes in mental status or mood. The most notable effect should be symptom relief. However, the absence of perceived effects can be unexpected or mistrusted by individuals who expect them. Patients who are accustomed to using drugs to change their state of mind or mood may continue to do. Practitioners should clearly point out to patients that substance use should be avoided. If this is not realistic, then the patient's continued substance use should be considered as a potential prescribing problem.

Cost

Cost is no small concern when prescribing medication, particularly SSRI anti-depressants. It is not uncommon for these medications to cost over $1 a tablet. Practitioners should routinely consult with dispensing pharmacists and benefits counselors to ensure that they know the cost of the medications prescribed. There are also sound clinical reasons for addressing the cost of antidepressants. Few people are willing to pay large sums of money for a medication that does not appear to be helpful, but premium prices imply that a medication may be significantly better than less expensive medications. Practitioners should work with patients to clarify any misunderstandings or assumptions they may have concerning the cost of their medication.

Maintenance treatment

The recommended course of treatment with most SSRI anti-depressants is 2 to 6 weeks for symptom relief and remission followed by 6 to 9 months of maintenance. Continual treatment with SSRIs to prevent future episodes of depression is a topic of serious debate that cannot be resolved here. Practitioners can expect to encounter individuals who have taken antidepressants for years and fully expect to continue doing so. There are also people who wish to take antidepressant medications to get through a stressful situation rather than to treat diagnosed depression. There are efficacy questions in using antidepressants to treat mild symptoms of depression. Until these concerns are clarified, practitioners will have to deal with them on a case-by-case basis, weighing benefits against risks (Fava and Davidson, 1996).

☎ Consultation and Referral

Practitioners should consult with a specialist when a depressed patient is suicidal but the risk of action cannot be calculated; when there is evidence of profound functioning impairment; when the patient requires more services than can be provided in primary care; when the patient may have multiple DSM-IV diagnoses; when atypical symptoms of depression are evident; when there are significant situational, interpersonal, child-care, or partner problems; or when there is a history of unsuccessful treatment with antidepressant medication. Depressed patients should be referred to a specialist when symptom relief and remission or full recovery will require aggressive or complex treatment; when there is a high or unpredictable risk of suicide; and when there is evidence of SMI. Practitioners with managed-care organizations may have very limited referral resources, but in these cases referral is indicated. If a referred patient has to wait weeks to see a specialist, the practitioner should arrange to continue with the patient until the referral is complete and should expect to encounter limits on the total number of appointments with a psychiatric specialist. Under these conditions, practitioners should refer to specialists for diagnosis, stabilization, and treatment recommendations.

References

Agency for Health Care Policy and Research: *Depression in primary care: Vol.2., treatment of major depression*, Rockville, Maryland, 1993, U.S. Department of Health and Human Services.

Beck AT, Rush AJ, Shaw BF, Emery G: *Cognitve therapy of depression*, New York, 1979, The Guilford Press.

Burke MJ, Preskorn SH: Short-term treatment of mood disorders with standard antidepressants. In Bloom FE, Kuper DJ (eds): *Psychopharmacology: the fourth generation of progress*, New York, 1995, Raven Press.

Coyne JC: *Toward an instructional description of depression*, Psychiatry 39(1):29-40, 1976.

Fava M, Davidson KG: Definition and epidemiology of treatment resistant depression, *Psych Clinics North Am*, 12(2):179, 1996.

Friedman RA, Kocsis, JH: *Pharmcotherapy for chronic depression*, Psych Clin of North Am 19(1), 1996.

Goldman H: *Review of general psychiatry*, Norwalk, CT, 1995, Appleton & Lange.

Hagerty, B: Advances in understanding major depressive disorder, *J of Psychosocial Nrsg*, 33(11):27-34, 1995.

Jarrett, RB, Rush AJ: Short term psychotherapy of depressive disorders: current status and future directions, *Psychiatry*, 57(2):115, 1994.

Keller, MB: Depression: a long-term illness, *British J of Psych*, 165(supple26)9, 1994.

Miranda J, Hohmann A, Attkisson C, Larson D: *Mental disorders in primary care*, San Francisco, 1994, Jossey-Bass.

Parry P: Mood disorders linked to the reproductive cycle in women. In Bloom FE, Kupfer DJ (eds): *Psychopharmacology, the fourth generation of progress*, New York, 1995, Raven Press.

Richelson E: Treatment of acute depression, *Psych Clinics North Am*, 16(3), 1993.

Spitzer R, Williams J, Kroenke K, Linzer M, Verloin D, Hahn S, Brody D, Johnson J: *Utility of new procedure for diagnosing mental disorders in primary care: The prime-MD 1000 study*, JAMA 272(22):12, 1994.

Zisook S: *Treatment of dysthymia and atypical depression*, Clin Psych 10(1):15, 1992.

Stress and Adjustment Disorders 5

Stress and adjustment disorders develop as reactions to internal and external events that threaten an individual's ability to cope. The risk of developing a stress or adjustment disorder is related to the nature of the stressors as well as the individual's coping resources and coping skills. The experience of severe stressors can have a pervasive effect on humans, producing significant biological, physical, psychological, and social disruptions that compel the individual to incorporate the stressors, adjust to the stress, or seek mastery. Mastery allows the individual to reintegrate and continue to grow and develop. This chapter presents a review of the assessment and management of acute stress disorder, chronic stress, adjustment disorders, and crisis.

➲ Who Is at Risk

Two individuals experience the same stressful event, yet one develops a stres disorder and the other does not. In most cases, individual differences can be attributed to variations in personal experience, appraisal style, coping skills, and coping resources. Each of these factors can significantly influence the individual's ability to cope effectively with the stressful event and, subsequently, increase the individual's risk of developing a stress disorder. Effective coping decreases the risk of developing a stress disorder.

The risk of developing a stress disorder is based on the nature of the stressful event, when it occurs in a person's life, the circumstances of the event, and the individual's psychosocial stage of development. Effective coping decreases the risk of developing a stress disorder by decreasing the biopsychosocial impact of the event, but the actual onset of a stress disorder should not be seen as the result of failure to cope. Many events commonly associated with stress disorders require effective coping and adjustment just to recover from them, much less prevent the onset of a disorder. High-risk factors for stress disorders are: sudden, chronic, and severely stressful life events; rigid personal appraisal style; emotionally focused rather than problem-solving coping skills; and inadequate coping resources. Risk factors are not only correlated with the onset of stress disorders but also with recovery from them. A significant decrease in risk may be necessary for recovery; otherwise the individual continues to be at high risk for recurrent stress disorders.

Each risk factor listed here could independently increase the risk of developing a stress disorder, but the overall risk, based on their combined effects, offers a more comprehensive approach to understanding individual variations. For example, experience may initially appear to be a more important risk factor, but in some stages of life appraisal style, coping skills, or coping resources could be more important. Decreased risk for stress disorder is also based on the individual's experience, appraisal style, coping skills, and coping resources.

Experience

Experience can be defined as positive and negative preparations for future stressful life events. ***Positive experience*** consists of mastery or resolution achieved with the use of effective coping skills and resources. When individuals have a positive experience related to a stressful event or problem, they can feel that they have mastered the event or problem. Experiences of mastery support positive self-concept and high levels of self-confidence and self-esteem that, in turn, motivate individuals to face new events and problems as challenges to be mastered.

Negative experience is defined in terms of an individual's effort to master the stressful event and one's response to it, as well as to maintain an adequate level of functioning. Negative experience also refers to the experience of events or problems so severe that most people would be overwhelmed by them. The inability to cope with a stressful event or problem can undermine self-confidence and self-esteem. When repeated and sustained effort does not lead to mastery, the individual becomes psychologically exhausted and feelings of defeat, demoralization, and self-doubt can develop, to the point of establishing avoidance reaction to future stressful events and problems. This risk is compounded by a quirk of human nature that causes people to place more importance on their negative experiences than on their positive ones.

Appraisal Style

Appraisal style refers to the pattern of thinking and the frame of reference an individual uses to understand stressful events and problems. An individual's frame of reference is influenced by strongly held personal beliefs and attitudes about life. For example, some people believe that ups and downs in life are normal and so people must simply do their best and never give up rather than win every battle. The opposite belief is that life is a game that can never be won, or life is a game and defeat must be avoided at all costs. These idealist, pessimist, and competitive beliefs act as cognitive frames of reference that directly affect the way an individual thinks about stressful events.

The individual's frame of reference is the basis for the first and second steps of appraising an event or problem; both are performed almost instantly. The first step, defined by Lazarus, Averill and Opton (1974) is ***primary appraisal***, asking whether the event or problem is a threat to oneself. The second step, ***secondary appraisal***, is asking what one's coping alternatives are. When conditions warrant, a third step, ***reappraisal,*** may be performed. Reappraisal is essentially a repeat of steps 1 and 2. How an individual responds and copes is in large part determined by this continual process of appraisal and reappraisal.

Beck, Rush, Shaw, and Emery (1979) developed a comprehensive cognitive model of thought patterns shown to be significantly related to depression, but these thought patterns also affect coping and therefore the risk of developing stress disorder. The most common thought patterns are referred to as the individual's cognitive triad, cognitive schemas, and cognitive errors. The ***cognitive triad*** is a negative view of the self, the world, and the future. ***Cognitive schemas*** are stable, self-defeating thought patterns. ***Cognitive errors*** are due to faulty information processing, usually caused by rigid thinking. Rigid thinking consists of overgeneralization, magnification or minimization, personalization, and absolutes (Beck et al, 1979). ***Overgeneralization*** is the process of using one event to draw conclusions about many others. ***Magnification*** and ***minimization*** refer to viewing an event as either more significant or less significant than it actually is. ***Absolutes*** is thinking of events in either-or terms so that, for example, a problem is viewed as either impossible or effortless to deal with, when actually both views may be true.

Coping Skills, Styles, and Resources

Lazarus, Averill, and Opton (1974) define coping as the problem-solving efforts of an individual who is faced with important demands that tax one's skills and resources. The advantage of viewing coping as a problem-solving skill is that the relation between coping and stress disorder is made clear. Coping skills and coping style should be distinguished. ***Coping skills***, like other skills, are learned or developed abilities. From childhood on, individuals learn from experience to use coping skills or problem-solving methods that have worked for them, whether or not those skills are positive and effective.

Coping style can be thought of as an individual's actual rather than potential use of coping skills. Coping style refers to the individual's usual way of handling stressful events or problems; most individuals have multiple coping styles. For example, a man's coping style with interpersonal conflict may differ significantly from his coping style with financial problems. The same man may have a fairly stable way of coping with problems when he is rested but have a totally different style when he is tired. His coping style will also vary depending on how threatened he feels and his perception of the nature of that threat (appraisals). For example, when his skill as a computer programmer is questioned, he may make jokes and laugh it off because he is confident in his talents as a programmer. If he did not feel confident he might perceive any questioning of his programmer skills as a threat, and his style of coping with threats is to directly challenge the person who he feels has threatened him.

Under extreme conditions, regardless of the individual's ability or skill, coping can become immobilized. This occurs when an individual is unable to address a stressful event or problem. Any number of factors can produce an immobilizing effect on coping. It may be helpful to think of the immobilized individual as being frozen or stuck. Although faced with immediate demands for coping, the immobilized individual takes no action. For example, a woman learns that her husband of 25 years has decided to file for divorce. She is deeply hurt by his decision and does not want a divorce, yet she has not talked to him about her feelings. Instead she continues with her normal routine of going to work, taking care of their home and their pets, and visiting her parents.

Coping resources are the supplies that make coping possible. Anything that supports the individual's coping effort is a coping resource, such as information, beliefs, a positive attitude, education, intimacy, a confidant, money, a car, friends, family, a dog, and prayer. More resources mean more coping options. Individuals with demanding events and problems but limited coping resources are less able to cope effectively. Additional resources can significantly improve an individual's ability to cope. However, in order for resources to support coping, the individual must use the resource effectively. For example, a woman has to pay her rent today or she will be evicted from her apartment. A relative gives her the money she needs but, feeling depressed about her chronic money problems, she spends half of it on new clothes. She did not use her resources effectively, despite her ability to do so, and her stressful problems will therefore continue (Solomon, 1995).

* Common Symptom Onset Patterns

Stress is as an intense, chronic, or accumulative biopsychosocial burden that can disrupt all areas of functioning. It is significantly related to numerous physical health problems (e.g., hypertension) in addition to the mental disorders reviewed here. Any number of events and problems can cause stress, but the actual biopsychosocial arousal that defines stress is essentially universal.

Robinson (1990) describes three pathways of stress symptom onset: direct effects, behavioral-coping effects, and self-care effects. The ***direct effects*** of stress are physiological arousal, specifically the autonomic, sympathetic, and pituitary-adrenal cortical arousal that partly define the physical experience of stress. These physiological changes, such as increased blood pressure, reduced immunosurveillance, and altered corticosteroid release, are directly related to disease and disorders. Severe physiological symptoms of stress can also cause severe emotional and behavioral symptoms, such as fear or aggression. The ***behavioral-coping effects*** of stress are less direct than the physiological effects but are no less troublesome. Stress can increase the amount of effort needed to engage in healthy coping behaviors such as physical exercise. Stress can lead to the use of effortless, unhealthy coping behaviors, such as the consumption of various substances: stimulants; CNS depressants; foods high in sugar, salt, and fat; tobacco; caffeinated beverages; alcohol; marijuana; or fast-foods.

With acute stress disorder, the stress response or symptom onset develops immediately and is clearly in response to an identifiable event or problem. Just the opposite is true for the symptom pattern of chronic stress. As with many chronic disorders, the true point of symptom onset may be difficult to ascertain. The chronic or recurrent nature of the symptoms distinguishes this disorder. Chronic stress usually implies chronic stressors; that is, the symptoms of stress are chronic because the cause of the symptoms is chronic. Crisis as a stress disorder is the experience of near or actual panic levels of anxiety, in response to an identifiable event or problem. Because the onset of the disorder involves severe symptoms, crisis is viewed as an emergency.

Symptom onset with adjustment disorders also follows an identifiable event or problem. A diagnosis of adjustment disorder includes specification of the individual's predominant symptomatology, such as mixed anxiety or depressed mood. Symptom duration of less than 6 months is classified as acute adjustment disorder and symptom duration of 6 months or longer is classified as chronic adjustment disorder.

Stress And Adjustment Disorders

Acute Stress Disorder

The defining symptom criterion for a diagnosis of acute stress disorder according to the *Diagnostic & Statistical Manual of Mental Disorders, fourth edition*, (DSM-IV) is symptom onset immediately following the experience of an extremely traumatic event. This disorder differs from post-traumatic stress disorder in that the symptoms of acute stress disorder do not become chronic.

Symptoms of acute stress disorder should last for at least 2 days but not longer than 4 weeks. Acute stress disorder symptoms are:

1. Experiencing, witnessing, or being confronted with a traumatic event
2. Responding with intense fear, helplessness, and horror
3. Exhibiting dissociative symptoms
4. Persistently reexperiencing the traumatic event
5. Avoidance
6. Anxiety

Traumatic events

These include actual or threatened death, injury, or harm to oneself or others. Each individual has a cutoff point for trauma, but this is not the bottom line. An event that might be traumatic in childhood may not be traumatic in adulthood. The cutoff point for trauma may be different when one is alone than when one is in a crowd or with significant others. In most cases, trauma involves actual or potential physical pain, suffering, or mutilation. Individuals may experience, witness, discover, or be told of the event. Trauma is a biopsychosocial explosion that scatters mind, body, and soul. Coping responses are aimed at helping individuals to reorganize or pull themselves together (Foster, 1994).

Fear, helplessness, horror

Fear may be presented as anxiety, trepidation, aversion, or physical symptoms such as tremor, and may or may not be limited to the traumatic event. The fear may be directly related to the trauma, but it is also possible for the individual to become generally fearful. ***Helplessness*** may be evident as either general inability or increased needs for assistance. The individual may be unable to carry out a necessary task, such as notifying significant others or authorities, and may feel susceptible and vulnerable. ***Horror*** is usually the intense physical and emotional experience of revulsion or disgust. The scene of common traumatic events, especially car accidents and assaults, may contain elements that are shockingly dirty or nasty. These images can make up a large part of the reexperience of trauma (Wise, 1993).

Dissociative symptoms

The diagnosis of acute stress disorder should not be made unless there is evidence of three or more dissociative symptoms that occur during or following the traumatic experience. Dissociative symptoms include numbing, detachment, a lack of emotional responsiveness, reduced awareness of surroundings or being in a daze, perception of events as not quite true or real (derealization), a loss of sense of self (depersonalization), and inability to remember aspects of the trauma. Dissociative symptoms are protective screens that decrease the individual's awareness of the trauma, much like a cognitive dimmer switch that reduces the conscious intensity of it. Dissociative symptoms create psychological distance between the individual and the traumatic event. Without dissociative symptoms the individual would be exposed to the full psychological force of the trauma.

Reexperience

With acute stress disorder, the individual has involuntary continual reexperiences of the trauma (e.g., recurrent mental images, dreams, or flashbacks). Whereas dissociative symptoms are mental mechanisms that reduce the impact of trauma, reexperience symptoms can be thought of as a semiconscious floating awareness of trauma. Individuals may describe upsetting images that pop in and out of their consciousness without warning. Although the actual reexperience may last no longer than a moment, that image may be enough to cause a repeat of the initial reaction to the trauma.

Avoidance

Individuals with acute stress disorder may go to great lengths to avoid contact with anything they believe will cause them to fully recall the traumatic event. Typically they try to avoid people, places, and objects that are connected to or somehow representative of the trauma. Avoidance can become global rather than focused, as though the world has become an immediate danger. The connection between what is being avoided and the trauma that was experienced may or may not be apparent. Avoidance may represent intentional efforts to try to regain a sense of cause-and-effect control in one's daily life. By avoiding, for example, public parking garages, an individual can feel more in control of the experience of having been robbed in a public parking garage. Avoidance allows individuals to feel there is something they can do that will benefit them. Avoidance may occur whether or not it is effective. However, eventually an individual may develop a strong need to return to the location of the traumatic event as a means of bringing the experience to closure.

Anxiety

Symptoms of anxiety associated with acute stress disorder are intense. The individual undergoes much of the biopsychosocial arousal described in Chapter 6.. This includes sleep difficulties, irritability, poor concentration, restlessness, and hypervigilance (Robinson 1990).

Chronic Stress

Chronic stress is not a DSM-IV diagnosis but it is a commonly diagnosed mental health condition. Chronic stress can be defined as cumulative and sustained states of biopsychosocial arousal that are physically, emotionally, and psychologically consuming, leaving the individual exhausted and empty. Commonly known as ***burnout***, the distinguishing features of chronic stress are functioning impairment or disability and failing health. Burnout is progressive, occurring as stages of increasingly severe symptomatology (Mitchell, 1981) as follows:

Stage 1. Early warning
Stage 2. Beginning burnout
Stage 3. Midpoint burnout
Stage 4. Complete burnout

The ***early warning stage*** of burnout is a disquieting listlessness. The individual may experience mild anxiety, fatigue, depressed mood, boredom, and apathy (Mitchell, 1981). ***Beginning burnout*** may also be experienced as vague, but compared to early warning signs these symptoms are more disruptive. Beginning symptoms include moderate anxiety, sleep disturbances, headache, backache, muscle aches, loss of energy, fatigue, social withdrawal, and nausea. In some cases these symptoms become disruptive enough to cause the individual to seek health care.

Midpoint burnout is defined by severe symptoms, including skin rashes, marked physical weakness, depression disorder, increased use of alcohol or cigarettes, high blood pressure, migraine headaches, irritability, isolation and withdrawal, dramatic emotional outbursts, irrational fears, rigid thinking, loss of appetite, loss of sexual interest, and gastric ulcers. ***Complete burnout*** has been associated with disabling physical and psychological conditions and symptoms. These include coronary artery disease, diabetes, cancer, heart attacks, severe depression disorder, low self-esteem, impaired occupational, academic, or interpersonal functioning, social isolation, episodes of uncontrolled crying, suicidal thoughts, muscle tremors, severe fatigue, hyperemotionality, agitation, uninterrupted tension, accidents, carelessness, and hostility. At this stage of burnout, there is increased risk of psychosis, which in turn increases the risk of behaviors that are potentially dangerous to self or others. With complete burnout, the individual is forced to make significant life-style changes, particularly in employment and important interpersonal relationships. At this stage the risk of disability or infirmity is significant.

Chronic stress implies chronic stressors, or an inability to decrease the biopsychosocial arousal caused by chronic stressors. For example, poverty generates multiple daily stressors that are nearly impossible to avoid or escape. Highly educated professionals with demanding jobs, homemakers, and students may also be exposed to more stressors and stress arousal than they can manage.

Crisis

Crisis can be thought of as an unforeseen struggle for reequilibrium and reorganization when an individual is faced with problems perceived to be insolvable. Much of who we are, both to ourselves and to others, is what makes up our personality. Personality is the psychological organization of many small personal characteristics. Crisis is experienced as a threat to this psychological organization and therefore to self-concept. Crisis events represent both danger and opportunity and can be classified as situational or maturational. A ***situational crisis*** is an event, such as losing a job or a significant other, becoming seriously ill, or being in a natural disaster, that causes disequilibrium and threatens to disorganize the individual's sense of self. A ***maturational crisis*** is an event that occurs as a normal part of growth and development but is extremely difficult and challenging. The major symptoms of crisis are the psychological and physical symptoms of anxiety, which occur in three stages:

Stage 1. Mild anxiety
Stage 2. Moderate anxiety
Stage 3. Severe anxiety

In Stage 1 individuals experience mild anxiety that alerts them to the need to activate their normal coping skills and mobilize their coping resources. Should these skills and resources resolve the crisis and restore equilibrium, the threat of disorganization decreases, thereby decreasing anxiety. Either the event is resolved or the individual has been able to protect oneself from the threat. If normal coping skills, coping resources, and psychological defenses prove insufficient to resolve the crisis or to decrease the threat of disorganization, anxiety will continue to increase. In Stage 2 moderate levels of anxiety can lead to defeat and resignation or to the adoption of new coping skills and resources. If at this stage the individual employs new skills and resources that resolve the crisis or protect the individual, the crisis can be considered a growth and development challenge that was successfully mastered.

If new coping skills and resources are ineffective, Stage 3 occurs. Here anxiety levels increase significantly and the risk of psychological disorganization becomes great. At this point severe anxiety precludes effective coping and escape may become the individual's sole objective. Individuals escape from crisis events in many ways, but escape is typically accomplished by engaging in behaviors that allow retreat from the event or regression into a state of psychological comfort (O'Connor, 1994). If effective help is obtained and the individual's anxiety is immediately addressed, coping rather than escape or comfort can once again become the focus of the individual's efforts. In this case the risk of long-term problems is decreased. If instead of crisis resolution the net outcome is retreat from the event or psychological regression, the individual may be worse off than before the crisis event. In this case the risk of long-term problems, such as chronic stress, substance abuse, and depression is significant (Cui, 1996).

Adjustment Disorders

Life demands constant adjustment. Humans seek stability and predictability in their lives but also need stimulation and challenge; therefore things change. To survive change individuals must be able to adapt. This is not to imply that humans are passive victims who are subject to any and all changes. Individuals can try to prevent or alter the nature of changes in their lives or they can draw needed resources from their physical and social environments to enable them to adjust. Individuals also tend to create much of the change they encounter. Desired changes, such as a different school, a new baby, or more responsibility at work can be just as stressful and difficult to adjust to as unexpected problems.

A DSM-IV diagnosis of adjustment disorder is made when an individual has experienced a stressor, has had a great deal of difficulty coping with the changes brought about by the stressor, and when this difficulty is manifested as distress and impaired functioning. Adjustment disorders differ from crisis in that crisis occurs over a period of days whereas an adjustment disorder is diagnosed within 3 months of an identifiable stressor. A diagnosis of adjustment disorder should not be made when symptoms fit better with a more inclusive disorder, such as major depression, or when symptoms are an exacerbation of another disorder, such as personality disorder. Adjustment disorder should not be diagnosed for cases of bereavement. When a diagnosis of adjustment disorder is made, and symptom duration is 6 months or less, the disorder is classified as acute. When symptom duration is 6 months or longer, the classification is chronic. A diagnosis of chronic adjustment disorder implies that the stressor and its consequences are chronic.

Adjustment disorder diagnoses are specified according to predominant symptomatology. These are (APA, 1994):

- Adjustment disorder with depressed mood
- Adjustment disorder with anxiety
- Adjustment disorder with mixed anxiety and depressed mood
- Adjustment disorder with disturbance of conduct

- Adjustment disorder with mixed disturbance of emotions and conduct
- Adjustment disorder, unspecified

Adjustment disorder with depressed mood is diagnosed when the predominant symptoms are depressed mood, tearfulness, and hopelessness. Adjustment disorder with anxiety is diagnosed when the predominant symptoms are mild anxiety, worry, nervousness, and apprehension. Adjustment disorder with mixed anxiety and depressed mood is diagnosed when the predominant symptoms are a combination of depressed mood and mild anxiety. Adjustment disorder with disturbance of conduct is diagnosed when the predominant symptoms are negative behaviors that violate social norms, laws or the rights of others. Adjustment disorder with mixed disturbance of emotions and conduct is diagnosed when the predominant symptoms are extreme emotions and negative behaviors. Maladaptive reactions to stress that do not fit these classifications are diagnosed as unspecified adjustment disorder (Akil & Morano, 1995).

A diagnosis of adjustment disorder generally implies that in the absence of the stressor the individual's functioning and well-being is intact but that something about the nature of the stressor (primary appraisal), the timing of the stressor (experience), the impact of the stressor (secondary appraisal), or the individual's response (coping skills, coping resources) caused the stressor to exceed the individual's ability to adjust. Examples of stressors commonly associated with a diagnosis of adjustment disorder are termination of a job, academic failure, or the unexpected loss of an intimate relationship. Stressors such as these can cause the individual to feel a great deal of anger, fear, pain, and other intense emotions that can affect coping ability. This is not to imply that intense feelings about a stressor prohibit adjustment. Initially the presence of flexibility and resilience can be more important than the presence or absence of intense emotions. As with all stress disorders, the ability to cope effectively with a stressor is influenced by the nature of the stressor, prior experience with similar stressors, access to and effective use of coping resources, and individual coping skills (Rosenbaum, 1990).

Management of Stress and Adjustment Disorders

➤ Counseling

The first assessment and management goal for stress disorders is to reduce symptoms. Once symptoms are reduced, counseling should address the patient's need to build biopsychosocial resilience to stress. The goals of counseling are to identify the patient's current stress response and to improve his or her coping skills. Most hospitals and clinics with health promotion and illness prevention services offer self-care, stress management, and relaxation training programs. These programs can help patients to develop effective methods of discharging stress and preventing chronic or cumulative stress. Stress management must teach physical activity or relaxation. In addition, most stress management programs also focus on seeking and using support, avoiding substance abuse, conserving energy, bringing balance to the demands and pleasures of daily and life, and self-awareness of early warning signals of stress.

Depending on the format of available stress management programs, a high level of patient motivation may be required. Rather than place an unmotivated patient in a situation that may be frustrating or unhelpful, the patient's motivation should first be addressed. It is not necessary for a person to feel enthusiastic, but one should be open to the idea and willing to commit to an agreed-upon period of participation. Long-term support groups can be very helpful when the patient with a stress disorder has limited coping resources that seem to be a factor in the ability to recover. Effective coping requires that the patient take action. Support groups that have a behavioral rather than an emotional focus can help the patient to become active.

Stress management theory holds that human response to stress is a highly complex process made up of three basic components: stressor, stress response, and recovery. The stressor is subject to the individual's appraisal and frame of reference but appraisal does not determine what is or is not a stressor. For example, a flood is a flood regardless of how it is appraised. Appraisal personalizes a stressor so that a flood is defined in terms of its impact on the individual. Therefore a flood may mean lost dreams to one person but be just a fact of life on the river to another.

Stress management is primarily the management of the physical state of arousal that defines the stress response. The goal of learning stress management is to develop the ability to discharge the stress response and safely and quickly reestablish feelings of control. To discharge stress is to reduce the state of biological arousal. This can be accomplished by engaging in strenuous physical exercise or total relaxation. Both conditions allow for the physical arousal to taper and deplete.

Recovery marks the end of the acute stress response but is perhaps the most difficult stage of the entire response process. As soon as the acute phase is remitted, the individual is driven to either make sense of the experience or forget it. The latter is never helpful. How one recovers from stress greatly determines the risk of chronic stress disorder. For the most part, making sense of the experience means the individual must clarify one's personal experience.

Action is important in counseling a patient with a stress disorder. A behavioral coping plan is vital to recovery and future stress management. Starting today, what is the patient willing and able to do that is helpful? Until the patient begins to confront the stressor, the stress can continue. Realistic actions rather than perfect plans should be the focus. This plan of action should include attending a stress management program. When possible, helpful family and friends should be identified and family counseling should take place. When effective, family counseling can be an invaluable source of resources, comfort, and motivation.

℞ Prescribing

Medications are prescribed for most stress disorders to relieve acute symptoms, decrease distress, and enable active coping. Comprehensive reviews of prescribing medication for the treatment of depression and anxiety are presented in Chapters 4 and 6. The medications of choice for acute symptoms of stress disorders are benzodiazepines and tricyclic antidepressants. Benzodiazepines can be prescribed for up to 1 week to provide immediate symptom relief and rest. Antidepressants can be prescribed when more than 1 week of medication is needed. Low doses of tricyclic antidepressants can produce the sedation of benzodiazepines and reduce depression, anxiety, and tension, and they can also safely be prescribed for longer periods of time (Hartmann, 1995).

When low doses of antidepressants are not effective, the first step should be to gradually increase the dose. Effective doses may nevertheless be lower than the doses needed to relieve the symptoms of major depression or generalized anxiety disorder. Antipsychotic medications may be needed when there are severe cognitive symptoms (e.g., delusions), or evidence of disorganization (e.g., disorientation). When cognitive symptoms are severe, a possible diagnosis of thought disorder or psychosis should be evaluated.

The prescribing goal for acute stress disorder, acute adjustment disorder, and crisis is symptom relief. Evidence of active substance abuse should be evaluated before medications are prescribed for symptom relief. The prescribing goal for chronic adjustment disorder or chronic stress is treatment. Medications should be prescribed at treatment-level doses for 3 to 6 months.

Whether prescribing for symptom relief or treatment, the specific strategy will vary among individuals. Close monitoring and follow-up is recommended. A potential pitfall of prescribing medications for the relief of symptoms of stress disorders is the reliance on medications and rejection of self-care. When benzodiazepines are prescribed, the potential of medication abuse and dependence can be significant.

When is symptom relief a valid reason for prescribing medication for stress disorders? Is improved coping a result of symptom relief? Is adequate functioning dependent on symptom relief? These are questions that practitioners should consider as part of the prescribing process. Consider the example of prescribing diazepam (Valium) for a man who is unable to board a plane without taking it. Prescribing for symptom relief is weighed against the risk of abuse, misuse, and dependence. A prescription of 10 mg 10 times a year, in the absence of request for higher doses or larger counts, may be appropriate if flying without premedication places the man at risk for panic, a more difficult disorder to prescribe for.

If, on the other hand, a man is unable to cope with his adolescent children, prescribing medication for symptom relief may not be appropriate. If interventions such as stress management, family therapy, or cognitive-behavioral counseling are not effective, treatment of a disorder (e.g., major depression) rather than relief of stress should be evaluated. Functioning and coping can be used as parameters for prescribing. Symptom relief should lead to restored or maintained functioning. For example, the man is able to travel by air without extreme distress. When symptom relief leads the individual to redefine the problem as a need for relief, prescribing limits should be placed.

A clearly stated plan of prescribing should be made and this plan should include start and stop dates, dose maximums, and total count maximums. There are cases in which medications are appropriately requested and used for symptom relief. Symptom relief alone is less appropriate when a patient is unwilling to participate in stress management training or counseling, or when symptoms are poorly defined. For example, a patient who is experiencing acute symptoms attributes them to her "job." She may take a morning and bedtime dose of a benzodiazepines for a week as prescribed. During that week, she cuts back on her responsibilities and takes a few days off from work. The following week she feels better and is satisfied with the primary care she received. The patient is informed of her risk for chronic stress. Stress management is recommended, which she may or may not accept.

☎ Consultation and Referral

Consulting with a specialist may be helpful when patients present vague complaints or there is reason to believe that another disorder (e.g., substance or personality disorders) may account for the patient's symptoms. Consulting could also prove helpful in assessing and planning care for patients in the midst of crisis who seem potentially unpredictable or are without meaningful support. In these cases, the patient could become overwhelmed and a consultant can help develop an emergency plan for the patient to follow.

Patients who are acting out, or who appear to be out of control, should be referred immediately. Patients who are in an emergency situation that is the source of their stress will require a great deal of time and services in order to avoid immobilization, and therefore should be referred to a specialist. When the patient's physical or psychological symptoms are severe, or a diagnosis of complete burnout (chronic stress), chronic adjustment disorder, substance disorder, or personality disorder is evident, referral is recommended. Patients who will require more time than is available in a primary care setting should be referred, unless an excessively long wait is likely. Practitioners can also consider referring patients to a specialist for assessment and stabilization. Individuals who, after an adequate course of medication and coping interventions, continue to decompensate or do not improve should be referred for reassessment.

Evidence of destructive coping or causing harm to oneself or others should also be evaluated by a specialist. This is particularly important when the patient with a stress disorder is explosive and reports being abusive to children or an adult. Practitioners need immediate access to a specialist for all the referral conditions described here except the chronic disorders.

References

Akil HA, Morano MI: Stress. In Bloom FE, Kupfer DJ (eds): *Psychopharmacology: the fourth generation of progress*, New York, 1995, Raven Press.

Beck AT, Rush AJ, Shaw BF, Emery G: *Cognitive therapy of depression*, New York, 1979, The Guilford Press.

Cui X, Vaillant GE: Antecedents and consequences of negative life events in adulthood: a longitudinal study, *Am J Psychiatry*, 153(1):21, 1996.

Forster P, King J: Traumatic stress reactions and the psychiatric imagery, *Psychiatric Ann*, 24:603, 1994.

Lazarus R, Averill J, Opton E: The psychology of coping: issues of research and assessment. In Coelho G, Hamburg D, Adams J: *Coping and adaptation*, New York, 1974, Basic Books.

O'Connor F: A vulnerability-stress framework for evaluating clinical interventions in sxhizophrenia, *Image: J Nurse Sch* 26:231-237, 1994.

Robinson L: Stress and anxiety, *Nurse Clin of North Am*, 25(4):935, 1990.

Rosenbum M: *Learned Resourcefulness: on coping skills, self-control, and adaptive behavior*, New York, 1990, Springer.

Solomon P, Draine J: Subjective burden among family members of mentally ill adults: relation to stress, coping and adaptation, *Am J Orthopsychiatry*, 65(3):419-427, 1995.

Wise MG, Rieck, SD: Diagnostic considerations and treatment approaches to underlying anxiety in the mentally ill, *J. Clin Psychiatry*, 54(5suppl):22-26, 1993.

Anxiety Disorders 6

Anxiety is similar to depression in that it encompasses a wide range of human experiences, from nervous feelings to stable personality traits and mental disorders. Anxiety disorders are unique because, unlike acute symptoms of anxiety, the disorders cause a great deal of distress and function impairment. Basic sources of anxiety disorders are (1) stressful events (internal and external) that undermine coping and adaptation and (2) alarming childhood experiences. Anxiety disorders are characterized by physical and emotional symptoms and behaviors intended to discharge or decrease anxiety. This chapter reviews basic concepts of anxiety, generalized anxiety disorder, obsessive compulsive disorder, panic disorder, and phobias. Adjustment, crisis, and stress disorders are reviewed in Chapter 5 and post-traumatic stress disorder is reviewed in Chapter 17.

Basic Concepts

State or Trait

Anxiety can occur as a temporary ***state*** or as a stable trait. Individuals experience ***state anxiety*** at fairly high levels of awareness. Although transitory, state anxiety is highly unpleasant. The individual is acutely aware of emotional and physical symptoms of physical arousal, physical tension, apprehension, nervousness, and worry (Craig, Brown, and Baum, 1995). ***Trait anxiety*** is a stable personality or dispositional characteristic. Individuals with trait anxiety often have a semiconscious view of the world as threatening and see interactions or relationships with others as potentially threatening. Trait anxiety undermines self-esteem and self-confidence, thereby increasing the individual's susceptibility to episodes of state (acute) anxiety (Craig, Brown and Baum, 1995).

Self-efficacy

Self-efficacy refers to the belief that one can control or develop mastery within important personal environments or in response to important events and experiences. Psychologically, individuals need to believe that their efforts can and will influence events and experiences in their life and that their efforts on their own behalf will not be in vain. Self-efficacy is directly related to anxiety; high levels of self-efficacy correlate with low levels of anxiety. Self-efficacy is an important focus of treatment for anxiety (Williams, Dooseman and Kleifield, 1984).

Stress and Anxiety

Stress is a total human response to stressors that is characterized by physical and psychological symptoms of arousal and distress. Anxiety can be thought of as one of the many possible forms of human stress response (Krantz, Grunder, and Baum, 1985; Lazarus and Folkman, 1984). ***Mild anxiety*** typically signals the individual to increase alertness and attention and prepare to expend the necessary energy and resources. ***Moderate to severe anxiety*** can have just the opposite effect, causing the individual to feel confused and exhausted and unable to take action (Baum, Cohen, and Hall, 1993; Sarason, 1980). The stressors most often associated with stress-related anxiety occur as external (e.g., disasters) or internal (e.g., feelings of abandonment) negative events.

➲ Who Is at Risk

Mild anxiety is a normal reaction to the health care visit. Anxious patients may be rushed and nervous or they may react to the strange environments of hospitals and clinics. Mild anxiety can also be directly related to the purpose of the health care visit, such as waiting for important test results or undergoing painful treatments and embarrassing procedures. For most people who live busy and hectic lives, just the possibility of a health problem can trigger mild symptoms of anxiety. If this is the case, then as soon as the individual leaves the health care setting, or one's good health is confirmed, mild symptoms of ***(state) anxiety*** will remit, whereas an undiagnosed anxiety disorder would threaten the individual's health and well-being and undermine psychosocial functioning. Most patients are at risk for transient symptoms of mild anxiety, but persistent moderate to severe symptoms of anxiety may indicate an anxiety disorder and should therefore be evaluated. General risk factors for anxiety disorders are (1) a family history of depression or anxiety, (2) a personal history of depression disorders or substance disorders, and (3) acute trauma or chronic stress. (Stein et al, 1996).

* Common Symptom Onset Patterns

Anxiety disorders significantly interfere with or impair functioning. Individuals diagnosed with an anxiety disorder can have difficulty meeting social role demands (e.g., parenting) or establishing and maintaining satisfying relationships, and they may be highly preoccupied with their anxiety symptoms. Each of the anxiety disorders reviewed in this chapter has a somewhat unique symptom onset pattern, based on whether the symptoms can be considered state, trait, or both. ***State anxiety onset*** is usually related to identifiable stressors; however, individuals may not be fully aware of internal stressors. ***Trait anxiety onset*** may also be related to internal and external stressors, but symptoms are persistent or recurrent.

❑ Common Assessment Problems

The assessment of anxiety can require the ability to sort through multiple, perhaps confusing, experiences and events that may or may not be obviously related to the onset of anxiety symptoms. In part this is due to the fact that, for many patients, anxiety symptoms can be difficult to put into words, or patients may be alarmed by their physical symptoms. Anxious patients can seem evasive during the assessment, especially if talking about their anxiety seems to increase their symptoms. As with any mental disorder, negative practitioner reactions to the anxious patient can be an assessment problem. Perhaps the most difficult assessment problem related to anxiety disorders is the unspoken assumption that "good" patients will make every effort to suppress rather than express their anxiety. Assessment of anxiety disorders is also highly complicated when patients purposely attempt to mislead the practitioner or claim nervousness with the expectation of receiving antianxiety or sleep medications.

Anxiety Disorders

Generalized Anxiety Disorder (GAD)

Three or more of the following *Diagnostic and Statistical Manual of Mental Disorder, fourth edition*, (DSM-IV) symptoms should be present for more days than not, in the past 6 months. Symptoms should cause significant distress or impairment in social, occupational, or academic functioning. Physical symptoms of generalized anxiety are mild to moderate symptoms of panic attack, as listed in that section.

The symptoms of generalized anxiety are (APA, 1994):

1. Worry and apprehension
2. Inability to control the worry/apprehension
3. Restlessness, feeling keyed up or on edge
4. Easily fatigued
5. Poor concentration or mind going blank
6. Irritability and frustration
7. Muscle tension
8. Sleep disturbances
9. Mild to moderate transient physical symptoms

Worry and apprehension

Worry practically seems normal under the unrelenting demands and hassles that make up day-to-day life for many people. Most individuals are more than a little worried about something. The total absence of day-to-day worries would be unusual. The feature used to distinguish normal worry from the symptomatic worry of GAD is ***the ability to limit or stop worrying on demand***. Uncontrolled worry and apprehension indicates the possibility of an anxiety disorder. Individuals with GAD have little or no ability to control their worrying. The choices of not worrying, delayed worry, or selected worry are unavailable. More days than not, the person with GAD is unable to use such internal controls. They experience high levels of worry about a wide range of concerns, such as being socially accepted, meeting performance expectations, or future events in general. As a symptom of GAD, worry is not easily altered or subdued and tends to be vague rather than specific. Practitioners should try to ascertain what if anything makes it possible for the patient to limit or control the anxious worrying. Even if nothing is effective, it is helpful to learn what methods of control have been attempted. Excessive worry can be indirectly assessed as part of the history and physical or in the disclosure of important life events; it may be directly assessed by asking the individual to describe one's personal routine as well as one's emergency methods of controlling worry.

Restlessness

Restlessness related to anxiety disorders appears to be the same as restlessness related to other disorders, but there may be more physical jumpiness and hyperactivity. Individuals may be in a chronic state of anticipation or on the verge of taking some unpredictable action. Like worry, restlessness as a symptom of anxiety is difficult for individuals to limit, alter, or control.

Easily fatigued

Easily fatigued is a rather obvious symptom of anxiety. GAD symptoms can be physically and emotionally draining, making even routine activities all the more fatiguing. The anxious person may describe this fatigue as feeling tired or being physically unable to perform at home, work, or school. The fatigue will be present for pleasurable as well as performance activities. Individuals may report attempting to engage in various activities but almost always becoming too tired to complete or enjoy them. Easily fatigued should be distinguished from apathy or lack of interest.

Poor concentration

Concentration is directly decreased by worry, the primary symptom of generalized anxiety. The individual who has more control over worrisome thoughts also has better concentration in other areas. To concentrate is to remain focused on something. Anxiety interferes with the ability to remain focused. Some individuals become alarmed by their inability to focus their thinking, fearing that they may have a thought disorder or a brain disease. Individuals with poor concentration may complain that their mind goes blank. Blanking out often occurs as a semiconscious defense mechanism of dissociation in response to anxiety.

Irritability and frustration

Irritability and frustration are important symptoms of anxiety because they can lead to significant changes in behavior. They are also easy symptoms to overlook because people ***expect*** the anxious individual to be fearful. The biological basis for irritability and frustration appears to be related to the significant increase in epinephrine and norepinephrine levels and the changes in serotonin activity that occur with anxiety.

Muscle tension

Muscle tension is a common symptom of anxiety. Driving in rush-hour traffic can produce a stiff neck and sore shoulders. Muscle tension can be a physical manifestation of other symptoms of anxiety. Although common, muscle tension caused by anxiety can be severe, adding significant pain and worry. Some individuals may not accept anxiety as a diagnosis for muscle pain, thereby ignoring an important symptom. Others may find psychological explanations of their physical symptoms insulting; they may insist that the problem is in their back and not their head. However, the connection between everyday stress and muscle tension and pain is commonly accepted by people.

Sleep disturbances

Sleep disturbances related to anxiety vary greatly, to the point where it is difficult to determine what if any significant changes have occurred. Therefore the assessment standard of restful sleep should be applied. Individuals may report difficulty in falling asleep, frequent waking, early morning waking, or disturbing dreams. Some anxious individuals may describe undisturbed sleep but complain of waking tired, as though they had not slept well or sufficiently. Sleep disturbance as a symptom of anxiety can be assessed if the individual attempts to sleep. Some anxious individuals routinely stay up most of the night and may occupy themselves with activities such as working, reading, organizing, watching television, or exploring the internet. Sleep changes can also go unnoticed by busy, anxious individuals who may not think that staying awake most of the night is a sleep disturbance. However, when they want to sleep they may have very specific methods that work for them, and this information can be helpful in understanding their anxiety-related sleep changes.

Obsessive-Compulsive Disorder (OCD)

DSM-IV symptom criteria for obsessive compulsive disorder are obsessions (thoughts) that produce anxiety and compulsions (behaviors) that are time consuming and interfere with normal routines, functioning, social activities, or relationships. Individuals with OCD may or may not recognize that their obsessive thoughts and compulsive behaviors are excessive or unreasonable. Over the course of a lifetime, approximately 3% of American adults will meet the symptom criteria for a diagnosis of OCD. Individuals with OCD can be highly skilled at concealing their disorder. About 25% of individuals who have been diagnosed with OCD have obsessive rituals only, without behavioral rituals.

The symptoms of obsessive-compulsive disorder are (APA, 1994):

1. Obsessions
2. Compulsions

Obsessions

Obsessions are recurrent, persistent thoughts, impulses, or mental images that are experienced as intrusive or inappropriate and cause anxious distress. Individuals with OCD do not attribute their obsessive thoughts to unknown, outside forces; they engage in purposeful attempts to ignore, suppress, or somehow inactivate their obsessions. Despite their efforts to do so, however, they are unable to defend themselves against the obsessions or the anxiety without performing compulsive behaviors. As the symptom of a disorder, obsessions are negative and distressing, completely unlike the popular use of the term, such as being "obsessed" (fascinated or preoccupied) with a well-written novel. Common obsessive themes are bodily waste, dirt/germs, harm to self or others, chemicals, illness, sex, embarrassment, physical symptoms, losing things, exactness, remembering, apologizing, counting, and checking (Rapoport, 1990). Individuals feel tormented and trapped by their obsessive thoughts, but over the years these thoughts can become semiconscious as the individual learns to automatically use compulsions (cognitive or behavioral) to decrease the anxiety. To be considered a clinical obsession, the individual must be unable to modify, limit, or dismiss the obsession.

Obsessions can be influenced by situations and circumstances. Individuals often conceptualize their obsessions as an anxiety tape that plays in their head without warning. The volume of the tape can range from loud to soft, the images may be clear or fuzzy, and the speed of the tape may be normal, slow, or fast. The intensity or impact of the obsessions and the amount of incorporated details can also vary. These characteristics of an obsession can be situationally sensitive; that is, the overall strength of an obsession may increase or decrease depending on the situation. Most individuals have difficulty disclosing their obsessive thoughts to others, including practitioners. They may feel embarrassed but also understand that talking about their obsessions increases their anxiety. Individuals with obsessions can feel helpless, vulnerable, and unable to cope effectively, especially when the obsessions have a dangerous content or the compulsions are related to obsessions that are potentially harmful. For example, a man has intrusive obsessions of being embarrassed that are worsened whenever he is in a performance situation or any kind of situation where others may evaluate him. It can be easier to disclose compulsions related to obsessions, since the compulsions tend to be more obvious and may be a source of potential or actual health problems.

Compulsions

Compulsions are exact behaviors (e.g., hand washing) or mental actions (e.g., counting backwards) that are performed with the expectation of preventing or reducing anxiety generated by obsessions. Compulsions provide helpful relief from obsessions and anxiety, but they are also draining and sometimes extremely irrational. The most common compulsions are cleaning/washing, checking/ confirming, health behaviors, avoidance and distraction behaviors, hoarding, arranging, repetitive questions/statements, and counting/checking. In theory, obsessions increase anxiety and compulsions decrease anxiety. The actual experience of this increased and decreased anxiety varies from dramatic changes to nearly imperceptible changes. The individual's need for relief from obsessions and anxiety is enough to ensure performance of the compulsion, regardless of its nature. The amount of relief obtained may wax and wane, depending on the circumstances and the strength of the obsessions. Consider the previous example of the man with the embarrassment obsession. This obsession and anxiety causes the individual to be self-conscious, so he has developed a touching ritual, or compulsive touching, that relieves his anxiety. With his left thumb he quickly rubs the hair at the lower tip of his left eyebrow, the hairline at his left temple, and the left corner of his mouth. The entire touching compulsion takes less than 30 seconds to complete. Years of this ritualized touching has removed all of the hair on the lower half of his left eyebrow and the skin at his left temple hairline and the left corner of his mouth is dry and chapped with small, red, open areas. These areas occasionally develop a localized staph infection, for which he obtains antibiotics from his primary care practitioner. He tells the practitioner that his skin problem is acne, which he has had since high school, and that the missing eyebrow hair is due to an accident as a infant.

Panic Attack and Panic Disorder

The primary DSM-IV symptom criteria for panic disorder without agoraphobia are recurrent (at least two) episodes of unexpected panic attack followed by a month or more of persistent concern about recurrence or dire implications, such as heart failure or insanity (APA, 1994). There may be specific and significant changes in behavior as a result of the fear of a panic attack, such as keeping a phone on hand at all times. Panic attacks occur without warning but, as with most anxiety disorders, they can be limited to or triggered by specific situations. The frequency of panic attacks varies significantly from person to person. The number of clinical symptoms experienced dictates whether the panic attack is diagnosed as full (more than four symptoms) or limited (fewer than four symptoms). The essential feature of panic disorder is a fear of having a panic attack (recurrence). A childhood history of anxiety disorder is not uncommon (Pollack, 1996).

The symptoms of panic attack are (APA, 1994):

1. Pounding heart, increased heart rate
2. Sweating
3. Trembling or shaking
4. Feeling smothered or short of breath
5. Feeling choked or a restricted air way
6. Feeling chest pains
7. Feeling nausea or abdominal distress
8. Feeling dizzy or lightheaded
9. Feeling disconnected from oneself (detachment)
10. Feeling that things are not real (derealization)
11. Fear of going crazy or "losing it"
12. Fear that death is imminent
13. Numbness or tingling sensations
14. Chills, shakes, hot flushes

Individuals experience panic attacks as severe physical symptoms caused by sudden and intense biochemical activation of multiple "fight or flight" stress response systems. The biochemical activation is a result of biological hypersensitivity. Individuals with frequent panic attacks have been shown to have hypersensitive reactions that cause sudden increases in stress hormone discharge (e.g., norepinephrine) and severe symptoms of stress (e.g., dramatic increases in blood pressure and heart rate). Researchers have successfully induced panic symptoms in hypersensitive individuals by exposing them to substances such as carbon dioxide, caffeine, or sodium lactate (Ballenger, 1994).

Early in the course of panic disorder, individuals are often convinced that their physical panic attack symptoms are life threatening. They may rush to a hospital or call for EMT services, believing that their cardiopulmonary symptoms of panic are symptoms of cardiac disease. About 90% of individuals with panic attack or panic disorder will insist that their symptoms do not have a psychological basis (Ballenger, 1996). Reassurances that they do not have cardiac disease may be suspected rather than welcomed. Some individuals may believe that practitioners have undisclosed reasons for failing to diagnosis their cardiac disease, while others suffer acute embarrassment when they are informed that their cardiac symptoms are not life threatening. Others may insist that they are not disturbed by a psychological diagnosis, but they remain convinced they have a cardiac condition that health care professionals are unable to diagnosis. There are many possible explanations for these patient attitudes, but fear of recurrence is a large factor in patient demands for treatment.

Two important psychological symptoms, detachment and derealization, signal severe levels of panic. An individual may feel removed or dissociated from one's physical and mental self and one's environment, as though one were observing the panic attack rather than experiencing it. Derealization is a dreamlike state in which the individual is uncertain of what is and is not real. These psychological symptoms can cause individuals to feel that they are having a nervous breakdown or developing a severe mental illness (e.g., schizophrenia). After one panic attack most individuals are able to think about the experience in such a way that it does not feel like an ongoing threat. After a second panic attack most individuals become focused on preventing future panic attacks and may go to great lengths to carry out plans they believe will be effective.

Individuals with a sustained history of panic attacks no longer view them as life threatening or as a possible onset of severe mental illness but may instead become focused on their panic attack symptoms (e.g., increased heart rate). Panic attack symptom patterns are highly individualized; no two people are likely to have the same symptom pattern. Some may have multiple symptoms, while others may have only one or two symptoms. The duration of a panic attack ranges from a few seconds to 10 to 15 minutes. A panic attack can occur unexpectedly or occur only in specific situations, or certain situations may predispose the individual to a panic attack. The predominant feature of panic attack disorder is the experience of unexpected panic attack and a significant concern about recurrence. The absence of unexpected panic attacks or a lack of concern may indicate an anxiety disorder other than a panic attack disorder. Individuals who report vague or subclinical symptoms of panic and anxiety with specific requests for medications should be carefully evaluated.

Phobias

The DSM-IV symptom criteria for phobia disorders are 6 months of excessive or unreasonable symptoms of anxiety or panic cued by actual or anticipated exposure to specific objects or situations (APA, 1994). Actual exposure to or contact with the phobic object or situation immediately causes symptoms of anxiety or panic. The individual with phobia disorder is able to recognize and acknowledge that one's anxiety in relation to the object or situation is excessive or unreasonable. Nevertheless, exposure to phobic objects and situations are routinely avoided. The individual's efforts to avoid or anticipate possible exposure to phobic objects or situations, and the anxiety experienced when exposure cannot be avoided, significantly interfere with or impair normal routines, relationships, and functioning.

The symptoms of phobia are (APA, 1994):

1. Anxiety
2. Panic
3. Avoidance

Symptoms of phobic anxiety must be directly related to clearly identified objects or situations. As a mental disorder, phobia is more than a fear or dislike of an object or situation. Significant symptoms of anxiety or panic and impaired functioning specifically related to avoiding exposure should be present. The actual levels of anxiety and panic experienced is usually related to level of exposure, potential for escape from exposure, and anticipatory anxiety related to potential exposure. Whether escape following exposure is an option can be a prime determinant of the level of anxiety and panic experienced. A diagnosis of phobia disorder is not appropriate when anxiety or panic is a reasonable response to an object or situation. The five DSM-IV categories of phobic objects and situations are (1) animals (e.g., cats, insects), (2) natural environments (e.g., storms, heights), (3) blood-injection-injury, (e.g., having blood drawn), (4) situational (e.g., enclosed spaces, public speaking), and (5) other (APA, 1994).

Phobia disorders may develop following the experience or the observation of a traumatic event (e.g., assault), an unexpected episode of panic, or by interpersonal transmission (e.g., phobic parent to child). Phobic disorders that develop following the experience of a traumatic event or panic attack can become severe and disabling. Phobias related to childhood fears (e.g., darkness) tend to improve as the individual matures but childhood phobias (e.g., spiders) that continue into adulthood often do not improve. Phobias not related to objects or situations, such as agoraphobia, require specialized psychiatric care. Mild phobias that do not significantly interfere with functioning are common. Many people have to force themselves to endure exposure to certain objects or situations (e.g., public speaking, flying); the key factor is that they are able to endure the exposure without severe anxiety, panic, or loss of functioning. Although phobia disorders can be dramatic and miserable, highly effective specialized brief treatments have been developed and the recovery rates for many phobias are excellent.

Management of Anxiety Disorders

➤ Counseling

Counseling the anxious patient need not require an excessive length of time, but this can be a factor. Comprehensive treatment for anxiety disorders generally involves a combination of cognitive-behavioral counseling and, when necessary, antianxiety medication to improve functioning and coping skills and relieve symptoms. Psychiatric primary care counseling can help patients to recognize and acknowledge their anxiety disorders and address their symptoms and functioning. However, some anxious individuals may focus on symptom relief only, with little motivation to apply cognitive-behavioral techniques to improve their functioning. When physical causes for the anxious patient's symptoms have been ruled out and the patient's symptoms are consistent with an anxiety disorder, teaching the patient about anxiety is vital. Individuals with anxiety disorders should fully understand the nature of their disorder and the effectiveness of cognitive-behavior treatment. In reviewing the disorder and treatment with patients, practitioners should make it clear that anxiety disorders are serious conditions but effective treatment is available. Specific treatment goals should be developed for each individual.

These goals should reflect the individual's symptom profile and behavior patterns.

Before starting treatment, practitioners should work with patients to develop a treatment contract or agreement that describes the goals of treatment and the steps to be taken to achieve those goals. Patients are expected to be active participants in the management of their anxiety disorders. Those patients who are not willing or able to actively participate in their treatment may require specialized care. Positive evidence of the patient's motivation to work towards long-term improvement is extremely helpful; however, patient motivation may be tied to symptom relief. Anxious individuals who seem unable to tolerate talking about their anxiety, or who are resistant to any treatment other than medication, should be referred to a specialist. Individuals with mild to moderate symptoms of anxiety and who seem able to benefit from psychiatric primary care should be referred to a specialist when there is evidence of multiple severe psychosocial problems or a concurrent severe thought, mood, substance, or personality disorder. Once diagnosed, individuals may begin to redefine their symptoms and behaviors. Being open to new ways of thinking about their symptoms is the essential first step of cognitive-behavior treatment for anxiety. Individuals who, for example, do not accept new evaluations of their symptoms or reject a diagnosis of anxiety disorder are less able to benefit from psychiatric primary care.

Cognitive-behavioral therapy (positive self-talk and self-care) is essentially a process of response prevention. Anxiety disorders improve with cognitive-behavioral therapy because anxious thoughts are highly associated with physical and behavioral symptoms of anxiety. Anxious thoughts, often rooted in mental images of danger that developed in childhood, maintain anxiety symptoms. With repeated exposure and relaxation training, individuals can gradually become desensitized to the source of their anxiety, thereby reducing their anxiety symptoms. This simple cognitive-behavioral technique has a 70% to 80% rate of effectiveness but requires considerable patient motivation.

Emotional support as a basic element of psychiatric primary care counseling can be effective in building and supporting the patient's motivation to use cognitive-behavioral techniques. However, emotional support does not replace teaching. The individual who is not facing major problems related to anxiety may require a great deal of information to become motivated to use cognitive-behavioral self-care. Excellent anxiety disorder patient education materials are available, as well as anxiety disorder support groups, self-help groups, and commercial self-help books. Information alone will not decrease symptoms or improve functioning, but very little can be accomplished without it. Information regarding relaxation techniques and training may be obtained from stress management clinics, patient education-training programs, self-help books, or less traditional alternatives such as yoga and meditation. Relaxation continues to be important after anxiety symptoms are under control.

℞ Prescribing

Benzodiazepines and, in some cases, antidepressants, anticonvulsants, or beta blockers can provide effective relief from anxiety symptoms (Hollister et al, 1993; Lucki, 1996; Wiborg and Dahl, 1996). Benzodiazepines produce pleasurable sedation and changes in mood and perceptions and may be prescribed for short periods of time to relieve acute symptoms but are not considered treatment for anxiety (Craig, Brown, and Baum, 1995). This caution applies to fast onset (e.g., lorazepam), intermediate onset (e.g., clonazepam), and slow onset (e.g., oxazepam) benzodiazepines. The well-known drawbacks of prescribing benzodiazepines for any reason are abuse, tolerance, dependence, and withdrawal (Shader and Greenblatt, 1995). At high doses, benzodiazepine dependence can develop within 2 to 3 weeks; with routine doses, dependence occurs in 6 to 8 months. In order to decrease the risk of severe withdrawal symptoms, benzodiazepines should not be prescribed for longer than 4 months (Wiberg and Dahl, 1996).

Busipirone is an atypical anxiolytic that alters cerebral serotonin, as well as nonadrenergic and dopaminergic activity, without sedation or addiction, but fewer patients find it to be effective. Patients who do benefit from this medication can expect to wait 4 to 6 weeks for full beneficial effects. Clomipramine, a potent serotonin reuptake blocker antidepressant, has been shown to be effective in the treatment of OCD. For some individuals fluoxetine, sertaline, or fluvoxamine, which are selective serotonin reuptake blocker antidepressants, may also be effective. Because OCD, like other anxiety disorders, is chronic, the need for long-term treatment presents prescribing problems; long-term use of medication is not recommended, but without cognitive-behavioral treatment, relapse occurs quickly when medication is discontinued (Craig, Brown, and Baum, 1995). Cognitive-behavioral therapy offers the best chance for long term remission. Prescribing for phobias does not differ significantly from prescribing for OCD. Medications such as clonazepam (anticonvulsant), fluoxetine, and buspirone are recommended. As with OCD and GAD, without cognitive-behavioral therapy, relapse can be anticipated within 3 to 6 months after discontinuation of medication. Clonazepam and beta blockers such as propranolol have been shown to be effective in the management of physical symptoms of panic attack and panic attack disorders (Pollack, Otto, and Rosenbaum, 1990). Because of the drug's gradual onset, Pollack recommends clonazepam for anxious patients who are prone to substance abuse.

Western social behavior norms of seeking instant relief from distress complicates prescribing for anxiety disorders. Individuals who do not have an anxiety disorder but may be experiencing physical symptoms of distress may seek prescribed medication. Second, the general population's use of stimulants, particularly nicotine and caffeine, can complicate the assessment of anxiety symptoms as well as the evaluation of medication effectiveness. Third, alcohol and marijuana consumption can complicate prescribing for the anxious patient who uses either substance (or both) for symptom relief. Finally, prescribing medication to relieve symptoms of anxiety is a highly individualized process that requires careful and continual assessment and evaluation. For example, a man who takes 10 mg of diazepam 25 minutes before boarding an airplane has no interest in learning to cope with his anxiety without the medication. Should diazepam be prescribed for him? The answer depends on the nature of the man's anxiety symptoms and how often he flies. The more he travels by air and the more disabling his symptoms of anxiety, the more important it is to offer him comprehensive treatment rather than sedation. On the other hand, if he flies once or twice a year and is willing to take 10 mg of diazepam at bedtime the night before, he can benefit from the sedation and anxiolytic effects of the medication without risking impaired functioning or psychological dependence. If he is willing to participate in a comprehensive treatment for anxiety, medication would be appropriately prescribed for temporary symptom relief while he learns cognitive-behavioral self-care skills.

A comprehensive approach to treatment is particularly important with GAD, since this disorder, unlike panic and phobia, is not defined by episode boundaries. Practitioners should note that individuals accustomed to using sedating substances for symptom relief may continue to do so while taking prescribed medications. Practitioners should inform patients of the hazards of taking nonprescribed psychoactive substances while taking prescribed medications. In prescribing medications for anxiety disorders, practitioners should consider symptom duration and intensity, what (if any) symptoms are object- or situation-dependent, symptom effects on occupational, academic, and interpersonal functioning, and the individual's routine methods of coping with distress. Factors that worsen or improve symptoms should also be noted. In most cases, anxiety symptom relief can be viewed as restorative, allowing the individual to regain mental and physical energy; however, the diagnosis of an anxiety disorder implies a need for comprehensive treatment.

☎ Consultation and Referral

Anxiety disorders can be difficult to diagnosis when the patient's personality or interpersonal style is distracting or dramatic. Consultants can be very helpful in discerning symptoms from style. Consultants are also helpful when patients present a history and symptoms that are confusing but also present specific episodes that are consistent with a diagnosis of anxiety disorder. Much of this confusion can be reduced by closely following DSM-IV criteria for a diagnosis of anxiety disorder as distinctive from acute subclinical symptoms of anxiety. A specialist should be consulted when diagnostic criteria are difficult to assess. Consultation can also be very helpful when the individual's history includes substance abuse, harmful behaviors, or unpredictable behaviors. Practitioners who have the resources to provide comprehensive treatment for anxiety disorders may consider consulting a specialist to develop long-range treatment goals and to try to anticipate potential treatment problems. Patients who are at risk for crisis or who report a history of crisis may be difficult to treat in primary care, and referral should be considered. Practitioners may find it difficult to respond to crisis quickly or to see patients often enough to observe subtle changes that might indicate the onset of a crisis.

Practitioners should refer patients with anxiety disorders to specialists for assessment and treatment when the patient appears to be unpredictable or impulsive, when there is evidence of severe substance abuse or harmful/dangerous behavior, or when the patient's treatment needs exceed the resources of primary care. In most practice settings the difficult patient is the one who does not improve, and patients with anxiety disorders tend to have chronic symptom profiles, highly ineffective coping skills, and very demanding natures. Sometimes the difficult anxious patient actually meets diagnostic criteria for a chronic disorder, such as a personality disorder, that may be difficult to assess within a primary care visit. These patients should be referred to a specialist for assessment, treatment, and management.

References

Ballenger JC: Unrecognized prevalence of panic disorder in primary care, internal medicine, cardiology, *Am J Cardiology* 60:39J, 1994.

Ballenger JC: Practical approaches to treatment of panic disorder, *J Clin Psych* 57(1):45, 1996.

Baum A, Cohen L, Hall M: Control and intrusive memories as possible determinants of chronic stress, *Psychosomatic Med* 55:274, 1993.

Craig KJ, Brown KJ, Baum A: Environmental factors in the etiology of anxiety. In Bloom FE, Kupfer DJ, (editors): *Psychopharmacology: the fourth generation of progress*, New York, 1995, Raven Press.

Hollister LE, Muller-Oerlinghausen B, Richels K, Shader RI: (Clinical uses of benzodiazepines, *J Clin Psychopharmacology* 13 (supple 1):1S, 1993.

Krantz DS, Grunber NE, Baum A: Healthy psychology, *Ann Rev Psychology* 36:349, 1985.

Lazarus RS, Folkman S: *Stress, appraisal, and coping*, New York, 1984, Springer.

Lucki I: Serotonin receptor specificity in anxiety disorders, *J Clin Psychiatry* 57(suppl 6):5, 1996.

Pollack MH, Otto MW, Sabatino BA, Majcher D, Worthington II, McArdle ET, Rosenbaum JF: Relationship of childhood anxiety to adult panic disorder: correlates and influence on course, *Am J Psychiatry* 153(3):376, 1996.

Pollack MH, Otto CMW, Rosenbaum JF et.al: Longitudinal course of panic disorder:findings from the Massachusetts General Hospital naturalistic study, *J Clin Psychia* 51(12 suppl A):12, 1990.

Sarason IG: Life stress, self-preoccupation, and social support. In Sarason IG, Spielberger CD (editors): *Stress and anxiety*, Washington DC, 1980, Hemisphere Publishing Corporation.

Shader RI, Greenblatt OJ: Use of benzodiazepines in anxiety disorders, *NE J Med*, 328:1398, 1993.

Stein MB, Walker JR, Anderson G, Hazen AL, Ross CA, Eldridge G, Forde DR: Childhood physical and sexual abuse in patients with anxiety disorders and in a community sample, *Am J Psychiatry* 153(2):275, 1996.

Williams SL, Dooseman G, Kleifeld E: Comparative effectiveness of guided master and exposure treatment for intractable outcome, *J Consul Clin Psychology* 52:505, 1984.

Wiborg IM, Dahl AA: Does brief dynamic psychotherapy reduce the relapse rate of panic disorder, *Arch Gen Psychiatry* 53(8):689, 1996.

Substance Disorders 7

Substance disorders are highly individualized blendings of physical, social, psychological, emotional, and behavioral symptoms that affect an individual and his or her significant others. These disorders are characterized by short-term impairments in functioning and significant risk of physical and psychiatric disability. This chapter reviews basic substance abuse concepts and substance disorders. Practitioners will routinely encounter patients with substance disorders and related psychosocial problems who can improve with psychiatric primary care, but individuals with substance dependence or dual diagnosis (a mental disorder and a substance disorder)(El-Guebaly, 1995a) should receive specialized care.

➲ Who Is at Risk

High risk for substance disorders is directly related to family substance-use history, substance availability, and learned stress response patterns and coping skills. Each of these risk factors is important, but family history tends to be the best single predicator of substance disorder, and availability and access are important social predictors. Traditionally, individual risk has been based on an individual's membership in high-risk social groups defined by gender, ethnicity, age, income, or education level and urban, suburban, or rural community. Today few if any social groups or communities can be said to have significantly limited availability or access to drugs and alcohol, but some groups and communities (e.g., adolescents, low income communities) are less able than others to influence substance availability and access.

Social groups and communities also act as individual risk factors by affecting individual psychosocial development demands and life circumstances (Alarcon, 1995; Tobler, 1992). An individual's risk for developing a substance disorder should be thought of as fluid, changing with demands and circumstances, but having predictable points of increased risk. Such points include exposure to acute or chronic negative personal events (e.g., divorce, poverty, illness) that cause psychological pain and are therefore difficult to cope with. Depression, schizophrenia, bipolar disorder, personality disorder, and severe psychosocial problems (e.g., divorce) are also significant substance disorder risk factors (Kaufman, 1996).

* Common Symptom Onset Patterns

Substance disorders tend to develop gradually over long periods with more than one substance. Individuals typically report substance use starting at an early age and may attach a great deal of psychological and social importance to their first smoke or the first time they got drunk or high, drawing elaborate connections between their early and current substance behaviors. Gradual advancement from substance use to abuse can be attributed to any number of risk factors, but basic paths of progression have been defined: (1) the addictive properties of the substance used, (2) the pleasurable experiences individuals have when using the substance, and (3) the escape from or alteration of reality and negative events that is provided by intoxication (Meyer, 1996). Unaltered, these paths of progression can lead to the use of more dangerous substances, more dangerous combinations of substances, more dangerous amounts of substances, or the continued use of a substance known to be dangerous. The progression experienced by individuals with mental disorders may be related to the course of the disorder and the individual's drive to obtain relief from its symptoms.

Like all behaviors, substance use and the onset of substance disorder are influenced by countless personal and social factors, such as psychological resiliency and learned social skills. Listed below are personal factors and skills that Krumpfer and Hopkins (1993) have identified as protecting the individual from the onset of a substance disorder. Although individual characteristics ultimately determine onset, social group expectations are critical. Social groups that define substance disorders as unacceptable tend to provide individuals with social resources that can protect them when they are faced with high risk developmental demands and life circumstances. Social groups that do not define substance disorders as unacceptable are less likely to support individual development of protective personal factors and social skills.

Protective personal factors

- Optimism
- Empathy
- Insight
- Intellectual competence
- Self-esteem
- Mission and purpose
- Determination and perseverance

Protective personal skills

- Emotional management skills
- Interpersonal (social) skills
- Intrapersonal (psychological) skills
- Academic and job skills
- Ability to restore self-esteem
- Planning skills
- Life skills and problem-solving skills

❑ Common Assessment Problems

Denial and rationalization are the two most commonly encountered substance disorder assessment problems. These powerful psychological defense mechanisms protect against painful anxiety, self-awareness, and the inevitable self-hate associated with substance disorders. In fact, it can be said that substance disorders *require* denial and rationalization. ***Denial*** is the refusal to recognize reality. Despite absolute evidence of a substance disorder, the individual either denies the disorder completely or is willing to recognize aspects of the disorder, such as frequency, amounts, and duration of use, but denies the disorder itself (Botelho and Novak, 1993). ***Rationalization*** is the formation of an acceptable explanation for that which is unacceptable. A well-rationalized substance disorder poses multiple assessment problems. A "reason" for a substance disorder seems irrational, but to the individual, being able to rationalize a substance disorder is a means of decreasing anxiety, self-awareness, and self-hate. Classic examples of rationalized substance disorders are: "I always drink when I watch the game," "I have more fun when I drink," and "Because of [fill in the blank], I drink." Rationalizations are endless circles of "yes-but" thinking that allow the individual to focus on concerns other than the substance disorder.

From substance use to substance abuse, any aspect of a substance disorder can be denied and rationalized. The personal cost of these defenses to the individual is great but rarely exceeds the immediate benefits. Denial and rationalization effectively ensure that substance behaviors continue despite immediate, recurrent, and long-term negative consequences. Paradoxically, years of substance disorder can strengthen rather than weaken denial and rationalization. Over time most people become much more sophisticated in their denial and rationalization. An individual who, for example, has been drinking alcohol for 8 hours may once have denied the behavior, insisting it was only "a few beers." After 15 years the same individual may simply insist that drinking for 8 hours is normal.

Individuals with substance disorders are rarely alone in their denial and rationalization. Significant others gain the same benefits as the individual with the substance disorder when they deny and rationalize any aspect of the loved one's disorder. For example, it is not unusual for an adult child of an alcoholic to reach one's forties before recognizing the parent's substance disorder. The overall effect of denial and rationalization is to render the substance disorder invisible. Practitioners will encounter significant patient denial and rationalization of, as well as ambivalence toward, an obvious substance disorder. Rather than insist that a patient admit to a disorder, the practitioner should help the individual to build the confidence and psychological will power needed to confront the disorder. One way of accomplishing this is to avoid talking about the disorder in ways that seem to increase the patient's anxiety and thereby compel him or her to continue to deny and rationalize.

Substance Disorder Assessment

The *Diagnostic and Statistical Manual of Mental Disorders, fourth edition*, (DSM-IV) defines substance disorders according to the stage of use behaviors (abuse or dependence) and the following use effects (APA, 1994):

- Intoxication
- Withdrawal
- Intoxication delirium
- Withdrawal delirium
- Substance-induced persisting dementia
- Substance-induced persisting amnestet disorder
- Substance-induced psychotic disorder with hallucinations substance disorder with delusions
- Substance-induced mood disorder
- Substance-induced anxiety disorder
- Substance-induced sexual dysfunction
- Substance-induced sleep disorder

Reliable assessment of substance disorders is comprehensive and includes biopsychosocial factors (Craig et al, 1996; Ries, 1995). ***Biological assessment factors*** include presence of alcohol (or other odors) on breath, positive drug tests, abnormal lab tests, physical injuries and trauma, evidence of toxicity or withdrawal, and impaired cognition or neurological changes. ***Psychosocial assessment factors*** include habitual patterns of intoxication, evidence of social isolation and conflict, manipulation of others, and denial and rationalization. Substance disorder assessment should include the individual's mental status, mood, and stressors or life circumstances. Two of the most important areas of assessment that are very likely to be overlooked are the individual's self-concept and self-esteem. Individuals with a substance disorder should also be assessed for underlying mental disorders, such as depression, anxiety, grief, stress, and personality disorders. When more information is needed or the individual seems unable to give needed information, collateral information from significant others is important. Friends and family members can provide helpful information about the individual's development and life circumstances, including family substance history. Assessment of the individual's social support resources—individuals and groups—is also important. Many primary care settings have begun to include substance abuse screening as a routine element of care for all patients.

The following questions should be asked in any substance abuse screening:

1. Do you use the following substances [list] in any amount?
2. Describe your first substance use, most recent substance use, and patterns.
3. Are there any changes you would like to make in your substance use?

Basic Assessment

All individuals who use drugs or alcohol, including tobacco products, should be assessed for their experiences with use, abuse, dependence, crashing, craving, bingeing, withdrawal, remission, and relapse. Accurate assessment of these experiences makes it possible to help patients work toward achieving desired or necessary changes in their substance use.

Use literally refers to the use of a substance. A substance either is used or it is not used. Amount, frequency, or duration of use are not considered.

Abuse is defined by the DSM-IV as recurrent substance use, with one or more of the following symptoms, over at least a year (APA, 1994):

1. Failure to fulfill important obligations at work, home, or school (e.g., through absence)
2. Recurrent use in hazardous situations (e.g., while driving)
3. Recurrent legal problems (e.g., arrest)
4. Continued use despite important social or interpersonal problems caused by it (e.g., partner conflict)

Dependence is defined by the DSM-IV as three or more of the following symptoms occurring over a year (APA, 1994):

1. Tolerance, defined as significant increases in the amounts of substance needed to achieve the desired

effect, or a significant decrease in effect without a decrease in the amount of substance used
2. Withdrawal, defined as the experience of substance-specific withdrawal symptoms, substance use to avoid withdrawal symptoms, or substance use to relieve withdrawal symptoms
3. Using larger amounts of the substance or using the substance for longer periods than intended
4. Persistent desire or unsuccessful efforts to decrease or control substance use
5. Large amounts of time spent obtaining the substance, using the substance, or recovering from having used the substance
6. Lack of participation in important social activities when the previous level of participation had been consistent
7. Continuation of use despite persistent or recurrent physical or psychological problems that are made worse when the substance is used.

An individual's experiences with crashing, craving, and bingeing are extremely important. Many of the severe psychosocial problems associated with substance abuse occur during these phases of substance use. More importantly, individuals who hope to change their substance behaviors need to be able to think of their behaviors in these terms. ***Crashing*** is the acute onset of withdrawal symptoms immediately following intoxication. The individual literally collapses, physically and emotionally, and is mildly to severely incapacitated. This experience is often compounded by lack of sleep or little or no food intake. It should be noted that experienced substance abusers frequently make arrangements in advance to avoid a severe crash following intoxication. One of the more common methods used is to take benzodiazepines, which smooth out the individual's transition from intoxication to complete withdrawal.

Craving is the experience of strong physical and emotional urges to use a substance, to obtain substance effects (e.g., euphoria, relaxation, confidence), or to avoid withdrawal symptoms. Cravings can take any form, such as fond recollections of intoxication, vivid flashbacks, reexperiences of intoxication, reexperiences of tastes, smells, and bodily sensations associated with intoxication, obsessive and intrusive thoughts about the substance, or anticipation of substance use and substance effects. Drugs, alcohol, and tobacco produce a range of generic cravings, mostly related to early symptoms of withdrawal, but individual differences can be significant. With some drugs, such as cocaine or nicotine, cravings can immediately follow use, but craving onset can also be cued long after an episode of substance use. ***Craving cues*** are internal or external stimulants that trigger an urge for the substance or substance effects. The more common and predictable craving cues are massive sensory experiences, strong mood states, negative events, observing others using the substance, engaging in nonsubstance behaviors that are similar to established substance use behaviors, and engaging in behaviors that normally precede substance use.

Sensory craving cues can be extremely powerful. Just as the aroma of warm popcorn sells popcorn, smells are powerful cues for alcohol, nicotine, marijuana, crack cocaine, and tobacco. Distinctive nonsubstance-related odors, such as the smell of frying food, can also cue cravings. Visual images and tactile simulations are also powerful cues. Mood states, negative or positive, cue cravings because a large part of substance effect and intoxication is the experience of changes in mood state. Stressful life events can cue cravings when the events induce strong mood states or the desire to escape, avoid, or alter unpleasant circumstances. One universal craving cue is observing the substance use of others. Watching others use a substance allows the individual to idealize the substance and its effects; it therefore activates denial and rationalization defenses. Nonsubstance-related behaviors can trigger cravings when the behavior includes actions and motions that are similar to the usually very precise behavior rituals of substance use.

Psychological symptoms of craving include anxiety, anger, irritability, sadness, agitation, obsessive thinking, and hyperactivity. Psychological symptoms of craving also include the idealization of previous experiences of intoxication. The biological process of craving is a neurodysregulation caused by recurrent substance use and the chemical properties of the substance being used. Sudden hard-hitting cravings can produce dramatic alterations in the individual's perceptions, thoughts, feelings, and behavior, leading to gross impairment of judgment as well as impulsive behavior (Mendelson and Mello, 1996).

Bingeing is the use of a substance until one is physically unable to continue or until the substance is no longer available. The individual has lost or relinquished control and feels physically and psychologically compelled to continue using. A binge is an all-consuming process that continues despite immediate and long-term negative consequences to the individual and others. Depending on the substance and the individual's physical stamina, the duration of a binge can be measured in hours, days, or weeks. Early on, bingeing can be the result of the chemical effects of the substance, particularly the effects of intoxication and disinhibition. Both conditions interfere with decision making, including the decision to stop consuming the substance. A binge can also be self-promoting; that is, bingeing simply leads to more bingeing.

Bingeing does not occur with all substances. Substances that do not produce dramatic mental and emotional changes or that have low overdose thresholds are not associated with binge consumption. For example, binge drinking of alcohol is common, but valium bingeing does not occur. A binge is a traumatic experience made even more traumatic by secondary "out of control" behaviors, such as unplanned sex and violent conflict. Bingeing is extreme behavior, but in many social circumstances it can seem ordinary. For example, at sporting events and college parties, binge drinking may not be labeled as bingeing. Individuals with well-established binge behaviors typically make statements such as, "I always use too much," "I never stop when I should," and "I always get into trouble when I use." Practitioners should be aware that binging always causes feelings of anxiety, guilt, and remorse that individuals may or may not be able to express freely.

The final areas of assessment to be reviewed here are withdrawal, remission, and relapse. Individuals with a substance disorder and substance-related psychosocial problems will have a significant history in each area. ***Withdrawal*** is the process of biological detoxification that begins the moment substance use ends. The amount of time required for complete detoxification depends on the substance, the individual's biological capacity to metabolize and excrete the type and amount of the substance, the addictive properties of the substance, and the individual's level of addiction. Despite the fact that withdrawal symptoms signal detoxification, withdrawal symptoms can also ensure recurrent substance use. The more awful the withdrawal, the more appealing withdrawal avoidance becomes. For example, after years of daily use, nicotine withdrawal produces multiple acute detoxification symptoms within minutes to hours. The individual experiences dysphoria, insomnia, irritability/frustration/anger, anxiety, loss of concentration, restlessness, decreased heart rate and increased appetite (Cocores, 1993). These symptoms are unpleasant enough to be an accurate predictor of continued smoking. To most people, withdrawal is worth enduring only when there is reason to believe that complete withdrawal will mark the end of substance use. Unfortunately, with most substances this is not the case, and individuals can expect to go through withdrawal more than once.

Remission is the recommended first goal of treatment for substance disorders. The DSM-IV defines specific criteria for remission associated with substance dependence, but except for the category of sustained partial remission, these same criteria are useful in describing remission related to substance abuse. ***Full remission (early)*** is diagnosed when there are no symptoms of abuse or dependence for at least a month but less than a year (APA, 1994). ***Partial remission (early)*** is diagnosed when less than full remission criteria (only 1 or 2 symptoms of abuse or dependence are present) is evident for at least a month but less than a year. ***Full remission (sustained)*** is diagnosed when no symptoms of abuse or dependence are present for a year or longer (APA, 1994).

Symptom remission does not imply recovery from a substance disorder. Individuals are "recovered" when they are physically, psychologically, and socially substance free and have achieved developmentally appropriate psychosocial functioning. ***Relapse*** is a predictable phase of remission and recovery from substance disorders. Regardless of the type of substance, approximately two thirds of all first episodes of relapse occur within 90 days of remission. Because relapse is a normal phase of remission and recovery, terms such as ***treatment failure*** or ***treatment noncompliant*** are no longer useful. Marlatt and Gordon (1985) conceptualize relapse as a process that centers around the individual's exposure to and ability to cope with high-risk situations or situations in which substance use is likely to occur. In their research, they observed that an individual's cognitive and emotional reaction to the first relapse can determine whether or not a full return of the substance disorder will occur. Thus, how an individual copes with one's first relapse is critical. The focus of Marlatt and Gordon's model of relapse prevention therapy is to improve the individual's ability to cope with high-risk situations and negative mood states. Accordingly, relapse is most likely to be prevented when the individual is able to manage personal thoughts, feelings, and behaviors in high-risk situations. The process of developing the coping skills and the mastery required for recovery from substance disorders begins with the first relapse.

Substance Abuse Disorders

Practitioners are referred to the DSM-IV for specific diagnostic information. This section is limited to a review of the common substance disorders.

Alcohol Abuse

Practitioners are expected to assess patient alcohol use. Approximately 13.8% of American adults will, in their lifetime, become dependent on alcohol or will abuse alcohol (APA, 1995). Alcohol intoxication is a factor in approximately 50% of highway fatalities and over 50% of domestic violence incidents. The frequency of suicide attempts and completed suicides among individuals with alcohol dependence is 3 to 4 times the rate for the general population. The high incidence of depression with alcoholism contributes to this suicide rate (APA, 1995). The peak age period for the development of alcohol dependence is 20 to 30. Female onset tends to be later in life and to occur in response to trauma (Kaufman, 1996; Quinby, 1993; Wheeler, 1993).

Alcohol is a central nervous system (CNS) depressant that produces sedation and relaxation, decreased anxiety, and changes in perceptions. Alcohol intoxication produces loss of psychomotor coordination, impaired judgment, aggression or passivity, disorientation, disinhibition, and negative mood states. The development of alcohol abuse can occur gradually, and relapse is a long-term treatment problem. The psychosocial problems related to alcohol abuse can be severe and include long-term unemployment, academic failure, and family violence (El-Guebaly, 1995b). In some communities alcohol abuse has come to be viewed as a predictable stage of individual growth and development. The social assumption is that young people will abuse alcohol, then outgrow the behavior. However, trends in middle school and high school students suggest that the growth and development stage during which alcohol abuse behavior starts has changed. Younger individuals are abusing alcohol, and because of their youth, they may be less able to "outgrow" the behavior.

Health and social behavior experts continue to debate the question of whether alcohol abuse should be viewed as a disease or as individual maladaptive behavior. For the sake of treatment, alcohol abuse is both. The assessment of alcohol abuse should include the individual's history of alcohol consumption and intoxication, physical and mental status exams, substance abuse treatment history, family substance history, and laboratory screens, including screens for infectious diseases (APA, 1995).

Effective assessment of alcohol abuse in primary care is not complicated, but unique assessment problems can be anticipated. Practitioner attitudes and patient motivation can be the source of many problems. Havassy and Schmidt (1994) warn that practitioner stereotypes of the alcohol abuser as difficult, demanding, and uncooperative can interfere with assessment and treatment. At the same time, this stereotype allows practitioners to fail to recognize alcohol abuse in patients with more socially acceptable substance behaviors. Poor patient motivation can be a source of problems when, for a variety of reasons, individuals who abuse alcohol are not be motivated to change. They may resist, deny, and rationalize or insist on being prescribed a medication that will do the hard work of remission and recovery for them. Practitioners should note that the most common reason for poor motivation is failed previous attempts at controlled drinking. Apathy can be an effective defense against semiconscious fears of more failure. Patients who meet the diagnostic criteria for alcohol abuse but who are in the early stages of the disorder and are motivated to change may benefit from primary care. Evidence of chronic alcohol abuse, alcohol dependence, dual diagnosis, severe psychosocial problems, or unpredictable behavior indicates a need for specialized care.

Nicotine Abuse

Nicotine is a CNS stimulant commonly consumed by smoking or chewing tobacco products. Every year 60% of all smokers make a serious attempt to stop smoking (Frank and Jaen, 1993). Nicotine produces a complicated array of immediate and long-term biopsychosocial effects across multiple body systems. The immediate effects of nicotine are a burst of short-duration stimulation, mild euphoria with an alerting effect, and enhancement of memory followed by relaxation and tranquilization (Carr, 1993; Cocores, 1993). Nicotine tolerance develops gradually and nicotine withdrawal symptoms are severe. Nicotine effects include electrocortical activation through the enhancement of cerebral glucose metabolism. Nicotine binds to multiple receptor sites throughout the nervous system and affects nearly every endocrine and neuroendocrine system. Nicotine produces skeletal muscle relaxation and significant cardiopulmonary effects at the hypothalamus, hippocampus, thalamus, midbrain, brainstem, and specific areas of the cortex. This causes the release of acetylcholine, norepinephrine, dopamine, serotonin, vasopressin, and growth hormone. Feelings of calm and well-being are the result of nicotine-induced alterations across the mesolimbic and dopaminergic pathways. The noticed effects of nicotine are momentary improvement in stress response, vigilance, and cognitive functioning (Frank and Jaen, 1993).

As with alcohol consumption, all patients should be routinely assessed for nicotine consumption, but effective early assessment is complicated by the fact that most lifelong smokers start smoking in their early teens, when they are less likely to have regular health care visits. According to Cocores (1993), new smokers and light smokers may be able to stop smoking through sheer willpower, but only about 10% of heavy smokers can stop smoking this way. This trend is therefore important. Because of severe withdrawal symptoms most heavy smokers who want to stop smoking find it difficult to do so. New smokers may find it less difficult to stop smoking, but they are less likely to try. Many smokers who are highly motivated to stop smoking find themselves unable to endure withdrawal symptoms.

Caffeine Abuse

Caffeine is a CNS stimulant consumed in beverages (coffee, soda, tea) or tablets. Caffeine abuse produces symptoms of intoxication, tolerance, and withdrawal. Symptoms of intoxication can occur following consumption of as little as 250 mg; these include restlessness, nervousness, excitement, insomnia, flushed face, diuresis, GI upset, muscle twitching, rambling thought and speech, tachycardia or arrhythmia, periods of inexhaustibility, and psychomotor agitation. Long-term hazards of caffeine abuse are becoming more of a health concern now that so many people routinely consume large amounts of caffeine. High-dose caffeine drinks (coffees and sodas) are always being developed and marketed and most people, particularly children and adolescents, are unaware of their daily caffeine intake. They are, however, fully aware of the withdrawal headache, nausea, and irritability that is relieved by consuming more caffeine. To date, most individuals who withdraw from caffeine do so for health conditions that are made worse by caffeine.

Cannabis (Marijuana) Abuse

Cannabis contains tetrahydrocannabinol (THC), a psychotomimetic agent contained in the leaves of the cannabis plant. THC effects and intoxication are determined by dose, setting, method of consumption, and the quality of the cannabis plant. The most common method of consuming THC is to smoke dried cannabis leaves rolled as a cigarette or in a pipe. The leaves may also be consumed by adding them to food or by brewing them into a tea. Because different species of the cannabis plant contain different amounts of THC, the THC amount or potency varies greatly from low-potency homegrown plants, which usually have less THC than high-potency cultivated plants.

THC produces sympathomimetic effects, sedative-hypnotic effects, euphoria, altered perceptions, and tachycardia. Consuming large amounts can induce hallucinations, paranoia, anxiety, or psychosis (Carr, 1993). Individuals who smoke high-grade cannabis and therefore consume large doses of THC report withdrawal symptoms and craving onset within 4 to 8 hours after the last dose. Multiple long-term effects of marijuana abuse have been identified (Pope, 1996). THC abuse can lead to amotivational syndrome or chronic apathy, which is indicated by severe psychosocial problems such as chronic unemployment, underemployment, or academic failure. Amotivational syndrome in turn can support continued consumption of THC.

As baby boomers become America's middle class, the consumption of marijuana is once again a topic of social debate. A significant percentage of this generation used marijuana in the 1960s, and these adults are less likely to be alarmed when their adolescent children try marijuana. Those who consume THC regularly compare themselves to those who use alcohol, drawing the conclusion that, compared to the health and psychosocial problems related to alcohol, THC is not harmful. THC consumers often compare themselves to nicotine users, a comparison that might lead to more negative conclusions.

Practitioners should note that marijuana is also used in conjunction with other drugs, such as powder heroin, cocaine, speed, and alcohol. Because of its sedating effects, THC is used to prevent crashing and to minimize the withdrawal symptoms of other drugs. As with all controlled substances, THC use is difficult to assess if a patient is reluctant to report illegal behavior.

Amphetamine Abuse

Amphetamines are CNS stimulants that produce immediate or prolonged feelings of energy and euphoria. Compared to alcohol, nicotine, caffeine, or THC, amphetamine abuse is less common, but is increasing in popularity. Although true amphetamines (e.g., methamphetamine) are controlled substances, they are easily purchased on the street. Amphetamines are consumed as a liquid, tablet, powder, or nasal spray that is swallowed, injected, inhaled, or smoked. The main effects of amphetamines are a speed buzz, a loss of appetite, insomnia, hyperactivity, and feelings of super competency. Long-term use and high doses of amphetamines cause acute and chronic symptoms of severe paranoia, psychosis, and impaired judgment. Amphetamine tolerance and withdrawal develop quickly, and amphetamine crashes and cravings are among the worst drug experiences. Following market demands for drugs that can be consumed by smoking, smoked amphetamines have become available, accessible, and popular. However the "blast" obtained from smoked amphetamines, such as "ice," leads to violent behavior often enough that the popularity of this drug has not reached the level of crack cocaine. Individuals who abuse amphetamines may also seek CNS depressants or use other drugs with sedating effects in an effort to offset the effects of the amphetamines.

Cocaine Abuse

Cocaine is a controlled CNS stimulant that is injected, inhaled, or smoked. With recurrent use, the amount of time between first use and addiction is from 2 to 4 years (Gawin, 1991). The form of cocaine that is consumed determines the magnitude of the initial impact and the duration of effect. The two most common forms are powder (loose) cocaine, which is primarily snorted, and crack (solid) cocaine, which is smoked in a pipe. Powder cocaine costs more than crack cocaine and delivers a less intense but longer-duration high. A dose of crack cocaine can cost as little as $5 and delivers a tremendous blast of simulation, the duration of which is measured in minutes.

Cocaine inhibits the reuptake of norepinephrine, serotonin, and dopamine, producing a state of arousal, elevated mood, and altered perceptions (Mendelson and Mello, 1996). Smoked or snorted, cocaine can produce a flawless sense of well-being and alertness. In the early stages of abuse, normal pleasurable experiences, including sexual pleasure, are magnified. The individual who is high on cocaine feels self-confident. At high-enough doses, powder or crack cocaine can produce feelings of invulnerability, superiority, and a sense of all things being limitless. Anxieties drain away instantly, social inhibitions are released, and hunger is suppressed. With recurrent use, neurodysregulation occurs when the drug is not present, causing tolerance, withdrawal, crashing, and cravings so severe that relapse can be anticipated (APA, 1995).

Highly motivated patients who wish to stop using cocaine will struggle with cravings and relapse. Long after cocaine stops providing superhuman feelings, the memories of such experiences can retain their allure and motivate continued use. Abuse and dependence alter the effects of cocaine, so that pleasurable feelings are significantly decreased and dysphoria rather than euphoria is experienced. This dysphoria is unique, because individuals seem to feel abandoned by the drug that had "given" them so much pleasure. Because of temporary improvements in self-concept and self-esteem resulting from cocaine use, the individual who has developed a tolerance to the drug or who is struggling with remission undergoes a very real sense of having lost something private and valuable. The deterioration in health and psychosocial functioning caused by cocaine abuse is dramatic. The motivation to face withdrawal and relapse often does not develop until the individual has encountered painful legal, financial, or health problems (e.g., asthma) that cannot be avoided.

Hallucinogen Abuse

Hallucinogens, such as lysergic acid diethylamide (LSD), mescaline, and psilocybin are psychotomimetic agents that produce distortions in perception and alterations in mood that are experienced as being transported to an alternative reality, or "tripping." Hallucinogens are organic (e.g., psilocybin mushrooms) or chemically manufactured and are consumed by swallowing or smoking the drug. Hallucinogens are often inexpensive, clean, and simple drugs that do not require frequent or repeated dosing to produce prolonged and varied effects. These drugs continue to have an appealing counterculture image for those who wish to be a member of such groups. Designer hallucinogens and pharmaceutical products taken for the purpose of "tripping" have become popular with young and exclusive counter-culture groups. In most forms, a single dose can provide multiple sequential episodes of silly euphoria, sedation, perceptual distortion, stupor, confusion, arousal, anxiety, fear, pain, depression, and impaired judgment. Individuals who abuse hallucinogens are more likely to receive emergency health care for psychosis or physical injury than primary care for health promotion or illness prevention. Unlike most drugs, the abuse or repeated use of hallucinogens may not induce withdrawal.

Inhalant Abuse

Volatile substances produce vapors which, when inhaled, dramatically alter mental status. The full range of products used for this purpose is difficult to define, but the typical products are paint thinners and toxic glues. Individuals also "sniff" aerosol sprays, cleaning fluids, gasoline, and other petroleum products. The process involves applying the substance to a piece of cloth, then holding the cloth over the mouth and nose or holding the cloth in the mouth. The immediate intoxication effects of volatile substances can be intensified by concentrating the vapors. This can be accomplished by containing the soaked cloth in plastic wrap, then holding both plastic and cloth over the mouth and nose. Containment can also be accomplished without plastic wrap, by placing a paper bag over the head while applying the cloth. Because the cloth is in contact with the individual's skin, chemical odors from the substance cling to the skin long after use. The high that is produced by inhalant intoxication is essentially disorientation and euphoria with reduced anxiety. The adverse effects include acute cardiac symptomatology, violent behavior, and paranoia. Tolerance and compulsive abuse of volatile substances can develop quickly, leading to severe psychiatric disability. Inhalant abuse occurs primarily among the very young (school age) and the very poor. Numerous inexpensive volatile products are available on most store shelves. Efforts to control children's access to these products often leads to their discovery of yet another product. As with all substances of abuse, despite the associated physical and mental health risks and psychosocial problems (including combustion and fire), inhalant abuse continues.

Opiate Abuse

Heroin is a controlled opiate narcotic (CNS depressant) that can be injected, snorted, or smoked. Initially, injected heroin produces an extremely seductive high of euphoria, pleasure, and altered perceptions. A heroin high is somewhat less intense when the drug is snorted or smoked. The death rate for opiate narcotic abuse and dependence is 10 deaths per thousand users per year (APA, 1995). Death is usually the result of overdose, accident, injury, or medical complications. Since the late '70s, injected opiate abuse has also been recognized as a primary source of infectious disease, including HIV and hepatitis.

Heroin tolerance and dependence develops relatively quickly, with ever increasing amounts of the drug needed daily in order to prevent painful withdrawal symptoms. Heroin withdrawal is so difficult and painful that preventing withdrawal soon becomes the individual's single goal in life. Dependence on oral methadone, an opiate substitute, is for many an acceptable alternative to heroin withdrawal. Smoking heroin reduces the risk of being discovered, and many people erroneously believe that smoking is less addictive or less dangerous than injecting the drug. Similarly, some individuals reserve heroin for use on special occasions, with the assumption that occasional use is safer than daily use. Injecting a mix of heroin and cocaine (speedball) or smoking heroin sprinkled on marijuana are also popular methods of consumption.

Heroin in a marijuana joint carries less social stigma and is viewed as less degrading, allowing individuals to feel they have more control of their substance intake. Abuse of pharmaceutical opiates is one of the most dangerous forms of opiate abuse and also one of the most difficult to detect. Pharmaceutical opiates such as meperidine, hydrocodone, and oxycodone are narcotic analgesics that can be swallowed, crushed and smoked, or dissolved and injected. Unlike street opiates, pharmaceutical opiates provide a reliable measure of narcotics, ensuring tolerance and dependence. There is a large street market for pharmaceutical narcotics, but abuse also occurs among health care professionals who divert patient medications for their own use, as well as among patients who "shop" for narcotic prescriptions for their own use or for resale.

Sedatives-Hypnotic-Anxiolytics (SHA) Abuse

The abuse of pharmaceutical sedatives-hypnotic-anxiolytics (SHA), or downers, is extremely common. At treatment doses, SHAs provide relief from acute symptoms of anxiety, stress, and insomnia. For this purpose these medications are appropriately prescribed for brief periods of time (6 to 8 weeks). New anxiolytics are being formulated to relieve these symptoms without producing the dramatic "downer" effects typically associated with substance abuse; however, there is a tremendous street market for SHAs that can produce downer effects, particularly benzodiazepines. "Benzos" are easily obtained by illegal street purchase, theft, fraud, and "shopping" practitioners. As drugs of abuse, benzos are free of the social stigma attached to street drugs and opiates, but tolerance and dependence can develop very quickly, even at prescribed doses. The complex health hazards of withdrawing from SHAs are such that hospitalization is warranted.

The street popularity of benzos can be attributed to the nature of the high they produce. These medications were developed to deliver feelings of comfort, safety, and relaxation. The appeal is obvious. SHAs are abused as "little helpers" during difficult times, taken in large single doses as party pills, and used as a method of controlling the crash and withdrawal from a stimulant binge. According to the DSM-IV, the longer SHAs are taken, and the higher the dose, the greater the probability of severe health hazards and complex withdrawal symptoms (APA, 1994). Practitioners should also note that lethal overdose, intentional and unintentional, with SHAs is a significant risk.

Management of Substance Disorders

➤ Counseling

Specialized substance disorder recovery programs and patient education materials are widely available and should be utilized (Crits-Christoph and Siqueland, 1996; Langenbucher, 1996). Ultimately, the treatment goals for substance disorders are remission, relapse prevention, and recovery. Primary care counseling cannot replace specialized substance abuse services, but primary care counseling plays a vital role in helping patients start the process of change that leads to recovery. No step in this process is too small to be taken. Psychiatric primary care counseling can help those who are ambivalent or discouraged to build the self-confidence they need to make changes in their substance behaviors. In many cases, psychiatric primary care counseling can prepare the patient for successful participation in specialized substance abuse programs (Fuller, 1994).

In this section, patient acceptance, confidence building, and recognition of personal benefits are presented as "getting-started" goals, followed by a review of relapse prevention. Practitioners can anticipate that most patients will have to start many times before they can make real progress, which is why "getting started" is so important. Patients with long-standing substance abuse which may involve multiple substances, substance dependence, dual diagnosis, or highly unpredictable behavior, require specialized care and should be referred to a substance disorder specialist. However, patients with long-standing substance disorders may be unwilling to accept specialized substance abuse care. Psychiatric primary care may be the only resource for these patients. The focus of psychiatric primary care counseling should remain the same, with the objective that the patient can improve and with improvement may be more willing to participate in needed specialized care. Practitioners should remember that each patient has already tried and failed to change his or her substance use and is looking for evidence to support trying again.

Acceptance

Realistic expectations promote acceptance. Individuals with substance disorders continually question whether or not their use of drugs or alcohol truly constitutes a substance disorder. Full acceptance develops slowly because questions and doubts are relentless. Questioning can be expressed in countless ways, the most common of which is half-hearted efforts to change the substance behaviors. Significant levels of doubt make changes in substance behaviors more difficult than they already are. It is, however, unrealistic and unnecessary to expect anyone to have no doubts. Practitioners can view patient acceptance and patient doubt as two separate lines of appraisal and focus on building acceptance. Paying a lot of attention to patient doubts can cause them to grow rather than yield. By focusing on acceptance, practitioners can also avoid getting into a power struggle with patients, which will only distract the focus away from what is important, the patient's substance use.

Big changes in substance use behavior are the cumulative results of many small changes. Unrealistic expectations, are a set-up for failure at any point in the process. Especially in the beginning, it can be very difficult for patients to even imagine living without the substance, and practitioners risk their credibility when they set unrealistic goals. The start of counseling is not the time to test a patient's resolve. Keeping expectations realistic also makes it easier for practitioners to avoid overreacting to a patient's struggle as he or she tries to accept behavior that the practitioner may view as apparent. By definition, a realistic expectation is a change that a patient can make today, tomorrow, or this week. Unrealistic expectations are changes made today for forever.

For the person with a substance disorder, substance use has become a routine if not acceptable part of life. Acceptance means helping the patient to build a new frame of reference, rather than trying to tear down the very powerful frame of reference that has supported substance use. Despite the fact that immediate success occurs with only a very small percentage of substance disorder patients, many patients hope to be one of the lucky few. Even those without such hope will find failure to be a powerful experience. Failure makes acceptance difficult. Practitioners should address patient's feelings and fears about failure but then move on.

Confidence Building

Along with the patient's need to develop acceptance, patients must also strive to develop confidence in their own abilities and the counseling process. The most meaningful source of confidence is positive experience, and the most positive experiences are some sign of progress. Progress supports acceptance, builds resolve and, most importantly, buffers the impact of relapse. Practitioners can immediately work with patients to identify opportunities for success. Positive substance abuse educational resources (e.g., videos, booklets) that the patient can refer to anytime and anywhere build confidence and are necessary components of psychiatric primary care counseling (Davis, Parran, and Graham, 1993). A full range of materials, including information on how others have handled their problems, should be available. Few people gain much from a single source of information or from materials that are gloomy or impersonal. Positive written materials are helpful because patients react to the information differently over time, and changes in their thinking are major signs of progress. Practitioners should beware of those patients who are not making process, but who are just using new words to express old thinking. In the final analysis, confidence comes from being in control rather than under the influence.

Unexpected personal problems, particularly financial problems, are a direct threat to a patient's efforts to change (Humphreys, Moos, and Finney, 1996). No one likes unpleasant surprises, but they are a fact of life. Individuals who are regaining their ability to handle life drug free can be extra sensitive to anything that suggests the opposite may be true. Practitioners can help patients to build their confidence by teaching them to anticipate, prepare, and plan how they will handle problems. The focus should be placed on how the patient will respond to potential problems and changes, not on the problem itself. Patients should be encouraged to adopt the belief that progress is important, but it is not perfect or trouble free. The aim is to help patients avoid using unexpected problems, such as an auto repair bill, as an opportunity or excuse for substance abuse.

Acknowledge benefits

Each patient must continually and factually identify how he or she will personally benefit from psychiatric primary care counseling and from changing his or her substance use. Vague global benefits such as "fewer arguments at home" or "a better life" are not sufficient to motivate early or long-term changes in behavior. Personal benefits must be unique to the individual, and as the individual's circumstances change, new benefits should be identified. For example, an early personal benefit might be attending the Monday morning staff meeting at work without a hangover. The patient will function better and participate more and not have to endure dirty looks from coworkers. A later benefit might be having the confidence to present a good idea to coworkers.

Many patients will resist the very idea of personal benefits, insisting that there are none. Sometimes this response is a reflection of the patient's need to avoid disappointment and fear of failure. To hope for nothing is a way to avoid disappointment and failure. When this is the case, a slight change in approach may be effective. Patients should think about aspects of their lives that are important to them and then define how changes in their substance use would be beneficial in these areas.

Relapse prevention

When the patient's goal is abstinence, the counseling goal is relapse prevention. Both require time, effort, and motivation, but relapse prevention is the key to abstinence. A sense of humor helps. Factors that increase the risk of relapse also threaten abstinence. Some of the most powerful relapse risk factors are boredom, isolation, relationship conflict, ambivalence, and low self-esteem (Sullivan and Hanley, 1992). Marlatt and Gordon (1985) view relapse risk in terms of high-risk situations that the individual is either able or unable to cope with effectively. They identify two categories of risk factors, internal and external. ***Internal risk factors*** are rationalization and denial, cravings, small decisions that put the individual into a high- risk situation, and impulsive testing of one's abstinence or control. ***External risk factors*** are relationship conflict and social pressure to use (defined as the substance use of others and their expectation that the individual will conform his or her behavior to theirs).

Relapse prevention is necessary both before and after a relapse has occurred. In the latter situation, the goal is to end an episode of relapse as quickly as possible. In both cases, the focus of relapse prevention is to master experiences that, if left unresolved, could lead back to full substance abuse. Marlatt and Gordon (1985) warn that to be effective, relapse prevention strategies must be individualized to fit each person and must be updated frequently. The patient's goal should be to recognize high-risk situations and be able to take effective coping action. In short, prevention means being prepared.

℞ Prescribing

There are three basic approaches to prescribing for substance disorders: (1) treatment of underlying mental disorders, (2) relief of withdrawal or craving symptoms in order to reduce the risk of relapse, and (3) prevention.

Treatment

Patients with substance disorders who meet the criteria for another mental disorder should receive appropriate medication for that disorder. In some cases, the underlying mental disorder may be the basis for the substance disorder, and improvement with the former can lead to improvement with the latter. However, mental disorders may also occur independent of each other, meaning that improvement in one does not produce improvement in the other. The most common undiagnosed and untreated mental disorders that are related to substance disorders are major depression, bipolar disorder, and generalized anxiety disorder (GAD). Improvement with these disorders often means improvement with a substance disorder. Post-traumatic stress disorder (PTSD) and personality disorder are also related to substance disorders, but improvement is more difficult because the boundaries between the two disorders are less well defined. In prescribing for mental disorders, the target symptoms of the disorder should be identified and used as indicators of treatment effectiveness. If possible, the target symptoms should also be meaningfully related to the substance disorder. For example, if a patient drinks more when depressed, then depression symptom relief should produce decreased alcohol intake as well.

Relief

When prescribing for the relief of withdrawal or craving symptoms, regardless of the type of substance, two rules apply: only nonaddicting medications should be prescribed, and the rationale and purpose of prescribing such medications should be clear. The most troubling risk associated with prescribing for the relief of withdrawal and craving symptoms is that the wrong message can be implied: namely, that if a substance is the problem, a substance is the solution. At the same time, if withdrawal symptoms and cravings make it so difficult to stop that the patient is unable or unwilling to try, medication can at least give the patient the opportunity to try. Patients who require a long complicated course of medical treatment for substance withdrawal should receive specialized care.

Prevention

Medications may be prescribed for the purpose of preventing relapse when the medication is one component of a comprehensive relapse-prevention program. Ideally, medication should be prescribed for the first 90 days following remission, the highest risk period for relapse. In most cases, the prevention treatment goal is to decrease or control cravings (e.g., nicotine withdrawal). A wide range of medications has proved effective in decreasing the cravings related to cocaine, nicotine, and opiates, but individual variations in effectiveness rule out any single drug as superior to another or effective for everyone. Currently, the medication of choice for alcohol disorder is naltrexone, but less experienced practitioners should work with a specialist when prescribing this drug. Naltrexone is an opioid antagonist that has been shown to be effective in reducing alcohol cravings. However, naltrexone may be less effective with alcohol abuse than with alcohol dependence, since in the former case alcohol use may not be daily. Medications that can decrease cravings related to cocaine abuse and dependence are those with significant serotonin (e.g., sertraline), dopamine (e.g., bupropion), or anticholinergic (e.g., amatadine) effects. Opioid cravings have traditionally been managed with substitute narcotics (e.g., methadone) that allow for improved psychosocial functioning, prevent cravings, and prevent a return to opioid abuse. Presently, the recommended medications for safe opiate narcotic withdrawal and remission maintenance are clonidine and buprenorphine. Prescribing for nicotine withdrawal has not proven to be as effective as was hoped, but nicotine gums and patches offer many long-time smokers an opportunity to stop that they would not have without the products (Cocores, 1993).

Consultation and Referral

Most primary care settings are in partnership with alcohol or drug abuse (AODA) services, 12-step recovery programs, and AODA specialists. If these professional services and community programs have not been arranged for the primary care services as a whole, the practitioner should place a high priority on arranging for access to a consulting substance specialist. Specialists can help practitioners to assess low motivation, substance dependence, exploitive drug-seeking behavior, chronic mental disorders, and dual diagnosis. They can work with practitioners to develop medication treatment plans, to meet patients' acute and long-term needs, and to reduce prescribing hazards. Unpredictable behavior is not an uncommon feature of substance disorders, including behaviors that are potentially dangerous to the patient and/or others. Practitioners should therefore not hesitate to consult a specialist to obtain a second opinion on diagnosis and treatment. Patients who are excessively hostile, unmotivated, or court-mandated to treatment are poor candidates for psychiatric primary care for substance disorders.

References

Alarcon R (editor): Cultural psychiatry, *Psychiatric Clin of N Am* 18(3), 1995.

American Psychiatric Association: Practice guidelines for the treatment of patients with substance use disorders:alcohol, cocaine, opiates, *Am J Psychiatry* 152(suppl 11), 1995.

Botelho RJ, Novak S: Dealing with substance misuse, abuse, and dependency, *Primary Care* 20(1):51, 1993.

Carr LA: The pharmacology of mood-altering drugs of abuse, *Primary Care*, 20(1):19, 1993.

Cocores J: Nicotine dependence: diagnosis and treatment, *Psychiatric Clin N Am* 16(1):49, 1993.

Craig TJ, Branchey M, Buydens-Branchey L, Bernstein D, Chapman B, Goldfarb W, Handelsman L, Ness R, Roy A, Wolfsohn R: Admission criteria for inpatient substance abuse/dependence rehabilitation: implications for managed care, *Ann of Cli Psychiatry* 8(1):11, 1996.

Crits-Christoph P, Siqueland L: Psychosocial treatment for drug abuse: selected review and recommendations for national health care, *Arch Gen Psychiatry* 53(8):749, 1996.

Davis AK, Parran TV, Graham AV: Educational strategies for clinicians, *Primary Care* 20(1):241, 1993.

El-Guebaly N: Substance use disorders and mental illness: the relevance of comorbidity, *Can J of Psychiatry* 40(1):2, 1995a.

El-Guebaly N: Alcohol and polysubstance abuse among women, *Can J of Psychiatry* 40(3):73, 1995b.

Frank SH, Jaen CR: Office evaluation and treatment of the dependent smoker, *Primary Care* 20(1):251, 1993.

Fuller M: A new day: strategies for managing psychiatric and substance abuse benefits, *Healthcare Management Review* 19(4):20, 1994.

Gawin FH: Cocaine addiction: psychology and neurophysiology, *Science* 251:1580, 1991.

Havassy BE, Schmidt CJ: Alcohol and other drug abuse disorders in primary care settings: current and future research. In Miranda J, Hohmann A, Attkisson C, Larson D (editors): *Mental Disorders in Primary Care*, San Francisco: 1994, Jossey-Bass Publishers.

Humphreys K, Moos RH, Finney JW: Life domains, alcoholics anonymous, and role incumbency in the 3-year course of problem drinking, *J of Nervous and Mental Dis* 184(8):475, 1996.

Kaufman E: Diagnosis and treatment of drug and alcohol abuse in women, *Am J Obstetrics/ Gynecology* 174(1):21, 1996.

Krumpfer KL, Hopkins R: Prevention: current research and trends, *Psychiatric Clin N Am*, 16(1): 11, 1993.

Langenbucher JW: Socioeconomic analysis of addictions treatment, *Public Health Reports* 111(2):135, 1996.

Marlatt GA, Gordon JR: *Relapse prevention*, New York, 1985, The Guilford Press.

Mendelson JH, Mello NK: Management of cocaine abuse and dependence, *NE J of Med* 334(15):965, 1996

Meyer RE: The disease called addiction:emerging evidence in a 200-year debate, *The Lancet* 347(8995):162, 1966.

Pope HG, Yurgelun-Todd D: The residual cognitive effects of heavy marijuana use in college students, *JAMA* 275(7):521, 1996.

Quinby PM, Graham AV: Substance abuse among women. *Primary Care* 20(1): 131, 1993.

Ries, R: *Assessment and treatment of patients with coexisting mental illness and alcohol and other drug abuse (treatment improvement protocol series)*, Washington, D.C., 1995, US Department of Health and Human Services.

Sullivan EJ, Hanley SM: Alcohol and drug abuse, *Ann Review of Nursing Research* 10:281, 1992.

Tobler N: Drug prevention programs can work: research findings, *J of Addictive Diseases* 11(3):1, 1992.

Wheeler SF: Substance abuse during pregnancy, *Primary Care* 20(1):191, 1993.

Eating Disorders 8

Eating disorders are chronic conditions with severe psychological, physical, and social symptomatology. Numerous eating disorder etiology models and treatment protocols have been developed, and important progress has been made in both areas. This chapter reviews anorexia nervosa, bulimia nervosa, obesity, and obsessive-compulsive overeating. Because of the difficulty of establishing symptom criteria, obsessive-compulsive overeating and obesity are not specific disorders in the *Diagnostic and Statistical Manual of Mental Disorders* (DSM-IV), *fourth edition*, but are included in this chapter because of the high incidence and prevalence rates for both conditions. Practitioners will find that individuals with eating disorders will vary in the amount and type of psychiatric primary and specialized care that is needed, but most people will require some combination of the two.

➲ Who Is at Risk

Anorexia nervosa and bulimia nervosa are diagnosed primarily among females, with bulimia being more common than anorexia (American Psychiatric Association [APA], 1993). According to the APA, 1% to 4% of adolescent girls and young adult women meet the diagnostic criteria for anorexia nervosa or bulimia nervosa. Obsessive-compulsive overeating and obesity are less related to gender and age. Eating-disorder risk factors range from biology to behavior, but acute or chronic stressful life events (e.g., victimization, poverty) may be the most powerful single risk factors. Between 20% and 50% of females diagnosed with mental disorders, including eating disorders, are survivors of childhood sexual abuse (APA, 1993). Eating disorders can develop concurrently with or in relation to depression, anxiety, and some personality disorders. Clinically, eating disorders are similar to substance disorders in that both conditions are characterized by compulsions, cravings, tolerance, withdrawal, denial, and rationalization. As with substance disorders, individuals with eating disorders may become unable to control their behavior despite the pain, suffering, and health risk that the behavior causes. A family history of eating disorders is a significant and highly complex risk factor, with genetic, social learning, and social environment components.

The fact that anorexia nervosa and bulimia nervosa are rarely diagnosed in males suggests that gender role socialization is a risk factor for some females. Females who are socialized to associate food with femininity, and thinness with sexual attractiveness, may be at increased risk for anorexia and bulimia (Heinberg, 1996). Because of this socialization, by puberty a young girl has learned to value women who shop for, prepare, and serve food without public displays of appetite or weight gain unrelated to pregnancy, since she has learned that such women have a higher social status than women who define their femininity differently. By her early teens, this girl may have also learned to express her appetite in private and to fear weight gain. At the same time, her body image, self-concept, and self-esteem can become attached to social symbols of femininity and sexuality over which she has little personal control. Just the opposite can be true for little boys who are more likely to be socialized to strive for the high social status awarded to the male, whose appetite for food is not subject to social controls. Individuals who have not had the "female socialization" experience may be less at risk for gender-related eating disorders.

Dramatic changes in eating behavior, with significant increase or decrease in appetite, can occur as symptoms of severe mental illness (SMI), such as schizophrenia or bipolar disorder. Individuals with SMI can become confused or disorganized and fail to act on their hunger; they may have no appetite or may overeat compulsively. Recurrent episodes of anorexia, bulimia, and obsessive-compulsive overeating can occur not only as a part of the individual's SMI symptomatology but also as a sign of SMI relapse. Medications for SMI can have a significant effect on appetite and weight. Learned coping skills and established coping patterns (e.g., avoidance), regardless of gender, can be related to the development of eating disorders, especially compulsive dieting, obsessive-compulsive overeating, and obesity. Families and cultures can act as indirect risk factors when they place extremely high value on food or eating as a source of physical or psychological comfort, recreation, celebration, status, or reward. Income level can directly and indirectly increase the risk of eating disorders. The stress of poverty can be a powerful psychological risk factor, and less expensive foods tend to be lower in nutritional value and higher in sugar, fat, and salt, thereby increasing the risk of overeating and obesity. Just as low income tends to be associated with overeating and obesity, high income tends to be associated with undereating and bulimia (Manson and VanItallie, 1996).

* Common Symptom Onset Patterns

Symptoms of eating disorders tend to develop along one of three basic patterns: (1) they may begin as mild or subtle behavioral changes that lead to serious and profound behavioral changes, which are difficult to alter; (2) they may develop in response to acute or chronic stressful life events; and (3) they may have no particular pattern of onset but may simply occur at critical stages of psychosocial development, so that there are significant periods of healthy as well as unhealthy eating. Onset patterns are important, but few people seek health care early in the course of an eating disorder. Most people are diagnosed with an eating disorder only after major changes in their behavior have become well established. Regardless of the type of eating disorder, individuals often report long-standing concerns about their weight, significant periods of weight gain, severe weight loss dieting, or all three. By the time alarming changes in weight and eating behaviors are recognized and acknowledged, the individual may have deeply established (but unrecognized or unacknowledged) negative thoughts and feelings that maintain maladaptive behaviors. The relationship of thoughts, feelings, and behaviors with eating disorders makes them similar to substance disorders in that it can be difficult to determine which changes occurred first. Even when the onset of an eating disorder appears to be sudden—such as the individual who one day induces vomiting after a large meal and thereafter continues to vomit after eating—negative changes in the individual's thoughts and feelings may have been established long before the first episode of vomiting occurred.

Common Assessment Problems

Full assessment of individuals with eating disorders should include developmental and sexual history; attitudes and beliefs about weight and food; body image and ideals; family history of depression, anxiety, and eating disorders; important adult relationships; self-inflicted starvation or self-induced vomiting; use of laxatives, diuretics, diet pills, and exercise; and history of traumatic or stressful life events (Yager, 1994). If possible, assessment of nutritional status by a nutritional specialist should also be obtained. Because of the long duration of eating-disorder symptomatology that may have preceded diagnosis, the assessment time frame should be measured in years. Many problems can greatly increase the difficulty of assessing individuals with eating disorders; these include the individual's reliance on denial and rationalization, semiawareness of symptoms, and strong feelings of anxiety, guilt, and shame.

Denial is a major problem in the assessment of eating disorders. Individuals may insist that they are not vomiting, undereating, or overeating, or that their behavior is not symptomatic. Direct confrontation of an individual's denial is not likely to be productive. In fact, individuals with eating disorders may be skilled at defending themselves against direct confrontation, since this approach is often used by family and friends. During the assessment it can be more effective to identify aspects of the individual's behaviors that do ***not*** activate denial, and start the assessment there. In most cases this means allowing the individual to start with behaviors about which he or she feels good. For example, a woman with obsessive-compulsive overeating may feel good about the fact that she never eats sweets.

Rationalization is as apparent as denial and just as revealing. The easiest form of rationalization of personal food and weight behaviors is to generalize them. For example, at any given time 25% of adult males and 50% of adult females are dieting, but few would meet the diagnostic criteria for anorexia (Bellows and Franke, 1994). Nevertheless, individuals who are malnourished from undereating routinely rationalize their weight as "successful dieting" and therefore socially acceptable behavior.

The same may be said for the rationalization of overeating. Whereas meals once held extremely important family, religious, and cultural meaning, in the late 1960s family meals became rare and then commercialized. Take-out and home delivery meals, oversized portions and overeating have become profitable and socially acceptable, but obesity continues to be socially unacceptable. Therefore the most ordinary rationalizations for overeating tend to be the most powerful. Statements such as, "I know I shouldn't eat this" or "I could be hit by a bus tomorrow, you have to enjoy life while you can" routinely precede and follow overeating. Self-awareness of maladaptive eating behaviors tends to decrease over time, to the point where the individual no longer has a sense of his or her behavior as being anything other than ordinary. ***Lost self-awareness*** is directly related to the chronic nature of eating disorders. Years of maladaptive eating lead to decreased awareness of the behavior, which in turn allows the behavior to continue. The individual's initial concern and self-awareness become silent. This numbness provides the individual with a much-needed psychological protection against anxiety and self-awareness. Later on, eating may be necessary to maintain the numbness that protects the person against anxiety and self-awareness.

Patients with eating disorders can become "experts" on their disorder—that is, they are able to provide detailed information about it as well as up-to-date health and food statistics. For some individuals, becoming an expert on an eating disorder makes it possible for them to talk about it but still avoid talking about anything personal. Assessment of eating disorders can be especially difficult when the disorder is a source of *shame*: the individual believes that he or she is bad or flawed as a human being. Shame is more severe than ordinary embarrassment. The behaviors related to eating disorders can feel extremely degrading even when performed in private. The assessment itself can feel degrading, thereby increasing the individual's use of denial and rationalization. Shame can be expressed in endless ways, including a reluctance to disclose personal information or the disclosure of misleading information. For example, a malnourished woman with anorexia who is also a successful business owner may feel that she should know better, and because she feels this way she gives misleading information about her anorexia. A basic strategy for these assessment problems is to listen for statements of shameful feelings and to respond to those statements by pointing out the importance of the individual's dignity and the intention to respect his or her feelings. At the same time, the message should be conveyed that feelings of shame are not a sufficient reason to continue to suffer the indignity of an eating disorder.

Eating Disorders

Anorexia Nervosa

Anorexia nervosa is characterized by extremely low body weight or efforts to produce weight loss in spite of low body weight. There are two types of anorexia behavior patterns: restricting and binge-purge. ***Restricting*** is literally the extreme restriction of total calorie intake to less than what is needed to maintain health. ***Binge-purge*** includes total calorie restriction, with episodes of binge eating and purging. In both types, body weight is the main preoccupation, marked by a seeming unwillingness (or, in the late stage of the disorder, an inability) to achieve and maintain a healthy body weight. Inadequate body weight is a physical symptom of anorexia nervosa, but it can also occur as an emotional, social, or psychological symptom.

Anorexia is more prevalent among females than males and among majority than minority females. According to the DSM-IV, fear of weight gain or weight phobia is a core symptom of anorexia nervosa; however, researchers have found that weight phobia need not be present for the diagnosis of anorexia nervosa. Hsu and Lee (1993) studied the interactions of culture and weight phobia and found that weight phobia is not a universal symptom of anorexia, but weight phobia with anorexia is common in industrialized cultures. The researchers draw on Brumberg's two stages of the development of anorexia, recruitment and career, to explain their findings. According to the Brumberg framework, anorexia nervosa almost always begins with severe dieting for social reasons (stage 1). Then the individual becomes adjusted to undereating and malnourishment, and both conditions become stable (stage 2). Weight phobia is only one of many social reasons for dieting. True loss of appetite does not occur until very late in the course of illness (Rock and Curran-Celentanao, 1994). Until this point is reached, undereating requires tremendous, deliberate effort.

One of the most striking clinical features of anorexia nervosa is the patient's strength, determination, and ability to maintain below normal body weight or to continue to produce weight loss. Individuals with anorexia are able to withstand extreme hunger for days at a time, during which extreme weight-reducing exercises may be performed. Calorie counting, weighing and measuring all foods, food-choice restrictions, hard exercise, hyperactivity, and fasting may define the individual's life. Obsessive thoughts about food and eating are common but usually lead to an increased need for food restrictions and controls rather than increased caloric intake. This ever growing need for control can manifest as rituals and rules that are aimed at mastering hunger at all costs, despite physical pain and discomfort. Typical food rules include rigid classification of all foods as either "good" or "bad," with few foods deemed as good; eating only at precise times and specific locations; eating strange or unpleasant food combinations so as to decrease their appeal; assigning long mealtimes to specific foods, such as 2 hours to eat one apple; and always eating alone.

Despite many food rules, individuals with anorexia may be highly involved in shopping for, preparing, and serving food to others. Despite food rules, rituals, and preoccupation, individuals with severe anorexia may gradually begin to lose what they believed were fail-safe behavior controls, which results in even more feelings of shame. In their study of anorexia and bulimia, Herzog et al,(1993) found that a patient's ideal body weight predicted recovery more than age, type of eating disorder, or comorbid mental disorders: the lower the ideal body weight, the more difficult recovery became. In this study, the 1-year rate of recovery for anorexia nervosa was 10%, whereas for bulimia the 1-year recovery rate was 56%.

Comorbidity with anorexia nervosa is common. Up to 60% of patients with anorexia nervosa also have major depression. Personality disorders and substance disorders are also fairly common comorbid disorders. Effective treatment of depression or substance disorders may lead to an improvement in the eating disorder, but an improvement in a personality disorder may ***not*** produce an improvement in anorexia nervosa. The typical duration of anorexia nervosa, before the individual seeks health care, is well over 4 years (Herzog et al, 1993). In this amount of time, significant physiological adaptation to starvation has occurred. Individuals adapt to semistarvation by developing lowered energy expenditures or decreased caloric requirements (Rock and Curran-Celentano, 1994; Pomeroy, 1996). This life protecting adaptation may be viewed by the patient as a reason to redouble his or her efforts to lose weight. When there is evidence that this adaptation has occurred, refeeding or weight regain must be gradual. The starting daily caloric intake should be 1000 to 1200 with increases of 200 calories every 2 to 3 days until a maximum of 4000 calories is reached (Solanto et al, 1994). Dangerous complications from too-rapid refeeding include congestive heart failure, gastric dilation, and malabsorption problems. Solanto et al, demonstrated weight gain, after 5 to 7 days of restabilization with no weight gain, at a rate of 0.20 to 0.36 lb per day. Regardless of the rate of regain, a target weight goal high enough to support healthy physiological functioning should be established, but treatment should also focus on the thoughts that are related to weight and weight loss as well as the individual's psychological defenses against anxiety (Yager, 1994).

Anorexia nervosa was once defined in psychoanalytical terms, with little emphasis on the biophysical nature of the disorder. Refusing to eat was believed to be a young girl's solution to the problem of growing out of the freedoms of childhood into womanhood, with its strict social rules, or a young girl's solution to severe family problems. Parent-child conflict and household conflict were viewed as causes of anorexia nervosa. Presently, more emphasis is placed on eating disorders as a maladaptive response to trauma, including childhood sexual abuse or sexual assault. Regardless of how anorexia is understood, the younger the individual, the more important it is to address parental or family problems, but parents and other family members need not participate in treatment (Robin, Siegel, and Moye, 1995).

By the time a patient with anorexia nervosa seeks health care, he or she will have experienced a great deal of interpersonal conflict. Well-meaning (***and*** less than well-meaning) significant others may have become determined to change or control the individual's behavior. Practitioners can assume that the individual with anorexia nervosa has already faced significant social pressure and personal confrontation, from accusing glances from strangers to family rejection and ridicule by peers. It is not always possible or necessary to work out these conflicts immediately. In some cases, as individuals begin to recover, they feel better and are then more able to explore painful relationships and conflicts. Of course, the most difficult thing anyone with anorexia will have to deal with is the prospect of weight gain.

Patients may initially view every measure of weight gain as a symbol of victory for the practitioner and defeat for themselves. This struggle, referred to by Zerbe (1993) as ***annihilation anxiety,*** rests in the patient's deeply rooted fear that, in wanting to destroy the anorexia, the practitioner also wants to destroy him or her. By refusing to play a role in the patient's psychological struggle, practitioners can continue to be helpful and avoid defining improvement as "victory" or "defeat." Practioners may find it difficult to be helpful when patients assign such threatening powers to them. Ideally, treatment includes helping the individual to contain this psychological struggle, ambivalence, and fear without blaming and accusing others. Another reason to avoid power struggles with patients is that the resulting anxiety or anger can scare them, so that they feel compelled to take more extreme and potentially harmful measures to win the struggle they believe is responsible for their anxiety. The patient may not realize that to defeat the practitioner is to lose to the disorder.

The DSM-IV criteria for anorexia nervosa (restricting and binge-purging) are (APA, 1994):

1. Refusal to maintain normal body weight (being less than 85% of normal)
2. Intense fear of gaining weight regardless of actual weight
3. Distortions in body image or denial of significance of severely low body weight
4. Amenorrhea (three consecutively absent menses)

Bulimia Nervosa

Bulimic bingeing is the uncontrolled, rapid consumption of large amounts of food or calories. Bingeing provides relief but may trigger purging or compensatory behaviors to get rid of the food or calories that have been consumed. Binge eating is almost always done in private and may be kept secret for years. The typical binge episode lasts from 1 to 2 hours (Agras et al, 1994; Yen, 1992). The frequency of bulimic episodes may be measured in hours, days, weeks, or months. Over the course of the illness, the frequency of episodes may fluctuate, with periods of significant increase or decrease.

The five common methods of purging after bingeing are (1) vomiting, (2) use of laxatives, (3) use of diuretics, (4) hard exercise, and (5) fasting. Vomiting can be accomplished by forcing the gag reflex or using emetics. Some individuals learn to vomit on command, without manual or chemical stimulation, so that it appears to be natural, spontaneous, or illness-related. Indicators of recurrent vomiting include edema in the hands and feet, headache, sore throat, parotid-and salivary-gland swelling, tooth-enamel erosion and caries, abdominal pain, lethargy, fatigue, dizziness, and dehydration (Leitenber et al, 1993). In one study of bulimia and purging, patients vomited an average of 8.5 times a week. The patients in this study also consumed 26 to 36 laxative tablets a week (Weltzin et al, 1995).

Whether a large amount of food (e.g., pizzas) or a large number of calories (e.g., candy) is consumed, the quantity can seem impossible. In severe cases, spending $100 or more on food in 1 day is not unusual. Individuals are able to eat large amounts of food very quickly because their loss of control is so great that they continue to eat despite severe physical pain. Bingeing is a frightening loss of control, usually followed by shame, concealment, anxiety, and dysphoria. Bingeing and purging can trigger overwhelming feelings of self-hate, which can lead to disinhibition and more bingeing or risk-taking behaviors, which may result in injury. The loss of control associated with bulimia cannot be overstated, although every episode may not reach the same level of frenzy (Abbot and Mitchell, 1993; Agras et al. 1992). Loss of control is manifested in many ways, such as mouth injuries caused by eating half-frozen foods or extremely hot food. When access to preferred binge foods is restricted, any available food may be consumed, from maple syrup to raw oatmeal. ***Preferred binge foods*** are foods (e.g., snacks or fast foods) that are designed to be eaten quickly and can be consumed in large amounts. They are usually extremely high in fat, sugar, or salt. Some individuals may have a favorite binge food (e.g., popcorn, cookies), but a binge is defined by uncontrolled eating and not by the type of food consumed. Individuals with extreme cases of the disorder may be involved in shoplifting food or in public bingeing and purging. Secondary problems associated with bulimia include serious financial problems, banishment from markets or restaurants, intense relationship conflicts, and misdemeanor legal charges, such as disorderly conduct, property damage, and theft.

Rorty, Yager, and Rossotto (1993) asked 40 women who had suffered from bulimia and purging for an average of 3 years how they were able to recover. These women said they wanted a better life and were tired of having their lives dominated by bulimia. They reported a wide range of effective treatment techniques, including psychotherapy, Overeaters Anonymous, and self-help books, but the most valuable help was the support of their families and friends. Almost all of the women indicated that the most difficult challenges they faced were intrusive thoughts of wanting to change their bodies and intense fears of becoming fat.

The DSM-IV criteria for bulimia nervosa (purging/nonpurging) are (APA, 1994):

1. Recurrent episodes of binge eating and inappropriate compensatory behaviors at least twice a week for 3 months:
   a. Eating large amount of food within 2 hours
   b. Feeling a lack of control during the binge
2. Compensatory behaviors that include self-induced vomiting; use of laxatives, diuretics, enemas, or other medications; fasting, and hard exercise
3. Self-evaluation that is strongly influenced by body shape and weight

Obesity

There is no single cause of obesity, nor has the condition been defined as a mental disorder. Promising genetic explanations for obesity continue to be developed and tested, but for the individual who is obese it is a complex problem with severe physical, social, and psychological symptoms (Ponto, 1995). Although it advocated a comprehensive biopsychosocial approach to the treatment of obesity, an NIH workshop in 1994 that reviewed content pharmacologic treatment of obesity strongly recommended treatment with medication (Atkinson and Hubbard, 1994). The NIH workshop defined ***obesity*** as a chronic syndrome with multiple causes and numerous health and well-being complications, but it concluded that certain types of obesity could be improved with medication. These conclusions were based on the observation that 95% of patients who are treated with diet, exercise, and behavior modification—without medication—regain the weight they lose. Researchers have speculated that serotonin, one of the neurotransmitters that regulate mood and behavior, is also an important determinant of body weight. Bray (1992) found that higher serotonin levels were significantly correlated with less food intake and recommended that treatment for obesity include the prescription of medications (e.g., antidepressants) that increase serotonin levels. Unfortunately, the most consistent research outcome in the study of medication treatment for obesity is that weight that is lost while taking medication is regained as soon as the medication is discontinued (Weintraub, 1992). The search for more powerful biological models of and medication treatments for obesity continues to hold promise.

Regardless of etiology or whether medication is prescribed, for the obese person obesity is much more than being overweight. One of the most important aspects is the mental health care needs of individuals who seek primary health care as their first step in obtaining treatment for obesity. When primary care is the first step, the practitioner's response can significantly influence whether a second step will be taken. The more comfortable it is to ask for treatment for obesity, the more likely the request will be made. Patients should not be made to feel uncomfortable or embarrassed; however, in Bellows and Franke's (1994) survey of health care providers' attitudes toward obesity, 87% of the providers believed that obesity is a product of self-indulgence, and 70% thought that obesity is an emotional problem.

Thinness as social status and a multibillion dollar weight loss industry have not reduced the weight of Americans; in fact, the median American weight continues to increase (Bellows and Franke, 1994). Keeping these trends in mind, practitioners may have negative attitudes toward individuals with obesity because they feel unable to provide successful treatment, or they may believe that their efforts will not actually improve the individual's health and well-being. In actuality practitioners can offer a great deal of benefit. Significant physical and psychological health benefits have been reported, by using a simple formula for a 10% reduction in body weight, by focusing on weight achieved rather than weight loss, and by meeting the individual's needs for emotional support. A 10% weight loss can be produced by normalizing the patient's eating pattern to three meals a day, gradually decreasing total dietary fat to 30%, and adding five 45-minute walks per week (Bellows and Franke, 1994).

What are the early emotional and psychological needs of the individual with obesity who is seeking treatment? The first need is to decrease negative feelings and expectations about seeking health care for obesity. Being able to explore and express these feelings can make it less difficult to focus on more important needs. Second, the individual needs to feel that his or her motivation to achieve a weight change, however weak or strong that motivation may be, is acknowledged and supported by the practitioner.

Confidence is an element of motivation, and practitioners who convey the opinion that the patient's condition is hopeless or that improvement will require superhuman feats will undermine the individual's confidence. Motivation grows slowly and must be handled gently. Finally, individuals need to start addressing their feelings and thoughts about their bodies. Feelings such as embarrassment, anger, and guilt should be identified, acknowledged, and discussed freely. Regardless of the type of treatment involved, the ability to talk about one's body is vital. All too often, individuals with obesity have learned to decrease their feelings of distress by becoming emotionally disconnected from their bodies.

Regardless of their weight, most people experience a range of strong emotional responses (e.g, comfort) to food and these responses motivate eating behavior. Most people have a favorite "comfort food," usually something with a large amount of fat and a pleasing texture, such as mashed potatoes or ice cream. Comfort foods can relieve stress and anxiety. However, when guilt and shame associated with weight gain develop, comfort foods can cause rather than relieve stress and anxiety. Individuals for whom food meets important emotional needs must develop nonfood alternatives to meet those needs.

Extreme psychological and social problems can be associated with obesity (Alger, Seagle, and Ravussin, 1995). Unlike many other chronic conditions (e.g., substance dependence), the individual with obesity cannot escape the stress and stigma of obesity by "passing" as a person of normal weight. It is socially acceptable to make fun of popular, powerful women who are obese. No other condition subjects an individual to such public torment and stress. Those who are unable to cope with the stigma of obesity may seek relief in self-destructive ways, such as substance abuse or social isolation, or they may develop stress disorders, such as depression or anxiety. In most cases, by the time an individual seeks professional health care for obesity, he or she has tried and failed to lose weight or tried and regained the weight that was lost. Practitioners should determine the type of weight-loss plans that may have been used and point out the methods that are potentially dangerous (e.g., liquid supplements).

Obsessive-Compulsive Overeating

Obsessive-compulsive overeating is a highly distressing condition not yet formally recognized as a disorder. The defining symptoms of obsessive-compulsive overeating are intrusive thoughts about food and a decreased ability to stop eating once one has started. The obsessions and compulsions associated with obsessive-compulsive overeating do not produce the extreme loss of control or frenzy associated with bingeing. Episodes of obsessive-compulsive overeating tend to last significantly longer than 2 hours, and obsessive-compulsive overeating does not necessarily include the consumption of massive amounts of food. Food consumption is largely determined by episode duration, but even long-duration episodes may add up to moderate consumption.

Some experts equate obsessive-compulsive overeating with uncompensated binge eating and obesity (Arnow, Kenardy, and Agras, 1992; Yanovski et al, 1992). Clinically, important distinctions between binge eating and obsessive-compulsive overeating can be drawn. In popular terms, obsessive-compulsive overeating is also known as ***anxious eating***, ***stress eating***, ***grazing***, or ***having a bad food day***. The individual is troubled by persistent thoughts of foods. Relief from food-thoughts tends to end the episode. Statements such as, "I'm not hungry, why am I still eating?" and "Why can't I stop eating?" are characteristic. The distinction between obsessive-compulsive overeating and binge eating may be one of degree, but both conditions are highly distressing. A woman with obsessive-compulsive overeating, for example, might eat a piece of cake with enjoyment. But when she stops eating it she becomes preoccupied with the cake, with the decision to eat the cake, with having actually eaten the cake, and with the amount of cake that remains. These obessions may continue as long as the cake is available. It may be hard for her to understand how others are able to be uninterested in the cake. Rather than bingeing, she is unable to stop eating and repeatedly has "one more bite." This behavior may continue until the cake is gone or until she physically leaves the area where the cake is located.

Individuals with obsessive-compulsive overeating put a great deal of effort into preventing food thoughts and are amazed by the nonchalant attitudes of those who are not obsessive-compulsive about food. Feelings of anxiety and stress are related to intrusive and persistent thoughts of food as well as to efforts to avoid food or to stop eating. Weight control and emotional coping tend to take the form of strictly adhered-to food rules and food plans, such as never eating in public, purchasing single-portion foods only, and avoiding food events such as potluck meals. Of all of the maladaptive eating patterns, this one may be the most common, but unless obesity, anorexia, or bulimia develops, obsessive-compulsive eating can remain unrecognized.

Management of Eating Disorders

Counseling

Patients with eating disorders should receive specialized care for the eating disorder and primary care for related health effects. Community and professional health care programs for undereating, overeating, and compulsive eating have become widely available. Specialized health care programs (inpatient, outpatient, and residential) should provide education and treatment specifically for the individual's disorder. Community self-help groups and support groups should provide emotional support and coaching. The range of community and professional eating-disorder programs now available is a direct reflection of the multiple-treatment and well-being needs of patients with eating disorders. The most effective professional health care programs emphasize weight goals, cognitive-behavioral change, and psychosocial well-being and functioning. Effective community programs are those with participants who are positive and committed to recovery, and includes individuals who are just starting out as well as long time participants. Actual community and professional options may be limited by availability and cost, but, as much as possible, a workable match should be made between patient coping style and program format (e.g., educational programs versus self-help groups). A single-method treatment approach should be avoided, because the long-term nature of eating disorders and long-term treatment requirements make it unlikely that any single method would be effective.

Psychiatric primary care counseling plays a vital role in meeting health care needs by helping patients with eating disorders to carefully consider and then prepare to participate in specialized community and professional programs. Recovery from an eating disorder requires considerable individual effort. Patients who are poorly prepared, who have treatment misconceptions (such as fantasies of being rescued or fears of being humiliated), or who simply do not know what to expect may react negatively to specialized care, spoiling what might otherwise have been an important opportunity. The ability to talk to a practitioner about difficult personal concerns before starting specialized care can give the patient the opportunity to sort out any mixed feelings about recovery. Treatment novices, as well as the experienced, can benefit from talking to a practitioner about their hopes and their fear of longstanding emotional pain, anxiety, and confusion. When the individual's physical health is stable, the goal of psychiatric primary care counseling is to build the motivation that is necessary to make a personal commitment to treatment. The emphasis is on committment to the process (treatment) rather than to any particular weight or food goals.

Motivation refers to the patient's level of (1) acceptance of the need for a change in eating behavior, (2) comprehension of why such change is necessary, (3) comprehension of the personal steps that are necessary to accomplish meaningful change, and (4) willingness to make the process a personal priority. Motivated patients are better prepared to cope with the anxiety and stress that accompany the initial phases of treatment and the challenges of learning to cope effectively with relapse. Practitioners can encourage patients to verbalize their hopes and fears, both realistic and unrealistic. Magical thinking or beliefs that treatment and recovery can be fast or effortless should be identified. It is highly unlikely that an individual will have no magical thoughts, but he or she will probably be reluctant to discuss them. Identifying such thoughts can serve an important purpose, because magical thoughts often represent unspoken hopes. When this is true, magical thoughts can be redefined as the individual's wish for improvement rather than as a wish to avoid the hard work of improvement.

Common wisdom of the past held that specialized care should be offered to patients with eating disorders if they were highly motivated and ready to put 100% effort toward improvement. In effect, patient motivation was used as a treatment screening tool. Rather than assuming that supermotivation is ideal, or that poorly motivated patients are poor candidates for treatment, practitioners should view the building of patient motivation as a basic component of psychiatric primary care counseling. Building motivation should be thought of as an initial, ongoing, and daily need, because patient motivation will certainly wax and wane. Patients should work to discover their own unique methods of building and rebuilding motivation. For many, building motivation begins with the identification of important personal needs. Motivation is a secondary concern when a patient's weight or behavior is life-threatening or self-injurious or there is evidence of acute substance abuse. In the absence of these contraindications, the longer the duration of the eating disorder, the more important and necessary it is to address the patient's need to build motivation. Both short-term and long-term goals should be identified, and all goals should be personally important to the patient.

Short- and long-term motivation goals can protect the patient from the ever-present fear of, and in some cases desire for, giving up—especially when improvement is slow, or when there are early failures or recurrent episodes of relapse. Multiple short-and long-term personal goals ensure that there will always be more than one measure of progress. In helping patients to deal with their needs for motivation, practitioners can also help them to think of how some of their personal needs can be met by confronting their eating disorder. Everyone with an eating disorder will have different personal needs, but for many, the most troubling needs are relief from the chronic stress, anxiety, and depression that are related to low self-esteem; ineffective coping skills; and unrealistic images of oneself, both psychologically and physically. The ultimate outcome of building motivation is for patients to begin to define their eating behaviors as no longer working for them, or as problems rather than solutions.

A word about community self-help groups and support groups: participation in such eating-disorder groups can decrease the difficulty of changing longstanding thoughts, feelings, and behaviors regarding weight and food. This benefit from group participation can be attributed to the fact that much of what we learn in life is acquired through membership in important social groups, beginning with the family. Groups are a vast source of both positive and negative information about who we are. Effective self-help and support groups can make it possible for patients to "try on" a positive self-concept. They can become comfortable with viewing themselves positively *before* they need to rely on such skills in difficult or stressful situations outside the group. Mature or established groups can provide this experience when group members share each other's success. Young groups, made up of mostly new members or individuals just starting out, may have too many members with the same vulnerable condition, and thus be unable to help an individual envision and embrace a positive self. Groups with members who share many negative characteristics can be very stressful and discouraging.

℞ Prescribing

Prescribing medication for the treatment of eating disorders continues to be a topic of controversy. Whereas biological models of eating disorders view medication as the single most important element of treatment, behavioral and psychosocial models take the view that, at best, medications provide short-term benefits or treatment for concurrent mental disorders. One point of consensus within this debate is that antidepressants or antianxiety drugs should be prescribed for patients with eating disorders *and* depression or anxiety disorder. Depression and anxiety disorders occur as antecedents or consequences of eating disorders, as well as being concurrent disorders. In some cases successful treatment of depression or anxiety produces improvement in the eating disorder. Remission of depression or anxiety disorder can also be beneficial as a precursor to the treatment of an eating disorder when depression or anxiety prohibits meaningful patient effort. When symptoms of depression or anxiety are an element of the eating disorder, symptom relief can result in improvement in the eating disorder, but this approach should be taken with caution. Depression or anxiety may be a way of denying or rationalizing the eating disorder, in which case their relief may prove difficult or produce little benefit.

Some experts assert that antidepressants and antianxiety medications can effectively treat anorexia nervosa or bulimia nervosa even in the ***absence*** of depression or anxiety disorder (Atkinson and Hubbard, 1994; Weltzin et al, 1995). A medication trial is usually considered with individuals who have chronic or severe eating-disorder symptoms that do not improve with other interventions. If antidepressants are used for the treatment of bulimia, they should be prescribed for at least 6 months and with specialized care (Abbott and Mitchell, 1993; Agras et al, 1994). Although some individuals with eating disorders may benefit from antidepressant medications, Herzog and Sacks (1993) found that one third to two fifths of bulimia patients treated with SSRIs may not respond. Sociocultural factors may also be considered when prescribing medications for patients with eating disorders. Discrimination based on obesity has led some individuals to advocate the position that obesity requires self-acceptance, not treatment or weight loss. Individuals who are overweight can experience depression or anxiety disorders that are unrelated to their weight. These individuals may seek treatment for depression or anxiety disorders and soundly reject offers of treatment for obesity. Overviews of prescribing antidepressants and antianxiety medications are presented in Chapters 4, 5, and 6.

Unlike antidepressants or antianxiety medications, fenfluramine is a sympathomimetic drug taken 3 times a day before meals for the treatment of obesity and bulimia nervosa. This amphetamine derivative, an antiappetite medication, can produce central nervous system (CNS) depression and sedation, but it is essentially serotonergic because it increases the release of and inhibits the reuptake of serotonin (Bray, 1992). Fenfluramine can be abused for the purposes of inducing a euphoric, relaxed, giggly state of intoxication. Adverse fenfluramine effects include nightmares, psychosis, hallucinations, and insomnia. Increased appetite and libido have been reported with extremely high doses. Abrupt discontinuation of fenfluramine can produce depression, so a gradual tapering off is recommended. Without concurrent cognitive-behavioral and psychosocial treatments, weight gain or binge eating returns when the medication is withdrawn (Leitenber et al, 1993; Weintraub, 1992). Medication as a treatment of eating disorders is an important subject of debate. Practitioners will find that some individuals may request a medication such as fenfluramine as a way of starting longer term treatments or in order to feel that they are not facing their problems unarmed. It can be desirable if the medication produces positive results with minimal side effects, and these results then motivate the individual. Prescribing medication for obesity or bulimia can lead to treatment problems, however, if the patient expects the medication to do all the hard work. This thinking can be a problem, but it does not automatically imply patient resistance; just the opposite can be true. After years of living with an eating disorder, the fantasy of normal eating becomes potent. The silent wish of many patients is to wake up one day without feelings of insatiable hunger, unrelenting fear, anger, or guilt, or obsessive thoughts about food or weight. Antiappetite medications may represent that wish and thus make it easier to start long term treatment. The risks and benefits of this approach must be weighed on a case-by-case basis.

Medication may also be considered when eating-disorder behaviors are out of control but hospitalization is not yet necessary. For example, if a patient with bulimia nervosa is vomiting several times a day, or a patient with anorexia nervosa is performing hard exercise several hours a day, antidepressant or antianxiety medications may be effective in treating an acute episode of severe symptoms, thus making it possible for the patient to regain partial control. Consideration of long-term alternatives and options may be impossible until the acute episode is over. Medication should not be considered for eating behaviors that do not meet eating disorder diagnostic criteria, such as wanting to lose a few pounds or trying to avoid weight gain during the holidays or while trying to stop smoking.

☎ Consultation and Referral

A wide range of consultation problems can occur in the assessment and management of patients with eating disorders. Many potential problems can be avoided by consulting with a specialist early on. When long-term specialized care for anorexia nervosa, bulimia nervosa, obesity, or obsessive-compulsive overeating is arranged, practitioners can continue with a case-management approach, which is very helpful to patients who may be involved with several types of treatment. Patients who have eating disorders that are secondary to substance abuse or who engage in self-harm or impulsive behaviors should be referred to a specialist for immediate assessment and evaluation. The practitioner's main dilemma may be determining with whom to consult. For example, in primary care settings, specialized care for eating disorders may be provided by a number of specialists such as nutritionists, psychiatric specialists, or primary care practitioners who have specialized their practice. Services may be centralized, and one referral or many referrals may be needed. Patient-education services, such as stress management, food and nutrition planning, and weight and well-being classes, are important resources for all patients with eating disorders.

References

Abbot DW, Mitchell MD: Antidepressants vs, psychotherapy in the treatment of bulimia nervosa, *Psychopharmacology Bulletin* 29(1):115, 1993.

Agras WS, Rossiter EM, Arnow B, Telch CF, Raeburn SD, Bruce B, Korna LM: One year follow-up of psychosocial and pharmacologic treatments for bulimia nervosa, *J of Clin Psychiatry* 55(5):179, 1994.

Agras WS, Rossiter EM, Arnow B, Schneider JA, Telch CF, Raeburn SD, Bruce B, Perl M, Koran LM: Pharmacologic and cognitive-behavioral treatment for bulimia nervosa: a controlled comparison, *Am J of Psychiatry* 149:82, 1992.

Alger S, Seagle H, Ravussin E: Food intake and energy expenditure in obese female bingers and non-bingers, *Inter J of Obesity* 19(1):11, 1995.

American Psychiatric Association: Practice guidelines for eating disorders, *Am J of Psychiatry* 150(2):212, 1993.

Arnow B, Kenardy J, Agras WS: Binge eating among the obeses: a descriptive study, *J of Behavioral Med* 15(2):155, 1992.

Atkinson RL, Hubbard VS: Report on the NIH workshop on pharmacologic treatment of obesity, *Am J of Clin Nutrition* 60:153, 1994.

Bellows RT, Franke AL: A second look at obesity, *Comprehensive Therapy* 20(1):3, 1994.

Bray GA: Drug treatment of obesity, *Am J of Clin Nutrition* 55(5):538S, 1992.

Heinberg LJ: Theories of body image disturbance: perceptual, developmental and sociocultural factors: an integrative guide for assessment and treatment. In Thompson JK (editor):*Body Image, Eating Disorders, and Obesity*, Washington DC, 1996, American Psychological Association.

Herzog DB, Sacks NR, Keller MB, Lavori PW, vonRanson KB, Gray HM: Patterns and predictors of recovery in anorexia nervosa and bulimia nervosa, *J of Am Acad of Child Adoles Psychiatry* 32(4):835, 1993.

Hsu LK, Lee S: Is weight phobia always necessary for a diagnosis of anorexia nervosa?, *Am J Psychiatry* 150(10):1466, 1993.

Leitenber H, Rosen JC, Wolf, Vara, Detzer MJ, Srebnik D: Comparison of cognitive-behavior therapy and desipramine in the treatment of bulimia nervosa, *Behavioral Res and Therapy* 32(1):37, 1993.

Manson JE, VanItallie TB: America's obesity epidemic and women's health, *J of Women's Health* 5(4): 329, 1996.

Pomeroy C: Anorexia nervosa, bulimia nervosa, and binge eating disorder: assessment of physical status. In Thompson JK (editor) *Body Image, Eating Disorders, and Obesity*, Washington DC, 1996, American Psychological Association.

Ponto M: The relationship between obesity, dieting, and eating disorders, *Nutrition* 10(7):422, 1995.

Robin AL, Siegel PT, Moye A: Family versus individual therapy for anorexia: impact on family conflict, *Inter J of Eating Disorders* 17(4):313, 1995.

Rock CL, Curran-Celentanao J: Nutritional disorder of anorexia nervosa: a review, *Inter J of Eating Disorders* 15(2):187, 1994.

Rorty M, Yager J, Rossotto E: Why and how do women recover from bulimia nervosa? The subjective appraisals of forty women recovered for a year or more, *Inter J of Eating Disorders* 14(3): 249, 1993.

Solanto MV, Jacobson MS, Heller L, Golden NH, Hertz S: Rate of weight gain of inpatients with anorexia nervosa under two behavioral contracts, *Pediatrics* 93(6):989, 1994.

Weintraub M: Long term weight control: the national heart, lung, and blood institute funded multimodal intervention study, *Clin Pharmacological Therapy* 51(5):581, 1992.

Weltzin TE, Bulik CM, McConaha CW, Kaye WH: Laxative withdrawal and anxiety in bulimia nervosa, *Inter J of Eating Disorders* 17(2):141, 1995.

Yager J: Psychosocial treatments for eating disorders, *Psychiatry* 57(2):153, 1994.

Yanovski SZ, Leet M, Yanovski JA, Flood M, Gold PW, Kissileff HR, Walsh BT: Food selection and intake of obese women with binge-eating disorder, *Am J Clin Nutrition* 56(6):975, 1992.

Yen JL: General overview and treatment considerations of anorexia and bulimia, *Comprehensive Therapy* 18(1):26, 1992.

Zerbe KJ: Whose body is it anyway? Understanding and treating psychosomatic aspects of eating disorders, *Bulletin of the Menninger Clinic* 57(2):161, 1993.

Part III

Psychosocial Problems

Psychosocial Problems Related to Functioning 9

The term ***functioning*** refers to how individuals interact with and within important environments. Individuals are in constant interaction with multiple biopsychosocial environments. Within this general framework, psychosocial environments are defined by their content, process, resources, stressors, demands, and duration. Of the many psychosocial environments, academic, occupational, and social relationship environments have been found to be particularly important in terms of overall psychosocial functioning. For adults, adequate overall psychosocial functioning implies the ability to interact effectively with academic, occupational, and social relationship environments and the ability to meet personal needs for self-esteem within and across these environments.

Severe mental illness (SMI), mental disorders, severe psychosocial problems, and medical conditions can directly and negatively impact functioning in these three important psychosocial environments (Hueston et al, 1996; Sartorious et al, 1993). Negative changes in academic, occupational, or social relationship functioning may also occur as a result of SMI, a mental disorder, psychosocial problems, or poor physical health. The *Diagnostic and Statistical Manual of Mental Disorders, fourth edition* (DSM-IV), addresses functioning change as cause and effect. The Axis IV diagnosis of psychosocial problems is used to diagnosis psychosocial problems related to functioning, and the Axis V diagnosis of global assessment of functioning (GAF) is used to indicate current and previous levels of symptoms (SMI, mental disorder, medical condition) and symptom effects on functioning.

Assessment of Functioning

Individuals with SMI, mental disorder, severe psychosocial problems, or medical conditions can find it difficult to function within important academic, occupational, or social relationship environments. SMIs such as schizophrenia, personality disorder, or substance dependence can lead to a significant loss of functioning in multiple environments, but in some cases individuals are able to minimize the loss of functioning, such as the individual with alcohol dependence who continues to work. This section is a brief presentation of the five DSM-IV Axis diagnoses as they relate to individual functioning. When functioning impairments are significant—the individual is disabled and unable to function independently or effectively within academic, occupational, or social relationship environments—specialized psychosocial rehabilitation care aimed at repairing and restoring functioning is needed.

In general, DSM-IV Axis I and Axis II disorders greatly increase the risk of acute or chronic impairment of functioning in the three central psychosocial environments. Axis III general medical conditions can also significantly impair functioning. Axis IV psychosocial problems are events or experiences that differ from those that normally occur in everyday life; they greatly tax the individual's coping resources and coping skills and negatively affect functioning.

Axis I: Clinical Mental Disorders

All Axis I disorders can potentially interfere with the ability to function effectively within important academic, occupational, and social relationship environments. For some individuals with mental disorders, functioning ability is directly related to the disorder, and improvement in the disorder produces improvement in functioning. In this case improvement in functioning is essentially a result of symptom relief: the individual is better able to function when free of mental disorder symptoms. However, when the disorder is partly defined by a severe loss of functioning, such as major depression or alcohol abuse, this clear distinction between symptoms and functioning can disappear. Axis I disorders can obviously make it difficult for individuals to meet the multiple complex demands of academic and occupational environments, but they also significantly affect the individual's ability to participate in important social relationships. Partner and family relationships are particularly vulnerable to the negative impact of mental disorders. Just as individuals with disorders may require a great deal of support to cope effectively with the many distressing experiences of the disorder, those who interact with the individual may also feel distressed. In either case, the risk of significant interpersonal problems is great.

Axis II: Personality Disorders

Axis II personality disorders negatively affect nearly every aspect of the individual's interactions, including those within academic, occupational, and social relationship environments, but the negative affects on social relationship functioning can be especially dramatic. By definition, a personality disorder (which differs from personality ***traits***), is an enduring pattern of thoughts, feelings, and behaviors that deviate markedly from social expectations (APA, 1994). This enduring pattern is manifested by two or more of the following characteristics (APA, 1994):

1. Rigid cognitive patterns or ways of perceiving and interpreting oneself, others, and events
2. Unstable emotions marked by a wide range of intense mood changes or by inappropriate emotional responses
3. Maladaptive interpersonal patterns
4. Poor impulse control

The psychosocial patterns associated with Axis II personality disorders are enduring and apparent across a broad range of personal and social environments. Evidence of this pattern should be present in all areas of functioning, although not all areas of functioning may be equally affected. An individual with antisocial personality disorder may be able to work in certain settings, for example, but may have very poor social relationships regardless of the setting. The enduring patterns of personality disorders may not necessarily cause significant levels of distress, but impairment in functioning is apparent. This impairment is generally referred to as the individual's pattern of relating or characteristic way of interacting with others. These patterns are recognizable beginning in early adolescence, although actual diagnosis usually does not occur until early adulthood, when performance expectations for the individual are likely to increase sharply. Personality disorders significantly increase the risk of Axis I disorders (e.g., depression, substance abuse) and chronic psychosocial functioning problems (e.g., academic failure).

Axis III: General Medical Conditions

General medical conditions can have direct and indirect as well as acute or chronic effects on functioning. Conditions such as diabetes or asthma can interfere with academic and social relationship functioning and severely limit occupational functioning. For example, a student with insulin-dependent diabetes would have to adapt his or her course schedule to allow for regular meals and self-monitoring. An individual with asthma might be unable to work in an office building that has poor ventilation. Individuals who are able to control their work environment or who have personally defined their academic expectations may find that their medical condition does not impose significant limitations on their ability to function in these environments. However, chronic conditions that are characterized by recurrent episodes of acute symptoms or frequent hospitalization can have a cumulative negative affect on functioning. Conditions that are by nature debilitating, such as Parkinson's disease or multiple sclerosis, may have different effects on psychosocial functioning, depending on the individual's unique biopsychosocial circumstances.

Axis IV: Psychosocial and Environmental Problems

The DSM-IV provides a comprehensive list of severe psychosocial problems that negatively impact functioning. Accordingly, evidence of these psychosocial problems places the individual at increased risk for functioning impairment and subsequent disability, particularly when these problems are related to an Axis I, II, or III condition.

Problems with primary support group

A ***primary support group*** is that group of people with whom the individual interacts daily or the group of relationships that are most important to the individual. Common problems include the death of a family/group member; health problems in the family/group; disruption of the family/group by separation, divorce, or estrangement; departure of a family/group member, remarriage of a parent; sexual or physical abuse; neglect of a child or adult; parental overprotection; inadequate parental discipline; conflict between siblings; birth of a sibling.

Problems related to the social environment

Social environment refers to important social relationships or interactions with important others. Common problems include the death of a significant other or the loss of a significant relationship; inadequate social support; social isolation; acculturation problems such as prejudice, harassment, or discrimination; stage-of-life adjustments such as retirement. Social environments can also be a direct source of problems for the individual when the environment or a relationship makes demands that exceed the individual's social and coping skills. Highly demanding interpersonal relationships can be extremely stressful but are easy to overlook as a source of distress.

Educational problems

Educational problems include academic performance and peer interaction problems, as well as such problems as illiteracy, academic failure, conflict with teachers or classmates, and inadequate or stressful academic environment. Educational and academic environments can become critical sources of psychosocial problems when achievement or failure takes on tremendous importance and therefore has an excessive impact on the individual's self-esteem.

Occupational problems

Occupational problems have long been a traditional source of stressful life events and problems. In the past, those who had good jobs could take pride in themselves and their work. Now, unexpected job loss, job loss anxiety, and chronic unemployment are becoming universal occupational problems. More people feel less secure about their work and their employment and, subsequently, less satisfied with both. In addition to employment and work stress and anxiety, modern occupational problems also include highly stressful work schedules, long workdays and workweeks, difficult work conditions, unpredictable changes in work demands and employment, personal conflict with employers and co-workers, and excessively competitive work environments.

Housing problems

Housing problems are issues that impact whether the individual has a residence or shelter, as well as issues directly related to living in the residence or shelter, such as adequate space, heat, and light, pests, or neighborhood crime.

Economic problems

Economic problems are a common volatile source of severe distress, largely due to the magnitude of the consequences generally associated with money problems and personal finances. The most powerful economic problems continue to be severe and chronic poverty or financial debt. Personal financial debt has now become a common yet powerful economic problem. For example, whereas individuals were once required to show their ability to repay a loan before they could borrow money, high-interest credit card borrowing, along with the high cost of durable goods (e.g., automobiles), has made severe financial debt much more common though no less distressing.

Problems with access to health care services

Access to health care services is defined as an individual's ability to locate and obtain necessary or desired health care services. Problems in this area have typically been poor transportation, inadequate health insurance, high cost, and language or cultural barriers. With the advent of managed care, access to health care services has for many become complex for reasons other than location, cost, language, or culture. For example, few people can afford to pay for necessary psychotherapy, but most managed care organizations have strict limits on access to, type of, and utilization of psychiatric specialist services.

Problems related to crime or to interaction with the legal system

Interaction with the legal system implies that the individual is already dealing with an important or difficult problem, such as being arrested for DUI, filing a petition for a restraining order against a violent partner, or being the victim of a crime. Legal system problems also include complicated or conflicted divorce, probate, and tort litigation. Individuals who are on parole or probation may have multiple ongoing problems in their interactions with the legal system.

Other psychosocial and environmental problems

Since it is impossible to fully list even the most common Axis IV problems, the DSM-IV includes the category of ***other problems,*** such as disasters, war, and conflict with family caregivers or health care professionals, such as counselors, social workers, physicians, nurses, or social service agencies (e.g., child protection services) A "problem" is broadly defined as an interaction that the individual perceives and responds to as a problem.

Axis V: Global Assessment of Functioning

The diagnosis of global assessment of functioning (GAF) is a useful measure of current and previous academic, occupational, and social relationship functioning. The DSM-IV measures GAF on a 100-point scale, with low scores indicating low levels of functioning. When a GAF score is included, functioning becomes an important element of the mental health diagnosis. Frequent use of the GAF score enables the practitioner to closely assess functioning in a manner that makes functioning losses and gains easy to observe. A GAF score of 50 on a 100-point scale is an approximate clinical cutoff mark for serious functioning impairment; it indicates serious symptoms, serious functioning impairment, or both. GAF scores of less than 50 indicate a profound loss of functioning and the need for comprehensive assistance, whereas a score of 80 indicates transient symptoms that are expected reactions to recognized stressors, causing no more than a slight impairment in functioning.

Assessment of Problems

Individuals with problems that affect their psychosocial functioning may seek out primary health care for help in coping with a problem more effectively or solving a problem (Tiemens, Ormel, and Simon, 1996). Individuals who are treated in primary care may have severe problems that affect their school, work, or social functioning, but they may seek primary care for what they view as a legitimate concern, such as sinus pain. Physical complaints are often just that—physical complaints—and not a pretext to speak with a practitioner about an academic, occupational, or relationship problem. If any of the following observations are made during such an appointment, however, there is an increased possibility that the individual may have a severe psychosocial problem that he or she may wish to discuss with the practitioner.

- Statements of feeling powerless, negative, critical, or out of control
- Statements of feeling hopeless about the future or desired goals
- Statements that are self-demeaning or that suggest significant anger toward or disappointment with oneself
- Statements of impending doom or possible negative life events that are viewed as unavoidable
- Statements of fear and mistrust of others, of fear that others will judge the individual harshly or harm, humiliate, shame, or violate the individual
- Statements of passivity of feeling unable to mobilize energy or effectively communicate feelings or needs
- Statements that show that the individual is easily irritated or excessively bothered by events and experiences such as noise, crime rates, the demands or expectations of others, or interpersonal conflict
- Statements that show that the individual has become socially withdrawn and feels ashamed or humiliated by specific situations or people
- Morbid preoccupation with specific themes, such as physical symptoms or safe drinking water

- Evidence of inappropriate social or sexual behaviors that are not congruent with the individual's verbal statements, such as flirting with the practitioner when talking about the death of a loved one or demanding special attention from the practitioner
- Expressed disregard for social conventions or laws or excessive blaming for a range of personal events and experiences
- Evidence of impulsive or self-defeating behaviors
- Poor social or communication skills, suggesting cognitive deficits, learning disability, extreme neglect, extreme poverty, or SMI
- Lack of interest in important areas (such as school or work) or decreased concentration in these areas, feeling that life has little meaning, or low self-esteem
- Reports or evidence of sudden major changes in behavior that are uncharacteristic
- Lack of goals or interest in the future
- Difficulty with age-appropriate tasks, such as peer friendships
- Inability to provide for basic food, clothing, and shelter needs
- Absence of a meaningful or satisfying close relationship with a friend or a sexual partner

These observations can suggest that the individual is experiencing significant problems that may or may not be related to SMI, a mental disorder, or a general medical condition. Individuals vary in terms of the point at which a problem becomes distressing or in how long they will continue to try to cope with a problem before seeking professional assistance. These observations are useful as indications that the individual is becoming, or has been, overwhelmed by problems. Although such observations can be fairly reliable indicators of problems, the actual individual presentation is subject to multiple factors that may not be apparent. For example, feelings of shame and stigma associated with alcoholism or partner violence can discourage or alter disclosures of problems that might otherwise reveal the alcoholism or violence. Therefore standard assessment of the three basic areas of psychosocial functioning (occupational, academic, and social relationships) should be considered for individuals with SMI, a mental disorder, or a significant general medical condition, as well as assessment of disability or impaired functioning due to SMI or a mental disorder (American Medical Association [AMA], 1993).

Occupational

Successful occupational functioning requires social relationship skills and work skills. Severe problems related to occupational functioning are indicated by poor self-care (e.g., hygiene, nutrition), poor concentration, reduced or absent persistence, decreased ability to pace work efforts, psychosocial deterioration in work settings, and poor social relationships with co-workers and/or employers. Decreased personal independence, inappropriate behaviors, and ineffective activities at work can also occur. ***Concentration***, ***persistence***, and ***pace*** in work environments refer to the ability to complete job tasks or to focus on the performance of job tasks. Problems with getting work done may be evident in current or previous jobs. Concentration is an important element of job performance. ***Deterioration*** in work environments is evidenced by repeated failures to adapt to or cope with the multiple stressors of work environments. Individuals may withdraw from the environment (e.g., chronic absence) or, if the individual has SMI, a mental disorder, or a medical condition, his or her symptoms may increase or intensify when in a workplace environment. Deterioration is typically associated with work demands, such as on-time attendance, decision making, schedule management, meeting task deadlines, and stressful interactions with persons in authority and co-workers (McGovern and Cossi, 1996).

Academic

Academic problems are usually gauged in terms of successful learning and significant peer relationships, based on consistent attendance and sufficient grasp of the material to allow the individual to fulfill class requirements. Academic peer relationships should be substantial, including significant interaction with peers and efforts aimed to become a member of a peer group. Social skills are important for the individual's ability to develop, maintain, and contribute to peer relationships, to meet the demands of academic authorities such as professors, and to meet performance expectations such as graduation criteria. Truancy, aggressive or disruptive behaviors, and apathy are common academic functioning problems. Academic functioning is a major area of concern for school-age children and adolescents. Many public schools are now staffed with professionals, such as psychologists, school nurses, and social workers, who try to identify children and adolescents who are at risk and arrange for appropriate diagnostic testing and (when necessary) appropriate therapy.

Social Relationships

This area of assessment has to do with the individual's capacity to interact effectively with others. Of particular concern is the individual's ability to communicate with others (Hagerty, et al, 1996). Social relationship functioning is a very broad area of assessment, but a general focus is placed on the individual's ability to get along with a range of people, such as family members, friends, neighbors, grocery clerks, landlords, and bus drivers. Problems related to social relationship functioning may be indicated by a history of interpersonal conflict or altercations, housing evictions, lost employment, fear of strangers, avoidance of close relationships, social isolation, and problems conforming to social and cultural norms. Effective social relationship functioning is indicated by the ability to initiate and participate in interactions with others effectively. Cooperation, reciprocity, the ability to show consideration for others, awareness of others, and social maturity are all evidence of effective social relationship functioning.

Disability

Physical or mental disability requires a great deal of adjustment, new skills, and determined coping. The years immediately following the onset of a disability are typically devoted to developing these psychosocial resources and to making important changes in various environments (e.g., physical, social) to accommodate maximum levels of functioning within the limits imposed by the disability. Individuals who are most likely to be able to make these enormous transitions are those who are by nature extremely resourceful, strong, self-reliant, knowledgeable and willing to make the many necessary changes to build a worthwhile lifestyle. Just about any loss of mental or physical functioning produces serious changes in one's self-concept and self-esteem and can decrease access to environments that might otherwise provide satisfying and rewarding experiences (Trieschmann, 1993).

Individuals with disabilities must be willing to accept personal responsibility for their lives, (***not*** their disabilities) and their daily needs as a way to continue to feel that their lives belong to them. For an individual with a disability, frustration is a constant problem, as are decreased levels of emotional and physical energy. Thoughts of suicide as an escape from disability are extremely common, particularly when day-to-day survival seems to require a great deal of energy and time with little satisfaction. Being able to develop and maintain the personal will to live becomes one of the most important indicators of psychosocial functioning with a disability. Some individuals with a long history of disability may have a highly assertive style of communicating with others, including practitioners, that is characterized by demands for full honesty and total rejection of insincere concern. There are some individuals who may become self-absorbed and develop an angry style of relating to others. Depression, as a secondary reaction to the multiple losses generated by disability, is also common.

The findings of a descriptive study of 56 disabled adults (Miller, 1993) indicate that individuals with disabilities tend to cope with problems in their lives by using either a direct approach or by trying to avoid problems. The direct approach requires that the individual confront problems and social expectations, whereas avoidance is just the opposite. According to the researchers, the direct approach to coping with problems actually requires numerous high-level coping skills, such as information seeking, spiritual faith, and the ability to distract one's attention in order to relax, express strong emotions, retain control of important areas of one's life, continue to set life goals and strive to achieve them, and take comfort in the company of others. Avoidant coping, on the other hand, is to evade dealing with the problem although it may still be a significant topic of conversation. Individuals use denial to minimize experiences, problems, and personal needs: to engage in social isolation, avoid talking about strong feelings, or maintain a fatalistic view of the future;

or to escape into sleep, drugs, alcohol, or television. Blaming others for problems and unmet needs, setting unrealistic goals, or manipulating others are also forms of avoidant coping.

Management of Psychosocial Problems Related to Functioning

➤ Counseling

There are several counseling approaches that can be used to assist an individual with psychosocial problems related to functioning or with impaired functioning due to SMI, a mental disorder, a medical condition, or a disability. The basic goals are to preserve current areas of effective functioning and to repair, restore, or replace damaged or lost functioning skills. Specialized psychosocial rehabilitation care will be needed when a significant loss of functioning occurs in relation to SMI, major depression, or substance dependence; in less severe cases, psychiatric primary care counseling can be extremely important to help individuals prevent or avoid loss of functioning and to effectively cope with occupational, academic, and social relationship problems. Regardless of the type or focus of counseling, the first and foremost concern must always be the individual's self-esteem (Evans, 1993). It is difficult, if not impossible, to engage in effective problem solving or to interact effectively with important school, work, and relationship environments with low self-esteem. At the same time, supportive psychosocial environments (academic, occupational, social) can be a critical source of support for high self-esteem.

People tend to measure their worth to themselves and to others according to their ability to achieve preset expectations, such as a course grade, job promotion, or marriage. Unrealistic expectations or psychosocial environments that undermine rather than support the individual's self-esteem can also have a significant negative impact on the individual's ability to function within those environments. Practitioners have much to offer in helping individuals to understand the importance of maintaining adequate levels of self-esteem as a starting point for addressing important psychosocial problems. Individuals who suffer from low self-esteem may be unable and unwilling to engage in meaningful problem solving.

Self-esteem is a critical ingredient in the process of recognizing personal strengths and skills and developing and implementing positive behaviors and effective problem solving. Psychiatric primary care counseling interventions aimed at supporting the individual's self-esteem are important and necessary. Individuals who make excessive self-derogatory comments or statements of feeling insignificant, worthless, or useless indicate a significant need for interventions that can help them to repair and restore their self-esteem (Ryan, 1993). Individuals who anticipate or have had a recent role loss or the experience of poor role performance at school, work, or in important relationships often express feelings of low self-esteem.

Psychiatric primary care interventions that target self-esteem help the individual to construct a positive view of oneself that is realistic, strong, resilient, and flexible and thus better able to sustain the individual's problem-solving efforts. To be ***realistic***, self-esteem must be based on the individual's acceptance and valuing of his or her actual characteristics. To be ***strong***, self-esteem must be based on many, rather than one or two, personal characteristics. To be ***resilient*** and ***flexible*** means that the individual's feelings of self-worth may decrease under certain circumstances (e.g., a poor exam grade), but the individual does not allow these feelings to persist or to carry over into other situations.

Practitioners can take an active role in identifying individuals who may be at risk for self-esteem losses or problems in work, school, or relationships and can intervene to help the individuals decrease their risks. This often means helping individuals to deal effectively with small problems rather than putting them off until they become large problems in the future. Family and community resources and support should be identified and utilized. Classes in such topics as positive social communication skills can be informative and self-validating. Practitioners should try to identify the major sources of low self-esteem that can be addressed, such as negative thoughts and feelings about oneself or criticism, verbal abuse, and rejection of significant others. Family counseling may be preferred by some individuals when a mental or medical diagnosis is the main source of decreased self-esteem and functioning problems. Family counseling allows practitioners to obtain current GAF information and to observe the family's coping style, problem solving skills, and tolerance for change.

Couples counseling, like family counseling, can make it possible to address an important social relationship as a potential problem that can be improved with specialized therapy. The couple relationship is one of the most powerful sources of positive and negative experiences that directly affects self-esteem and functioning, particularly occupational and academic functioning. Any type of confiding relationship can be an important source of self-esteem (Brown and Harris, 1978). Group experiences (e.g., self-help, support, therapy) are excellent resources for addressing problems related to self-esteem and functioning. A cohesive group can provide a psychosocial environment that allows the individual to work through various psychosocial problems with the active support of others. According to Yalom (1985), groups offer a wide range of therapeutic factors, include building hope, universality or the experience of not feeling alone in distress, emotional expression and relief, giving and receiving helpful information, a positive experience of altruism, and other positive interpersonal experiences.

References

American Medical Association: *Guide to the evaluation of permanent impairment 4th Edition*, Chicago, 1993, American Medical Association.

Brown GW, Harris T: *The social origins of depression*, 1978, London, Tavistock.

Evans IM: Constructional perspectives in clinical assessment, *Psychological Assessments* 5(3):264, 1993.

Hagerty BM, Williams RA, Coyne JC, Early MR: Sense of belonging and indicators of social and psychological functioning, *Archives of Psychiatric Nursing* X(4):235, 1996.

Hueston WJ, Mainous I, Arch G, Schilling R: Patients with personality disorders: functional status, health care utilization, and satisfaction with care, *J of Fam Practice* 42:1, 1996.

McGovern PM, Cossi DA: Work and family: policy and program options affecting occupational health, *Am Assoc Occupational Health Nurses* 44(8):408, 1996.

Miller JF:*Coping with chronic illness,* 2nd Edition, Philadelphia, 1993, F.A. Davis Company.

Ryan P: Facilitating behavior change in the chronically ill. In Miller JF (editor): *Coping with chronic illness,* 2nd Edition, Philadelphia, 1993, F.A. Davis Company.

Sartorious N, de Girolamo G, Andrews G, German G, Allen G, Eisenberg L, (editors): *Treatment of mental disorders*, Washington DC, 1993, American Psychiatric Press.

Tiemens BG, Ormel J, Simon GE: Occurrence, recognition, and outcome of psychological disorders in primary care, *Am J Psychiatry* 153(5):636, 1996.

Trieschmann RB: *Aging with a disability*, New York, 1993, Demos Publications.

Yalom I: *The theory and practice of group psychotherapy,* 3rd Edition, New York, 1985, Basic Books.

Psychosocial Problems Related to Sexuality 10

Sexuality is defined here as the physical, emotional, and social drive for self-discovery, attachment, expression, self-esteem, social identity, and personal identity (Levine, 1995). Sexuality is fundamental to life and affects all areas of psychosocial functioning; thus it is an ever-present, potential source of psychosocial problems. For centuries, sexuality has been—and most likely it will continue to be—the focus of uncompromising public debate between advocates of moral, social, cultural, scientific, legal, political, or religious standards of sexuality. Although the concept of "standardized" sexuality is interesting, from reproduction to orientation, sexuality is personal. What should sexuality mean and what should it mean to be sexual? Individuals, couples, families, and communities will continue to struggle with both questions. Given that sexuality-related problems are highly distressing to the individuals involved, practitioners can expect to be viewed as an important source of information, expertise, and support. This chapter reviews sexual dysfunction, the process of "coming out" as a homosexual man or a lesbian woman, distress related to infertility, poststerilization regret, and distress related to receiving a diagnosis of a sexually transmitted disease (STD).

➲ Who Is at Risk

Psychosocial problems related to sexuality are defined here as secondary, psychological (e.g., depressed mood) or social (e.g., relationship conflict) problems that affect the individual's identity and behavior. Given the possible range of psychosocial problems, it is impossible to identify specific risk factors. Therefore for the purposes of this discussion, individuals who are sexually active (i.e., who experience sexual desire and arousal or who participate in sexual activity) can be considered to be at risk for sexuality-related psychosocial problems.

Although specific risk factors cannot be defined, important social changes regarding sexuality and sexual behavior, identity, and relationships have occurred, and these changes can impact individual risk for psychosocial problems. In 1974 the risk of psychosocial problems related to sexual identity was reduced for many people when the American Psychiatric Association removed homosexuality and lesbianism from its list of mental disorders. Second, until the late 1960s, socially acceptable sexuality was defined as heterosexual marriage and children. By the 1990s, sex was no longer synonymous with marriage and children, the average age for first sexual contact for females had dropped to the early teens, and adult males and females were reporting significantly higher numbers of sexual partners (Turner, Danella, and Rogers, 1995). Younger age, more partners and fewer marriages indicate that more people are sexually active and more likely to be involved in short-term sexual relationships.

Third, there has been a sharp increase in the incidence and prevalence of viral STDs across all population groups. Instead of the short-term, acute psychosocial problems (e.g., relationship conflict) associated with bacterial STDs before effective treatment became available, the psychosocial problems associated with viral STDs tend to be chronic (e.g., social isolation) (Keller, Egan, and Mims, 1995). Fourth, despite the fact that the incidence of infertility has been stable for decades, advances in fertility and conception research, as well as improved diagnosis of and health care options for reproductive problems, seems to have increased rather than decreased the identity anxiety among those who wish to have children but cannot (Meyers et al, 1995). Finally, many of the social changes that have occurred over the last few decades impact individual sexuality and thus the risk of related psychosocial problems. The most powerful social changes include the return to the stress of long workdays and workweeks, increased social isolation, and renewed depersonalization of sexuality.

❑ Common Assessment Problems

For many reasons, sex can be a difficult topic of conversation for sex partners, let alone patients and practitioners. Since the 1960s, people have become more accustomed to superficial conversations about sex, but many people are still uncomfortable discussing their personal sexuality. Personal sexuality continues to be a source of intense feelings of vulnerability and conflicting biopsychosocial needs versus wants. Nevertheless, sexuality assessment can be accomplished effectively and need not be traumatic to the patient or the practitioner. The most common assessment problems experienced by patients are disclosure anxiety, privacy concerns, and fears of interpersonal rejection.

Not knowing what to say or how to express oneself is a common assessment problem for patients, regardless of the nature of the assessment. Practitioners can make the assessment of sexuality significantly easier for patients by starting with a clearly worded introduction, stating the purpose or goal of the assessment, the expected benefits of the assessment for the patient, and the topics that will be covered. An equally valuable benefit of starting a sexuality assessment with a brief introduction is that the patient has the opportunity to preview the practitioner's interpersonal style and to observe the practitioner's comfort level. A well-stated introduction conveys the message that the practitioner is prepared to be helpful. Rather than trying to anticipate practitioner reactions and viewpoints, the patient can focus on collecting his or her thoughts about personal sexual information. Regardless of the patient's age or gender or the nature of the health care visit, practitioners can be very helpful by taking the initiative and encouraging patients to disclose at a pace and level of detail that is comfortable for them. Letting patients know that their comfort is important can decrease their anxiety.

There are individuals who will not feel comfortable no matter what the practitioner does. Practitioners may also encounter exhibitionists who seem to take pleasure in disclosing sexual information or who compulsively disclose such information. When a simple answer is expected, the exhibitionist may insist on giving lurid details. In this case it may be best to respond by interrupting and starting again with a specific question (e.g., "How old were you when you had your first sexual experience with a partner?") rather than an open-ended question (e.g., "Tell me about your first sexual experience."). In the absence of such problems, disclosure anxiety may also be decreased by asking the individual how he or she would like to proceed with the assessment.

Privacy becomes an assessment problem when the individual is concerned that the assessment may be overheard, recorded, or reported. In most cases privacy also has to do with the intimate nature of sexual thoughts, feelings, and behaviors. Sexuality assessment requires the disclosure of highly personal information, including intimate details about significant others. By informing patients in advance of policies (e.g., notification of sexual contacts) or practices that will affect the confidentiality of the assessment, serious problems (e.g., misleading information) may be avoided. A less obvious issue of privacy is the fundamental reluctance to say more than what is necessary. Trying to figure out in advance exactly what information is necessary can itself be a significant assessment problem. Practitioners routinely end up with more assessment information than they can sort through. Both practitioners and patients have an interest in staying within certain bounds during the assessment, but it can be difficult to know where the boundary lines are or how to proceed without crossing them. One approach to this problem is to clearly state what information is and is not necessary. Clearly stated boundaries are not guarantees against assessment problems. Patients may still mislead, withhold important information, or present unnecessary details, but clearly defined boundaries can be useful in helping the individual to view the assessment as beneficial.

Fears of interpersonal rejection are often the product of not knowing what to expect from the practitioner. Today more people of all ages have a great deal of generic sex information, but sexuality assessment includes more than sex. A comprehensive sexuality assessment reveals a great deal about the individual's self-concept, self-esteem, body image, and self-ideal. Fear of interpersonal rejection can be related to psychological as well as sexuality disclosure. Anticipation of the pain of interpersonal rejection can be a significant assessment problem. Practitioners should respond to individuals who feel personally threatened by affirming that their dignity as human beings will be respected. Should practitioners be held to this standard when individuals disclose sexual thoughts, feelings, and behaviors that are not criminal or symptomatic but are professionally or personally unacceptable to the practitioner? The answer is yes. People are more than their sexuality, and professionals should be able to acknowledge this fact and interact with the individual without undermining his or her self-concept and self-esteem.

The following sexual history and sexual functioning assessments developed by Risen (1995) cover a wide range of sexual concerns and problems. Both assessments are fairly lengthy and could require 30 to 60 minutes to complete. In most cases the entire assessment is not necessary. By selecting relevant assessment items, it is possible to customize a sexuality assessment that will be useful and effective. Practitioners who have strong beliefs about sexuality, who become remote or distant when discussing sexuality, or who have difficulty setting boundaries should consider consultation and referral.

Sexual History Assessment

1. Family relationships (adults, parents, relatives)
2. Childhood development (e.g., sex education from parents)
3. Learned male and female roles
4. Affection displayed in the home while growing up
5. Religious norms and regulations for sex
6. Age at which one first started to have sexual feelings
7. Age at which one first started to masturbate (and feelings about this experience)
8. Childhood sexual contacts (children and adults)
9. Age at onset of puberty
10. Adolescent attractions and sexual contacts
11. First sexual experience (age, partner, behavior, effects)
12. Sexual behaviors that make one uncomfortable
13. Significant adult sexual relationships
14. Meaning of sexuality to the individual
15. Sexual problems or relationship problems
16. History of STDs
17. Safer sex practices

Sexual Functioning Assessment

1. Current sexual activity (male and/or female partners)
2. Current sexual problems
3. Troubling aspects of gender or sexual identity
4. Sexual attraction and orientation
5. Troubling sexual behavior
6. Types of sexual behavior engaged in
7. Problems related to sexual desire, arousal, orgasm
8. Duration of problem and uniqueness to a setting and/or a person
9. Recent major additions, losses, or changes in life, health, and well-being
10. Feelings related to sexual problems (e.g., guilt, anxiety, depression)

Sexuality-Related Psychosocial Problems

This section is a brief overview of sexual dysfunction, coming out, infertility, poststerilization regret, and STD diagnosis. A basic description of each is presented, and related short-term and long-term psychosocial problems are identified.

Sexual Dysfunction

Sexual dysfunctions are disorders of sexual desire, arousal, or pleasure. The most common sexual desire dysfunctions are absent, low, or hypersexual desire; sexual aversion; and sexual incompatibility. Disorders of arousal are indicated by emotional and/or physical inability to achieve or maintain a state of sexual arousal. Sexual pleasure disorders refer to the absence of, or inability to achieve or experience, sexual satisfaction. The *Diagnostic and Statistical Manual of Mental Disorders, fourth edition,* (DSM-IV) defines specific sexual disorders and subtypes of sexual disorders according to symptom onset, context, and etiology. ***Onset*** is defined as lifelong, (present since the onset of sexual functioning) or acquired (beginning after a period of normal functioning). ***Context*** is defined as generalized (not limited to a specific type of sexual stimulation, situation, or partner) or situational (occurs only with specific types of stimulation, situations, or partners). Etiology is defined as psychological when psychological factors alone are the cause of the dysfunction, and physical and substance-related causes have been ruled out. When it is not psychological, etiology is defined as (1) combined factors (psychological and physical), (2) due to a general medical condition (e.g., diabetes), or (3) substance-induced. DSM-IV sexual dysfunction disorders are defined by the predominant symptom and by a marked distress or interpersonal difficulty (psychosocial problem) that is not better accounted for by another DSM-IV disorder.

DSM -IV Sexual Dysfunction Disorder	Predominant Symptom
1. Hypoactive sexual desire	Persistently or recurrently deficient or absent sexual fantasies or desire for sexual activity
2. Sexual aversion	Persistent or recurrent extreme aversion to, and avoidance of all or almost all genital sexual contact, with a sexual partner
3. Female sexual arousal disorder	Persistent or recurrent inability to attain, or maintain until completion of the sexual activity, an adequate lubrication-swelling response to sexual excitement
4. Male erectile disorder	Persistent or recurrent inability to attain, or maintain until completion of the sexual activity, an adequate erection
5. Female orgasmic disorder	Persistent or recurrent delay in or absence of orgasm following a normal sexual excitement phase
6. Male orgasmic disorder	Persistent or recurrent delay in or absence of orgasm following a normal sexual excitement phase

7. Premature ejaculation	Persistent or recurrent ejaculation with minimal sexual stimulation before, on, or shortly after penetration and before the person wishes it
8. Dyspareunia	Recurrent or persistent genital pain associated with sexual intercourse in either a male or a female
9. Vaginismus	Recurrent or persistent involuntary spasm of the musculature of the outer third of the vagina that interferes with sexual intercourse

Medications with Sexual Dysfunction Side Effects

Antianxiety
Antidepressants
Antiemetics
Antifungal drugs
Antihypertensives
Appetite suppressants
Cholesterol-lowering drugs
Gastrointestinal drugs
Hormone agents
Muscle relaxants

Common Sexual Dysfunction Medication Side Effects

Breast swelling in men
Ejaculation inhibition
Impotence
Loss of desire
Lower sperm count
Testicular swelling

Psychosocial problems related to sexual dysfunction

Dysfunctions of sexual desire, arousal, and pleasure, regardless of etiology, can be associated with a number of cognitive, psychological, social, behavioral, developmental, or interpersonal factors. The prevailing cultural assumption is that adults will experience sexual desire and sexual arousal and that their desire and arousal will not deviate from defined norms. Sexual desire dysfunction (absent, low, hyperactive, incompatibility, or aversion) can cause significant psychosocial problems for individuals and their partners. The prevalence rate for ***low sexual desire*** among adult males and females is about 20% (Rosen and Leiblum, 1995). The prevalence rate for ***hypersexual desire***, also referred to as sexual addiction or compulsive sexual behavior, tends to be greater due to the wider range of behavior criteria. Hypersexual desire is classified as either nonparaphiliac or paraphiliac. ***Nonparaphiliac hypersexual desire***, such as promiscuity or prostitution, is similar to other compulsive behaviors that follow a pattern of increased anxiety that is relieved by the performance of specific behaviors, which then leads to a negative mood (Travin, 1995). ***Paraphiliac hypersexual desire*** also follows compulsive behavior patterns but includes sexual behaviors that meet DSM-IV criteria for a paraphilia diagnosis, such as pedophilia. Psychosocial problems related to nonparaphiliac sexual desire and sexual arousal disorders (i.e., female sexual arousal disorder and male erectile disorder) include intimacy intolerance, chronic feelings of guilt, chronic stress and anxiety, relationship conflict, low self-esteem, negative self-concept, and negative body image.

Sexual pleasure dysfunctions (i.e., orgasmic disorder, premature ejaculation, dyspareunia, and vaginismus) are among the least-reported sexual dysfunction disorders. The experience of sexual pleasure can be decreased by any number of psychosocial factors, including time and place of sexual activity, personal definition of sexual pleasure, how sex is initiated, personal goals and needs related to sex, and fears of being out of control. In the absence of physical or substance-related explanations for desire, arousal, or pleasure dysfunction, the dysfunction is attributed to psychological causes, and it can then be difficult to discern between psychological etiology and related psychosocial problems. Take, for example, the highly self-limiting stereotype of male sexual pleasure as effortless desire, erection, penetration, and orgasm. When this stereotype is the foundation of a male's self-concept and self-esteem, it can become a psychological cause of sexual dysfunction and a source of psychological distress (e.g., anxiety) and psychosocial problems (e.g., relationship conflict).

The overlap of a psychological etiology for sexual dysfunction with psychosocial problems also occurs with the individual's anticipation of sexual pleasure as a psychological component of sexual desire and sexual arousal. Desire and arousal may be diminished when little or no pleasure is anticipated. For example, a self-limiting female stereotype of sexual pleasure has been based on emotional and social criteria without physical criteria. Problematic sexual beliefs can be a psychological basis for sexual dysfunction or a psychosocial problem related to sexual dysfunction. When sex is thought of as an obligation, a privilege, a scored performance, a sleep aid, a measure of personal power, or a method of interpersonal control, this can lead to sexual dysfunction or related psychosocial problems. Individuals who are in a sexual relationship for reasons that interfere with satisfying, consensual sex (e.g., convenience, convention, social status) may also be more vulnerable to problems (Rosen and Leiblum, 1995).

Individuals vary in their beliefs about true indicators of sexuality-related problems. For example, personal definitions of sexual desire typically include sexual thoughts and fantasies, awareness of sexual cues from others, or frustration by a lack of sexual activity (Schiavi and Segraves, 1995). The individual who believes that he or she should have daily sexual thoughts but does not might become distressed. Short-term negative changes in sexual functioning often precede, follow, or occur with acute stress or day-to-day strains. An individual who is under significant work-related stress might experience decreased sexual desire, arousal, or pleasure, but in a stress-free situation (e.g., vacation) may experience full sexual functioning. Because of the psychological complexity of sexuality it is recommended that practitioners initially focus on the two most common psychosocial problems related to sexual dysfunction: loss of self-esteem and relationship conflict.

Coming Out and Related Psychosocial Problems

Coming out is a term used to describe the process of adopting a personal and social identity as a homosexual man or a lesbian

(Eliason, 1996; Mattison and McWhirter, 1995). In terms of sexuality-related psychosocial problems, the process of coming out, rather than homosexuality or lesbianism itself, is the focus of concern. Socially, to come out as a gay man or a lesbian means that the individual must come to terms with the majority social status of heterosexuality and the minority status of male homosexuality and lesbianism. This includes redefining what norms of sexuality are personally acceptable and unacceptable. Coming out also requires developing a homosexual or lesbian sense of self (self-concept, self-esteem, body image, self-ideal) that is personally acceptable.

The process of coming out can take a few moments or last a lifetime. Coming out to oneself is usually a one-time occurrence, but coming out to others can be ongoing, since there will always be new people or new situations that necessitate disclosure. Whom individuals come out to also varies: some come out to close friends only or friends and family only. To many, it is important to come out in both their private and public lives, including to their health care practitioners. The process of coming out may include a long-term internal struggle with childhood and religious teachings against homosexuality and lesbianism as well as with negative stereotypes. Regardless of the individual's ethnicity, age, gender, education, or income, coming out automatically defines one as a minority and therefore makes one subject to prejudice and discrimination. Discrimination against gay men and lesbians occurs in employment and housing, and harassment and violence are also common.

Gay and lesbian communities endorse widely divergent opinions about coming out. Some communities have taken the position that the best way to end prejudice and discrimination is for all gay men and lesbians to publicly declare their sexual orientation. A recent trend in some communities is to "out" individuals who the community has decided should publicize their sexual orientation. Once individuals start the process of coming out, invariably they and their significant others speculate about the development of an individual's homosexual or lesbian orientation. This question represents one of many social debates about sexuality: is sexual orientation freely chosen or biologically determined? For many the answer to this question is not particularly important, but some individuals feel that their sexual orientation has greater legitimacy if they have early-childhood self-awareness. Coming out may also mean that, after years of unhappy relationships and psychosocial problems, an individual becomes better able to build a stable relationship with an appropriate partner.

As presented here, coming out is more than the personal and public statement of sexual orientation. How well the individual copes with this complex process depends in large part on his or her age and circumstances and whether coming out was voluntary. The experience of coming out for an adolescent minority female will differ significantly from the experience of a middle-age majority male. Similarly, someone who is married with small children or who is alone in a rural community will have a different coming out experience than a college student who joins a gay and lesbian student organization. Prior to the mid-1970s, severe psychosocial problems among homosexual men and lesbians were not uncommon. Advocates attributed these psychosocial problems to the stressful experience of being "in the closet." Prior to the gay and lesbian civil rights movement, homosexual men and lesbians kept their sexual orientation private. Under these conditions, advocates believe that it was all too easy for individuals to begin to believe that no one else was like them and there was therefore something wrong with them. Depression, suicide attempts, and substance abuse were common. Political, social, legal, and religious debates about homosexuality and lesbianism continue, but for many individuals the psychological benefits of coming out of the closet exceed the psychological cost of remaining hidden from social view. For example, domestic partner laws make it possible for homosexual and lesbian couples to provide for each other and their families. These stable relationships and homes are significant sources of psychological well-being that in turn can significantly decrease the risk of mental disorders such as depression, and psychosocial problems, such as relationship conflict.

The process of coming out is complex, but in some cases it can be uneventful. Depending on the nature of the parent-child relationship prior to learning of a son or daughter's homosexuality or lesbianism, the most common problem associated with coming out is often a harsh negative reaction from parents. The most serious psychosocial problems are discrimination and violence. Practitioners should avoid making assumptions about sexual orientation, keeping in mind that sexual dysfunctions and related psychosocial problems occur independent of sexual orientation. When coming out is a primary source of interpersonal conflict, anxiety, or stress, specialized care may be indicated. Individuals with strong and persistent cross-gender identification and persistent discomfort with being male or female by birth should be referred to a specialist.

Infertility and Related Psychosocial Problems

Reported prevalence rates for infertility range from 1 in 6 to 1 in 12 U.S. couples (Meyers et al, 1995; Jirka, Schuett, and Foxall, 1996). According to Meyers et al, about 80% of these couples will be able to conceive within 5 years. Infertility has been subtyped as a primary or secondary condition. A diagnosis of ***primary infertility*** is used if a couple has not had a child, and ***secondary infertility*** is used if the couple has one child but has not been able to have a second child (Jones and Toner, 1993). Common causes of primary infertility are (1) multiple causes, (2) endometriosis, (3) semen factor, and (4) unexplained infertility (Jones and Toner, 1993). Fertility and infertility are significantly related to age and life-style. The peak age of fertility for women is about 22, after which fertility decreases quickly; the fertility rate for women in their early 40s is about 30% (Meyers et al, 1995). Other factors that affect fertility rates are the incidence and prevalence of STDs and the trend among married couples to wait a number of years before having children (Trantham, 1996). Publicity surrounding the introduction of fertility clinics as a routine part of health care has created the impression that infertility rates have increased greatly, but the percentage of infertile couples has actually remained stable for the last 25 years (Meyers et al, 1995).

Most people assume that they will be able to have children when they decide to do so. Infertility is a shock, a disappointment, and, to some, a serious threat to self-esteem. A diagnosis of infertility can suddenly bring into conscious awareness the buried longing for children and the experience of parenthood, thus precipitating a psychological crisis. When a diagnosis of infertility is a crisis for an individual or a couple, the usual phases of crisis occur: disbelief, denial, anger, and acceptance. Acceptance can be more difficult for couples who do not have a specific explanation for their infertility. Unresolved crisis related to infertility increases the risk of severe psychosocial problems, including relationship conflict. Men and women attach different personal and social meanings to having children, but it would be of little value to define a "typical" male or female reaction to infertility, since few people would fit such a general description. All that can be said is that males and females differ in their reactions to infertility, and for some couples this difference can become a source of severe relationship conflict (Boxer, 1996). For example, a woman may react with feelings of self-blame, but her male partner may react by withdrawing and isolating himself. Both reactions indicate psychological distress, but the profound difference between them can become a source of conflict that is sufficient to threaten the couple's relationship. Women more than men may avoid social activities that include children or friends with children, despite the fact that such behavior causes them to feel lonely and isolated (Jirka, Schuett, and Foxall, 1996). Golombok (1992) defines the following high-risk profile for extreme psychological distress related to a diagnosis of infertility: a young woman who identifies with a religion that emphasizes childbirth and child rearing, whose husband is not a confidant for her, who is trying to cope with other difficult problems in her life, and who does not have a specific infertility diagnosis.

Experts note that however severe the couple's psychosocial problems may be initially, their reaction should modify over time (Sandelowski, 1994). Psychological problems that continue unrelieved or that become more severe, with increasing loss of functioning, may indicate the onset of a disorder (e.g., acute stress disorder, major depression, obsessive-compulsive disorder, alcohol abuse). If the couple already has one child, practitioners should be alert for maladaptive changes in attitude or behavior toward that child. If there appears to be severe tension between the partners, or one or both of them abuses alcohol, practitioners should assess the risk of domestic violence. In the absence of these severe problems, most couples are able to move beyond their infertility diagnosis to focus on deciding their next step. Whatever the couple's choice, ideally it will not interfere with the process of bereavement that helps them deal with the many losses that infertility represents for them.

Practitioners offer important expertise in helping couples to pursue the choices that are right for them. Couples may choose to accept the fact that they cannot have children and make different plans for their life together, or they may find alternative ways to be parents, such as through adoption or foster parenting. Couples who choose to adopt or foster-parent may still experience stress as they make the transition to adopt life goals that they may not have previously considered. At the opposite extreme are couples who choose assisted conception and channel all of their energy and resources into trying to have a child. Fertility clinics offer some hope, but practitioners should be well informed of a clinic's methods, reliability, and safety before referring a couple (Copperman et al, 1996). Most fertility clinics use a formula to calculate a couple's "statistical" chances for conception. Without using a formula, the pregnancy rate for in vitro fertilization and donor-surrogacy for women under 40 years old is 15% to 20% (Meyers et al, 1995). Regardless of the couple's decision following a diagnosis of infertility, psychiatric primary care can help the couple to cope with the distress and psychosocial problems related to infertility.

Poststerilization Regret and Related Psychosocial Problems

Tubal ligation and vasectomy are increasing popular methods of birth control. People choose them because of circumstances or because of a certainty that they do not wish to have children. If an individual's circumstances change, or the certainty about not having children diminishes, he or she may experience regret. This regret may be experienced as feelings of guilt, remorse, or despair, or, because the procedure is available, regret may also take the form of surgery to attempt to reestablish fertility. Chi & Jones (1994) have identified age, marital status, and undue influence of others as common reasons for a reversal-surgery request. Age and parity at the time of tubal ligation or vasectomy are important factors in regret: the younger the age, or the younger the age at the birth of the first child, the greater the probability for regret. Marital status can become a factor if, after divorce and remarriage, the person's new partner wishes to have children. If tubal ligation or vasectomy was done under pressure from a partner or family members, the probability of regret is also increased. Finally, the death of a child can cause parents to seek reversal surgery.

Poststerilization regret is less likely to occur when the individual has enough time between the decision and the procedure to fully consider the many short-term and long-term effects, but preparation and time are not guarantees against regret. Regret can develop as a totally unexpected reaction in individuals who were originally confident of their decision. There are also people who are uncomfortable with making a decision of this magnitude and are therefore unlikely to feel sure of any decision. More often, however, regret occurs due to unexpected changes in circumstances. Regret with or without reversal may take the form of numerous psychosocial problems. The more obvious ones are anxiety and depression, in which case the individual may be confident that the decision to have a tubal ligation or a vasectomy was wrong. Regret can also be expressed as extreme ambivalence or uncertainty, in which case the individual is unhappy but unable to make a decision about reversal surgery. In the absence of clearly stated reasons for regret and reversal, the individual should have the opportunity to work with a psychiatric specialist and sort through the original decision and the subsequent feelings.

STDs and Related Psychosocial Problems

Individual reactions to an STD diagnosis are influenced by a variety of factors, including the type of STD diagnosed (bacterial or viral), the sexual contact believed to have caused the infection, and the individual's defense style and coping skills (Biro and Rosenthal, 1992). Viral STDs have a chronic or recurrent course that makes adaptation extremely difficult (Quinn, Zenilman, and Rompalo, 1994). For example, with the genital herpes virus, the individual may feel fine when the virus is dormant, highly distressed during recurrent outbreaks, and chronically distressed by the anticipation of unpredictable outbreaks. Regardless of the outbreak pattern, because of asymptomatic viral shedding, individuals with this diagnosis must consistently take precautions to prevent transmission. The initial psychosocial impact of receiving a diagnosis of the genital herpes virus may be relived with each outbreak or each time a new partner must be informed.

Newly diagnosed individuals may become preoccupied with the sexual contact that exposed them to the STD. They may ruminate about how they would behave differently if they had the chance, and they may have strong feelings of victimization. Those who are uncertain about how they were exposed may be troubled by this lack of information. However, full knowledge may not lead to decreased stress or improved coping. Regret, guilt, and anger related to an STD diagnosis can become increasingly difficult to cope with when the individual is convinced that he or she alone could have prevented the exposure. An STD diagnosis can tax the most mature defense style and the most effective coping skills. Those with less-developed psychological foundations can become vulnerable to feelings of self-hate and rage and may find it difficult to function in daily life.

Although there is no standard course, there are phases of coping and adjustment that newly diagnosed individuals may experience. The individual may become concerned with the possibility of an STD diagnosis, and this anxiety may lead him or her to seek testing (Godin et al, 1993). An STD diagnosis can also be an unexpected finding of routine health care or screening. Concern and anxiety about the possibility of an STD diagnosis may also lead to a delay in seeking health care or, in rare cases, rage and deliberately exposing others to the STD. Because an STD diagnosis represents a crisis and a serious threat to self-concept and self-esteem, individuals may try to cope by using denial and bargaining, which are both common responses to crisis. Regardless of how one felt before, once a positive diagnosis of STD is made, the individual may feel extremely vulnerable. At this time the individual's immediate and long-term defense style and coping skills become important determinants of his or her risk of developing major psychosocial problems. A mature defense style, effective coping skills, and active problem solving can protect the individual's self-concept and self-esteem, thereby increasing the probability that the individual will be able to cope responsibly with the STD diagnosis. For example, a single woman in her 40s becomes extremely anxious when she receives a diagnosis of the genital herpes virus. She immediately employs her usual coping skills, which is to learn as much as she can about the virus, the treatment options, and support resources, and she looks to her practitioner for support and guidance. For her, information is a powerful coping resource that helps her to adapt to her diagnosis, manage her anxiety, and maintain a satisfying life-style.

Keller, Egan, and Mims (1995) found that the psychosocial problems related to viral STDs include low self-esteem, feeling that one is being punished for sexual activity, embarrassment, feeling dirty, guilt, depression, relationship stress, self-blame, blaming others, doubts about a partner's fidelity, and concern about future sexual relationships. The researchers found that the most troubling psychosocial problems were informing new sexual partners, determining what to say or when to inform them, coping with social rejection and fear of sexual rejection, fear of transmission, and concern about future pregnancy and childbirth. Many primary care settings now have STD counselors who are skilled at recognizing distress and at providing support and crisis counseling for newly diagnosed patients.

Practitioner recognition of and response to the individual's psychosocial needs upon receiving an STD diagnosis can significantly impact his or her short-term and long-term coping, including the commitment to safer sex practices that can reduce immediate and future risks of transmission. In the absence of primary prevention options, secondary prevention and tertiary prevention (to reduce physical and psychological morbidity) should be the focus of care, with equal consideration for the individual's physical and psychosocial needs (Quinn, Zenilman, and Rompalo, 1994). When practitioners inform patients of positive STD test results, they should also initiate secondary and tertiary preventive care, which is specifically intended to support and protect the patient's self-concept and self-esteem.

Sexually Transmitted Diseases

Bacterial vaginosis
Chlamydia trachomatis
Genital herpes virus
Hepatitis B virus
Hepatitis C virus
Human immunodeficiency virus
Human papillomavirus
Neisseria gonorrhea
Pelvic inflammatory disease
Trichomonas vaginalis

Management of Psychosocial Problems Related to Sexuality

➤ Counseling

Emotional support is the core intervention of psychiatric primary care counseling for individuals with sexuality-related psychosocial problems. Those with related mental disorders, such as major depression or anxiety, along with sexual dysfunction, infertility, or an STD should receive the appropriate treatment and specialized care. Counseling should address psychosocial needs that might otherwise be overlooked. Emotional support is recommended because time can be the key in dealing with sexuality-related problems. It takes time to understand sexual dysfunction, for example, and then to decide if sex therapy is appropriate, and if so, how to obtain such therapy. Being able to express one's feelings and concerns to a practitioner can help a great deal when, for example, a patient needs to inform his parents of his homosexuality or tell her new partner about her viral STD diagnosis. Emotional support can help individuals to take important necessary actions, including seeking specialized care if necessary.

☎ Consultation and Referral

Many professional and community resources are available for consultation and referral for sexual dysfunction, coming out, infertility, poststerilization regret, and STD diagnosis. The problem can be finding a ***suitable*** resource. Consultation and referral for sexual dysfunction should involve a credible specialist or a sex therapist with a documented practice. This recommendation is easier said than done; even when such a resource can be located, patients may not wish to participate but may instead request medication such as an antidepressant or an antianxiety drug. Consultation and referral for infertility should take into consideration the couple's chances for pregnancy and the expense of specialized care. An excellent way for couples to evaluate their choices is to attend self-help or support groups with couples who have experience with both infertility and infertility health care. Relaxation training, stress management training, and massage therapy can be extremely helpful when stress is a factor. Individuals with paraphilia disorders require specialized care.

References

Biro FB, Rosenthal SL: Psychological sequelae of sexually transmitted diseases in adolescents, *Pediatric and Adolescent Gynecology* 19(1):209, 1992.

Boxer AS: Images of infertility, *Nurse Practitioner Forum* 7(2):60, 1996.

Chi IC, Jones DB: Incidence, risk factors, and prevention of post-sterilization regret in women: an updated international review from an epidemiological perspective, *Obstetrical and Gynecological Survey*, 49(10):722, 1994.

Copperman AB, Tanmoy M, Shaer J, Patel D, Sandler B, Grunfeld L, Bustillo M: A cost analysis of in vitro fertilization versus tubal surgery within an institution under two payment systems, *J of Women's Health* 5(4):335, 1996.

Council on Scientific Affairs, American Medical Association: Health care needs of gay men and lesbians in the United States, *JAMA* 275(17):1354, 1996.

Eliason MJ: Lesbian and gay family issues, *Journal of Family Nursing* 2(1):10, 1996.

Godin G, Fortin C, Mahnes G, Boyer R, Nadeau D, Duval B, Bradet R, Hounsa A: University students intention to seek medical care promptly if symptoms of sexually transmitted diseases were suspected, *Sexually Transmitted Diseases* 20(2):100, 1993.

Golombok S: Psychological functioning in infertility patients, *Human Reproduction* 7(2):208, 1992.

Jirka J, Schuett S, Foxall M: Loneliness and social support in infertile couples, *JOGNN* 25(1):55, 1996.

Jones HW, Toner JP: The infertile couple, *NE J of Med* 329(23):1710, 1993.

Keller MJ, Egan JJ, Mims LF: Genital human papillomavirus infection: common but not trivial, *Health Care for Women Inter* 16(4): 351, 1995.

Levine SB: What is clinical sexuality? *The Psychiatric Clinics of North Am* 18(1):5, 1995.

Mattison AM, McWhirter DP: Lesbians, gay men and their families, *The Psychiatric Clinics of North America* 18(1):123, 1995.

Meyers M, Diamond R, Kezur D, Scharf C, Weinshel M, Rait DS: An infertility primer for family therapist: Part I Medical, social, and psychological dimensions, *Family Process* 34(2):219, 1995.

Quinn TC, Zenilman J, Rompalo A: Sexually transmitted diseases:advances in diagnosis and treatment, *Advances in Internal Med* 39:149, 1994.

Risen C: A guide to taking a sexual history, *The Psychiatric Clinics of North Am* 18(1):39, 1995.

Rosen RC, Leiblum SR: Hypoactive sexual desire, *The Psychiatric Clinics of North America* 18(1):107, 1995.

Sandelowshi M: On infertility, *J of Obstetric Gynecologic Neonatal Nursing* Nov/Dec:749, 1994.

Schiavi RC, Segraves RT: The biology of sexual function, *The Psychiatric Clinics of North America* 18(1):7, 1995.

Travin S: Compulsive sexual behaviors, *The Psychiatric Clinics of North America* 18(1):155, 1995.

Trantham P: The infertile couple, *American Fam Physician* 54(3):1001, 1996

Turner CF, Danella RD, Rogers SM: Sexual behavior in the United States, 1930-1990: trends and methodological problems, *Sexually Transmitted Diseases* 22(3):173, 1995.

Death and Divorce 11

Death or divorce involve the traumatic loss of a person, relationship, or attachments that triggers reactions of grief and mourning. Individuals may grieve or mourn their losses in ways that are predictable and characteristic for them or in ways that are uncharacteristic. The actual experience of grief and mourning is influenced by many factors, and one of the most important is the nature of the loss to the individual. Coping with death and divorce, as with other types of losses, also requires coping with multiple changes and secondary losses that can greatly magnify the traumatic impact of the death or divorce. Regardless of the nature of the loss and the individual's coping skills and coping style, grief takes many paths, but the journey is fundamentally the same. This chapter reviews grief and mourning, death and divorce, and related psychosocial problems.

Who Is at Risk

Risk, in relation to death and divorce, refers to individual characteristics and circumstances that increase the traumatic impact of death and divorce or decrease the individual's ability to effectively cope, grieve, or mourn, thereby increasing the risk of psychosocial problems and mental disorders. Gender is a significant determinant of how individuals view, respond to, and subsequently recover from a loss, but there are no formulas that apply to all males or all females. Of the many possible gender distinctions that can be made, practitioners note gender influences on the individual's relationship-attachment style and expression of grief and mourning. For example, males may be emotionally avoidant and may react to the loss of an important person or relationship by trying to avoid dealing with it.

Although absolute gender distinctions are beginning to fade as male and female gender roles become less rigid, it is still more common for males to maintain a fairly high degree of emotional and psychological distance within their important relationships. Moreover, socially acceptable expressions of loss for females, such as crying or requests for support, are easy to recognize. Male expressions of loss (e.g., withdrawal) or request for support can be less easy to recognize or seriously ineffective (e.g., alcohol abuse). Despite the fact that gender is not a predictive risk factor, it should be considered when determining the individual's attachment to the person or relationship that has been lost as well as the individual's ability to express the experience of loss so that others can recognize and therefore respond to it.

Age is another risk factor: loss affects the young in ways that it does not affect adults and elders, and vice versa. Age-based differences in coping styles and coping skills are also important. Young people who face the loss of an important person or relationship will have less experience and fewer coping resources. An individual's appraisal of loss is also associated with age and developmental stage: how one defines the personal and social meanings of a loss partially determines one's coping response and the impact of the loss. Although age is not a good predictor of the importance that a loss may hold for an individual, it is an important determinant of how the individual will appraise the loss. A very young child, for example, may be as alarmed and saddened by the death of a parent as an adolescent or a spouse, but the loss will have different meanings for each person. Each will grieve and mourn differently, and in some households this difference may become an additional source of distress. The key point regarding age as a risk factor is that it influences the individual's ability to make sense of the loss and, subsequently, to grieve, mourn, and recover.

Loss occurs when an attachment has been broken. Humans can become attached to just about anything, from ideas, people, and places to objects, emotions, and goals. Attachments lend meaning, value, and purpose to life and are vital sources of emotional satisfaction and social identity. With little effort one can learn a great deal about a person simply by identifying his or her important attachments. Visible attachment objects, such as people and possessions, are obvious to the individual as well as to others; other equally powerful but invisible attachment objects can be difficult to recognize. Conscious awareness of the attachment may not occur until the attachment is threatened or lost. In this case the individual's reaction to a lost attachment is complicated by the individual's sudden conscious awareness of that attachment.

For example, a woman may be attached to her house, on which she has spent a great deal of time and money and in which she takes great pride. This attachment to her possession is obvious both to the woman and to others. However, only when circumstances threaten her ownership of the house does she become aware of her attachment to it as a symbol of the home she never had and has longed for since childhood. The loss of her house is complicated by reawakened childhood emotional attachments to the ideal home. The woman will react to the threatened loss of her possession *and* to the ideals her home symbolized for her. Prior to the threat of losing her house, she may not have been fully aware of her attachment to an ideal home, symbolized by the house. ***Silent attachments*** such as this can occur with any attachment object, including people and relationships.

Grief and Mourning

Grief and mourning are responses to loss. Rando's (1993) definitions of these three concepts are comprehensive, allow for a great deal of individual variation and thus are very useful. According to Rando, loss can be classified as ***physical*** or ***psychosocial***. Psychosocial loss includes change. The extent to which a loss is apparent (i.e., can be recognized by others) is also an important element in understanding the individual's experience of loss. The fewer explanations needed, the more "legitimate," or socially accepted, the loss. If a person loses something intangible or has psychosocial loss, he or she may have to work hard to make that loss understandable to others in order to receive support. Unlike physical losses, such as a death or a house fire, psychosocial losses (e.g., lost social identity) may not be viewed as losses by others, thus setting up a potential area of interpersonal conflict if significant others fail to validate the loss. The inability to obtain social validation for a loss can have a troubling influence on grief and mourning. Social validation and support are important resources for the individual who is trying to cope with a loss. However, social norms may control the definitions of valid (true) and invalid (false) loss events.

Rando (1993) defines bereavement as the experience of deprivation caused by ***primary losses*** (physical and psychosocial) or by related ***secondary losses***. For many, secondary losses can be as difficult, if not more so, than the primary loss. Secondary losses can occur concurrently with or following the primary loss. With death and divorce, secondary losses are numerous and can occur long after the primary loss, thereby increasing the difficulty of recognizing and validating the loss. For example, the loss of a partner due to death or divorce will bring about the loss of intimacy and social purpose, but neither secondary loss may be experienced immediately. Secondary losses can also be potential as well as actual. The loss of a potential or hoped-for attachment can be just as painful as the lost of an actual attachment. In fact, the loss of one's dreams can be one of the most painful losses that individuals experience.

Compared to bereavement and primary and secondary loss, grief and mourning are more universal experiences. Everyone grieves and mourns in a unique fashion and at one's own pace; individual and cultural variations in grieving and mourning are extensive. Experts, family, and friends may say that an individual is free to mourn a loss in ways that are personally meaningful and useful, but this social allowance is quickly withdrawn if others become impatient. No matter how an individual mourns, there is likely to be someone who will question the amount of time or the actions taken or some other element of the individual's mourning. The usual demand is an insistence that the individual get on with life. Another example is that if a person does not appear to be upset enough, others may ask why. Criticism is common and should be anticipated. In most cases, people think they are being helpful by giving the individual a little shove back into life. But grief is a total experience that involves many changes over time (Rando, 1993). Mourning is the conscious and unconscious process that makes it possible for a grieving individual to cut the many attachments to what was lost in a way that makes new attachments possible. As implied by these terms and definitions, the goal or hoped-for outcome of mourning is recovery, but the goal of grieving is to experience grief. To ***grieve*** is to feel a loss; to ***mourn*** is to recover from a loss.

Rando's Processes of Mourning (1996):

1. Recognize the loss
2. React to separation
3. Reexperience the attachments
4. Relinquish the attachments
5. Readjust to changes
6. Reinvest in living

Personal characteristics significantly influence how an individual will mourn a loss. Age, gender, and cultural identity form the basis for important elements of mourning, such as the individual's world view, one's coping resources, and socially acceptable mourning behaviors. Individual factors can be particularly important in terms of one's customary attachment style and the attachment that has been lost. For example, individuals with an ambivalent, controlling, or dependent attachment style will each react differently to the death of a loved one or to divorce. It is impossible to understand an individual's mourning style simply by knowing the person, relationship, or possession that has been lost. Silent attachments can account for much of an individual's response to loss, especially when a response seems uncharacteristic, such as a usually easygoing person who becomes aggressive and withdrawn. Personal characteristics, attachment style, and the specific attachment that has been lost are all important influences on the ability to mourn and the manner of mourning.

Previous experience with important losses significantly influences mourning: whether the current loss is the first major one in the individual's life or the most recent of many will be a factor. Ideally, previous experience with loss will mean increased self-awareness, self-understanding, and self-acceptance, and this insight will be a positive influence on mourning. Such a person might be better able to recognize, and then act to meet, his or her personal needs, thereby easing the transitions of mourning. An example would be members of a community with a high incidence of HIV-related deaths who have learned to anticipate their needs in mourning the loss of their loved ones.

However, those who have had major or multiple losses can become emotionally, physically, and socially exhausted and at increased risk for mental disorders, such as depression, anxiety, or chronic stress, rather than better prepared to mourn new losses.

The number and nature of concurrent and potential losses should always be considered. People differ in their tolerance levels, but everyone has a point at which one becomes overwhelmed. The number of concurrent losses obviously affects the individual's ability to mourn, but when there are multiple losses over brief periods or multiple concurrent losses, there is increased risk of severe distress or incomplete mourning. When mourning is incomplete, individuals struggle more and may carry around their loss like a heavy suitcase. Ultimately, how a person mourns a loss is influenced by numerous factors.

Complicated Mourning

The *Diagnostic and Statistical Manual of Mental Disorders, fourth edition,* (DSM-IV) describes ***bereavement*** as the normal process of grief and mourning following loss. The process of mourning can become complicated in many ways, but the term ***complication*** should not be used to imply that an individual is mourning incorrectly. Such harsh judgements are not likely to be helpful or accurate. Instead, complicated mourning should be thought of as personal needs that have interfered with the process of mourning. Complicated mourning implies that the individual is unable to move forward with the process of mourning. It implies that mourning is absent, delayed, inhibited, distorted, conflicted, unanticipated, or chronic (Rando, 1993). Mourning requires that individuals face the pain associated with the loss. Some people are surprised, if not alarmed, by how much psychological and emotional pain their loss has caused, and in severe cases their immediate goal may be to avoid or decrease this pain rather than mourn the loss.

Complicated mourning differs from ***pathological grief***, which is a severe disturbance requiring specialized care. Rando (1993) defines three types of pathological grief: fear, rage, and deflation. With each type, the individual's extreme reaction is related to the fact that the loss is viewed as a personal threat. This response occurs because much of our identity first develops within the context of important childhood relationships. Early traumas to a child's sense of self that occur within an important relationship can establish negative views of oneself in relation to others. Adult compensatory relationships can cover up this negative self and allow the individual to have a more positive and less painful sense of self. The negative self is then kept in the emotional and psychological background until loss (perceived or actual) of the much-needed compensatory relationship allows the negative self to reemerge. Self-hate in response to the loss of a valuable relationship can cause intense fear and sadness as well as rage at having been betrayed, abandoned, made to feel worthless, or unmasked (Rando, 1993). An increasingly common example of pathological grief is pathological self-hate and rage in response to the loss of a compensatory marriage through divorce.

❑ Common Assessment Problems

The goals of assessment are to determine the nature and significance of the person's loss as well as his or her current needs in mourning that loss. Although both goals can present assessment problems, continual changes in the individual's thoughts, feelings, and behavior are the most difficult. Change is a necessary element of mourning, but thoughts and feelings can range from moments of severe psychological distress to hopeful optimism. These dramatic changes may cause some people to feel they are out of control or that something awful is happening to them. This doubt and confusion becomes an assessment problem when participation in the assessment feels like a lot of work with little promise of benefit. Changes in the individual's definition of his or her loss, gradual recognition of secondary losses (expected and unexpected), and the reactions of important others who do not share the loss can also present assessment problems.

In some cases the duration of the loss itself can be a problem. For example, a person can lose loved ones, a home, and employment in an instant, as a result of a natural disaster such as an earthquake or a flood. The short duration is disproportionate to the magnitude of the multiple losses and leaves the individual in a state of shock. On the other hand, a divorce or a terminal illness that continues for years can complicate assessment because the individual's primary loss occurs in degrees. One way to decrease the problems related to the transitions that occur with loss is to focus on the individual's current perceptions, circumstances, and needs and reassess them frequently.

Crisis may be the most difficult assessment problem because the crisis itself (e.g., money problems) rather than the loss can become the focus. Finally, individuals who shut down when overwhelmed pose a unique assessment problem because the individual is essentially unable to participate.

Death

Death as a loss is, in large part, given meaning by the survivor's beliefs about life. There is growing concern that the increased social tolerance of death as news and entertainment has devalued life. At the same time, the introduction of assisted suicide, living wills, and organ transplants gives the unspoken message that death is negotiable. The devaluation of life and societal ambivalence toward death has removed many of the absolutes that once served as psychological guideposts for the living. Both of these powerful social trends are counter-balanced by the notion that however death and dying is defined by society, individuals may be more vulnerable than ever to the experience of lost attachments simply because more people have fewer attachments. Much of what is understood about loss, grief, and mourning is based on studies of individuals, families, and generations that have survived the deaths of significant others (Horowitz et al, 1996). To this day, the baby boomer generation is partly self-defined by the violent deaths of John Kennedy, Martin Luther King, Robert Kennedy, and the images of young men who came home from Vietnam in body bags. Since the 1960s, new generations have lived with equally powerful images of violent death but without the benefit of national mourning. When social definitions of life and death seem unreliable or unhelpful, individuals must develop personal definitions. This brief overview addresses the unique needs of children and the concepts of family grief and self-transcendence as an indicator of completed mourning.

Children are somewhat more predictable than adults in their responses to death and divorce and in the types of psychosocial problems they are likely to experience. The death of a parent and a divorce can feel like the same experience to children, since in both cases the child no longer has a loved one as part of daily life and may have to look to an adult for support who is also trying to cope with the loss (Trimm, 1995). Stage of development is a significant factor in children's reaction to and expression of their needs in relation to the death of an important adult. Children under the age of 2 do not comprehend death. From ages 2 to 7, children tend to believe that death is temporary, and they may develop strong feelings of egocentric self-blame when the loved one does not return. From ages 7 to 12, children understand that death means loss, and they are likely to engage in a search for causes and explanations. Over the age of 12, children have the same understanding of death as adults, but they do not have an adult frame of reference to help them cope with the loss (Trimm, 1995). Unlike adults, children may be more direct in their concern for their own safety and well-being, and they may become very demanding and uncooperative as a way of expressing needs of which they are aware but that they cannot articulate.

Families have a direct and powerful influence on how individuals experience and recover from loss due to death or divorce. The less adaptive a family's response is, the more difficult the experience can be for individual family members (Kissane, Bloch and Dowe, et al, 1996; Kissane, Bloch, and Onghena, et al, 1996). There are many ways in which a family can engage in maladaptive mourning that interferes with adaptive individual mourning. The family can avoid dealing with the loss, distort the meaning of the loss, or can prolong grief to the point that mourning is prohibited (Kissane and Bloch, 1994). Families have many ways to avoid dealing with death that can negatively impact individual mourning, such as disapproving of or disallowing expressions of grief. Families can also define the death of a relative in a highly negative way, resulting in family conflict or guilt. For example, a death may be defined as a punishment or as a warning to the family. Rigid families, those with little or no tolerance for individuality or change, may also have to struggle to find a way to grieve and mourn a death. The best evidence that a family is unable to grieve and mourn a death is that the experience of loss persists without relief. As pointed out by Kissane and Bloch (1994), families who are unable to grieve and mourn a lost relative may assign that lost relative a silent family role that maintains the attachment rather than allowing them to accept the loss. The family may feel duty-bound to keep the deceased alive. Keeping a place (rather than memories) in the family for the deceased interferes with grieving and mourning, whereas family rituals that allow members to talk about their attachments to the deceased is a helpful step in letting go.

However death is perceived, experienced, or mourned, for adults the ideal end stage of mourning is ***self-transcendence,*** which is the ability to extend oneself beyond personal needs and to experience relief by reaching out to others (Joffrion and Douglas, 1994). This goal may be difficult for many people, but the purpose is to better define the possible benefits of mourning, not add another hurdle to it. Self-transcendence is conceptualized as the sixth stage of Kubler-Ross's five stages of grief (denial, anger, bargaining, depression, and acceptance). Self-transcendence is less vague than acceptance and possibly more meaningful for of psychosocial functioning. Survivors may have less trouble understanding and personalizing self-transcendence, and a clear understanding of the goal of mourning can make it easier. Self-transcendence does not mean substituting new attachments to replace the lost attachment. However, substitution is not uncommon, especially if the individual was dependent on the lost relationship as a basis for a highly valued role, such as father or husband. Rather than trying to replace a lost attachment or avoid feelings of emptiness by filling the void with a new person, self-transcendence is accomplished by becoming part of life, such as joining a self-help group or a support group that advocates self-transcendence as a shared goal. A potential drawback of adopting self-transcendence as a goal of mourning is that it can invite people to skip the more painful stages of grief to become advocates or mentors for others. Another drawback is that those who are naturally sociable will find self-transcendence more appealing and easier than those who have a more private nature.

Divorce

Although the rate of divorce in the United States appears to have stabilized, it continues to be high. Currently, about 50% of first marriages end in divorce, but about 50% of divorced women and men remarry within 5 years of their first divorce (Emery and Coiro, 1995). These statistics suggest that most people value marriage, but that day-to-day married life is very demanding.

Social changes, since the 1950s, such as women working outside the home full time, have clearly altered married life but do not appear to have had the equivalent impact on the romantic ideal of marriage. The romantic ideal of marriage, symbolized by stories such as the princess who escapes danger by marrying a prince or the notion that a man's home is his castle, still have a strong social, psychological, and emotional appeal. In fact, the romantic ideal of marriage can be as important as actual married life in understanding how individuals cope with divorce (Jockin, McGue, and Lykken, 1996).

As with other psychosocial problems, coping with divorce can be understood through one's thoughts, feelings, and behavior. Since marriage is now more a choice than a cultural or biological necessity, people who marry are more likely to have specific reasons for doing so. These reasons partly define the psychosocial benefits that the individual hopes to obtain from marriage as well as the psychosocial problems that he or she hopes to avoid. Many people continue to marry for practical and personal reasons, such as raising children and growing old together, but marital relationships and married life have never been more complex. The difficult idealism, solutions, and problems that individuals bring to a marriage are critical elements of the increased complexity of marriage. For example, an individual may view marriage idealistically as a solution to personal loneliness and low self-esteem but, because of the hectic pace and multiple demands of actual married life, is not able to obtain either benefit. That individual may then reevaluate the decision to marry rather than reevaluate his or her unrealistic expectations.

Because more people draw on their marital relationship for support and comfort that in the past were provided by extended family and friends, it is not uncommon for couples as well as individuals to need more from a marriage than they bring to it. Few marriages are able to serve as the primary solution to personal psychosocial problems and as a substitute for family, friends, and community. For example, a romantic "conquest" that culminates in marriage is a common escape from feelings of inferiority or low self-esteem. But when marriage is viewed as the solution to personal psychosocial problems such as this, the individual's attachment may be to marriage as a symbol rather than as a day-to-day relationship with another person. This attachment may be so intense that the individual must remain relatively unaware of it until, when faced with the loss of it through divorce, he or she becomes flooded with anxiety. Coping with divorce thus requires coping with the loss of powerful attachments, both actual *and* symbolic.

Like marriage, divorce is a highly complex, intimate relationship. Despite the determined cynicism of the 1980s and 1990s, few people are emotionally prepared for or unaffected by the end of a marriage and the loss of the attachments that defined the marital relationship. The experience of divorce is a series of lost attachments, actual and symbolic, marked by significant changes. Some of these changes are expected but many are not, and each change requires personal adjustment. The more changes, the more the individual must adjust. For some individuals, gradual change is easier to adjust to than sudden change. Until the couple actually begins to discuss divorce, they may be able to avoid dealing with more change in their relationship than they can cope with. Legal divorce ends only one of the countless attachments that make up a marriage. Without the benefit of laws and social rules, couples must also find a way to divorce psychologically, emotionally, intellectually, economically, socially, spiritually, sexually, and behaviorally (Emery and Coiro, 1995). As difficult as this may be, the divorcing couple will also have to confront the powerful symbolic attachments they have to each other and to their marriage. At the same time, other extremely powerful attachments, such as children, family, friends, property, community, and money, may tie the couple together in ways that can never be changed. The divorcing individual or couple faces all of these changes and lost attachments while undergoing a myriad of emotions, from rage to emptiness.

When divorce is conceptualized as ending multiple interconnected attachments, ending the legal attachment of the relationship can seem easier to cope with, since this level of divorce is well defined and expert help can be obtained. In fact, the point at which the couple initiates a legal divorce can be very revealing as to how they cope with the end of their marriage. For example, filing for legal divorce immediately may mean that the couple hopes to benefit from the authority granted by divorce laws when they confront the end of their marriage. It is also not unusual for couples to easily end all but one or two of their attachments.

Perhaps they continue their sexual relationship or their financial relationship. When the couple has children, the parental relationship undergoes serious changes but is not ended. An interesting social phenomenon today is the common usage of the term "my child's father (or mother)" in place of " my husband (or wife)." For the benefit of children, this is also used for parents who were never married.

Divorce, like marriage, is also subject to symbolism and personal psychosocial problems, the most troubling of which are strong feelings of entitlement or claims regarding the ex-spouse. Although most couples divorce, end their attachments, and go on to live separate lives, some are unwilling or unable to relinquish their claims on a person to whom they have been married. These feelings can be the source of serious confusion and conflict. For as many reasons as there are divorces, there are individuals who act out various attachments to an ex-spouse, claiming their behavior is the privilege of a husband, wife, or parent. Hollywood images of "attached divorce," such as the film *The War of the Roses*, comically exaggerate violence and death associated with divorce, but in real life this situation is without humor. Most divorces take place without violence, but a 50% divorce rate increases the probability of divorce-related violence that is associated with powerful psychosocial losses for which the individual was not prepared.

One of the basic methods of coping with and enduring the process of divorce is to identify acceptable reasons for divorcing. Most people need to be clear about why they are leaving a marriage before they can act on leaving. Those with a strong emotional, rather than problem-solving, coping style may attribute their decision to divorce to an emotion, but because emotions fluctuate they are apt to always feel unsure about the decision. For most people, vague feelings of disquiet or unhappiness are not an unacceptable reason for such an important decision. Individuals who are certain about the decision to divorce but are not able to put a reason into words may eventually say the reason was unhappiness. Unacceptable new behaviors (e.g., a sexual affair) on the part of a spouse or discovering that old behaviors by the spouse are now intolerable (e.g., impulsive shopping) can also serve as a stated reason to divorce. In this case, the decision to divorce is more important than the reason given for the decision.

However, couples, family, and friends will probably have to struggle with whether the reason is good enough to act on, no matter what the reason is.

In their study of newly separated or divorced couples, Fishel and Samsa (1993) asked participants who initiated a divorce what their reasons were. They found that women initiated divorce more than twice as often as men, and their most common reasons were (1) the husband's unacceptable behavior, (2) incompatibility, (3) constant conflict, and (4) the wife's involvement with another man. The researchers then asked the same questions of men who said their wives initiated the divorce. Two men said they did not know their wives' reasons for divorce. A few said their behavior was the reason, but the majority of the men said that their wives had become dissatisfied with their roles in the marriage. Fishel and Samsa (1993) concluded that rigid male and female gender roles may have interfered with the marital relationship. Their findings suggest that fewer women may be willing to stay in marital relationships that do not meet their needs. Because many of the most dramatic social changes in the previous decades have happened in women's lives, more women may be less willing to live with unsatisfying marital gender roles.

Numerous psychosocial problems are experienced by individuals and couples who are divorcing, but conflict, violent and nonviolent, is a problem of particular concern. The conflict issues associated with divorce tend to be the same issues that produce conflict in marriage: money, children, sex, and power. In intimate relationships, power refers to control, or one person's ability to rule the thoughts, feelings, and behavior of the other. A fifth critical source of conflict, which is easy to overlook but is always present and is an important influence on coping ability, is hurt feelings. As the saying goes, hurt people hurt people. Hurt feelings can lead to hurtful behavior toward oneself or others. They can be difficult to define or explain to others, but few people can tolerate severe or prolonged emotional pain for very long. In divorce, which can become a contest allowing only one winner, hurt feelings can also be used as a tit-for-tat weapon when partners try to cause each other emotional pain. Oddly enough, hurt feelings can also maintain rather than end the relationship.

Emotional pain also occurs in relation to the consequences of divorce. For example, after a divorce women are more likely than men to become depressed, but women are also more likely to experience serious secondary problems (Aseltine and Kessler, 1993). In particular, the researchers found that financial problems and less time spent with supportive friends are two secondary problems of divorce that are significantly related to depression and more likely to be experienced by women. Women more than men have to cope with poverty and isolation in addition to the end of the marriage (Garvin, Kalter, and Hansell, 1993; Nelson, 1994). Similarly, studies of sexual activity following divorce indicate that males more than females, and younger more than older adults, are slightly more likely to be sexually active within the first year after divorce (Stack and Gundlach, 1992).

Not all adult psychosocial problems related to divorce are experienced by adults. One adult problem in particular is a troubling experience for children: ***parental alienation***. As defined by Price and Pioske (1994), this is the systematic denigration of one parent by the other with the intent of using the child to inflict pain. When adults employ parental alienation as a means of coping with a divorce or its secondary problems, they do so at the child's expense. When divorce becomes war and the children are enlisted, they end up being exposed to adult behavior and emotions that may be ***difficult*** for adults to endure, but are profoundly ***harmful*** to children. Telling young or adolescent children what Mom said or what Dad did indicates a need for specialized psychiatric care in order to protect the children and help the adults to better meet their children's needs. Specialists can help parents to define and maintain an emotional boundary between adults and children. Divorcing parents who treat their children as confidants or who go to their children for emotional comfort do so at the child's expense. The parent may gain a friend, but the child loses a parent (Grossman and Rowat, 1995).

Management of Psychosocial Problems Related to Death and Divorce

➤ Counseling

Practitioners should focus on three goals when counseling adults who are coping with the death of a loved one or a divorce: acute symptom relief, support for mourning, and prevention of functioning impairment. Symptoms of depression, anxiety, and stress are commonly associated with death and divorce. Acute episodes of alcohol abuse and interpersonal conflict, as ineffective methods of coping with loss, may also occur. These experiences usually motivate individuals to seek health care and may be their main concern initially. Individuals tend to be more willing to focus on difficult problems when they see that the practitioner is willing and able to be of real help. For example, a man who has been irritable, anxious, and unable to sleep since the death of his only child could benefit from talking about his child and his loss, but he may not want to do so. He may not be able to talk about his loss without being overcome by his feelings of grief or his symptoms of irritability and anxiety, or he may be unwilling to talk about his loss until he is convinced that the practitioner is willing to listen.

Symptom relief is an important first goal and a place to start in psychiatric primary care counseling. A basic symptom assessment is usually sufficient to find out the patient's immediate needs and to initiate conversation. If a disorder is diagnosed (e.g., depression), treatment should be initiated, but treatment for a disorder is not appropriate when the individual's symptoms are better described as distress. There is always a concern that by focusing on symptoms too soon, much-needed grief and mourning may be interfered with, prevented, or delayed. Treatment for a disorder does not replace mourning. Practitioners can help patients by educating them about grief and mourning and by supporting their efforts to address the loss. Patients who are unable to talk about anything other than their distress may require specialized care for symptom relief as well as mourning, to reduce the risk of chronic or complicated mourning.

Mourning the loss of a loved one due to death or divorce takes time, energy, and support. Most primary care settings have patient information pamphlets and videos that can provide very helpful information and direction, but social support tends to be the most helpful resource. People react to death and divorce in many ways, but social isolation and negative coping behaviors can undermine functioning quickly, thereby increasing the likelihood of secondary losses. Grief and loss support groups and self-help groups are extremely effective for most people and should be used as soon as possible. These groups provide a safe environment for the expression of the anger, hurt, and fear that is associated with early stages of mourning. Groups also allow the individual to "see" the mourning process by viewing people at different stages of the process.

☎ Consultation and Referral

Immediate consultation and referral should be arranged if dangerous behavior toward oneself or others is a concern. Painful emotions can disinhibit behavior, and individuals may act on feelings that they might not have otherwise. All statements of harming oneself or others must be treated seriously. Survivor suicide following a death and violence between divorcing partners should always be in the back of the practitioner's mind as a possibility. Dealing with death or divorce is a long process and most individuals will have more than one moment of distress. Individuals who react to death or divorce by refusing to acknowledge the loss should receive specialized care. This response is more likely with divorce than with death, but when absolute denial is used as a method of coping with loss it is often because the individual is unable to mobilize other defenses. When this is the case, a specialist should work with the individual to establish alternative defenses and coping skills before questioning the individual's use of absolute denial.

References

Aseltine RH, Kessler RC: Marital disruption and depression in a community sample, *J of Health and Social Beh* 34:237, 1993.

Emery R, Coiro M: Divorce: consequences for children, *Ped in Review* 16(8):306, 1995.

Fishel AH, Samsa GP: Role perceptions of divorcing parents, *Health Care for Women International* 14(1):87, 1993.

Garvin V, Kalter N, Hansell J: Divorced women: individual differences in stressors, mediating factors and adjustment outcome, *Am J Orthopsychiatry* 63(2): 232, 1993.

Grossman M, Rowat KM: Parental relationships, coping strategies, received support, and well-being in adolescents of separated or divorced and married parents, *Research in Nursing and Health* 18(3):249, 1995.

Horowitz M, Sonneborn D, Sugahara C, Maercker A: Self-regard: a new measure, *Am J Psychiatry* 153(3):382, 1996.

Jockin V, McGue M, Lykken DT: Personality and divorce: a genetic analysis, *J of Personality and Social Psychology* 71(2):288, 1996.

Joffrion LP, Douglas D: Grief resolution: facilitating self-transcendence in the bereaved, *J of Psychosocial Nursing* 32(3):13, 1994.

Kissane DW, Bloch S, Dowe DL, Snyder RD, Onghena P, McKenzie, Wallace CS: The Melbourne family grief study, I: perceptions of family functioning in bereavement, *Am J Psychiatry* 153(5):650, 1996.

Kissane DW, Bloch S, Onghena P, McKenzie, Snyder RD, Dowe Dl: The Melbourne family grief study, II: psychosocial morbidity and grief in bereaved families, *Am J Psychiatry* 153(5):659, 1996.

Kissane DW, Bloch S: Family grief, *British J of Psychiatry* 164:728, 1994.

Nelson G: Emotional well-being of separated and married women: long-term follow-up study, *Am J Orthopsychiatry* 64(1):150, 1994.

Price JL, Pluske KS: Parental alienation syndrome, a developmental analysis of vulnerable population, *J of Psychosocial Nursing* 31(11):9, 1994.

Rando TA: *Treatment of Complicated Mourning*, Champaign, IL, 1993, Research Press.

Stack S, Gundlach JH: Divorce and sex, *Arch of Sexual Behavior* 21(4):359, 1992.

Trimm RF: Divorce and death: helping children cope with family loss, *Comprehensive Therapy* 21(3):135, 1995.

Psychosocial Problems Related to Pain 12

Although physical pain is a universal experience, there are several confounding aspects of the experience that increase the difficulty of helping individuals who are in pain. First, the experience of physical pain includes the expression of pain. The actual mechanism of physical pain may not be apparent, and if the cause of pain is not an obvious injury it may be difficult to pinpoint. Therefore the expression of pain is a significant aspect of the experience of pain. Second, any number of social, psychological, and cultural factors can affect a given individual's expression of pain, and as these factors change, the individual's expression of pain may also change. Just as no two people are likely to have the same expression of physical pain, one individual's expression can also change over time or with circumstances.

Variations in pain tolerance can be a source of conflict and confusion because individuals, significant others, and health care providers rely on social, psychological, and cultural norms to determine expected levels of pain as well as acceptable expressions of pain. Another troubling aspect of physical pain is that severe or chronic pain has traditionally been controlled with narcotic medications, which have an extremely high risk of dependence and abuse. Finally, the experience and expression of physical pain is confounded when pain leads to the development of psychological symptoms that are then incorporated into the experience of pain. With these factors in mind, this chapter briefly discusses the *Diagnostic and Statistical Manual of Mental Disorders, fourth edition,* (DSM-IV) pain disorders; issues related to gender, culture, and mood; chronic pain in children; and pain and HIV disease.

Definitions of Pain

Pain is defined as an unpleasant sensory and emotional experience that is associated with actual or potential tissue damage or described in terms of tissue damage (Benoliel, 1995).Pain is commonly defined as acute or chronic, predictable or unpredictable, and may or may not be associated with obvious pain-inducing events, such as surgery or trauma. Pain that continues for longer than 6 months is defined as ***chronic pain***. The more apparent the source of pain and the more acute the pain appears to be, the more likely it is that ***pain relief*** will be the goal of treatment. The goal with chronic or unpredictable pain is ***pain management***. In Western culture pain relief is assumed to be an achievable goal regardless of the source of pain. Over-the-counter (OTC) analgesics make up a large portion of the OTC medication market, and each new pain medication promises to be stronger, more efficient, and more reliable than all the others.

Recurrent acute pain (e.g., headaches, backaches, dysmenorrhea) and recurrent pain associated with chronic conditions (e.g., arthritis) differ from chronic pain unless the recurrence pattern is stable, the recurrence rate is frequent, and the individual experiences many of the same physical, psychosocial, and behavioral changes as in chronic pain syndromes. Severe chronic pain, such as the pain associated with cancer, combines the organic experience of physical pain with the added dimension of suffering.

Loss of physical functioning, loss of important social roles, severe money problems, and psychological and spiritual distress are all factors that can have a cumulative effect that compounds the experience of physical pain. Under these circumstances the pain is described as invasive because it is affecting multiple areas of biopsychosocial functioning. Effective pain management will require interventions that can lead to improvement in impaired areas of biopsychosocial functioning (Portenoy, 1993). Chronic pain due to progressive diseases, such as sickle cell anemia, can also have a cumulative effect because this type of pain is likely to be associated with progressive negative changes in the individual's expression of pain. This progression is a reflection of the fact that an individual who has lived with physical pain for years is unlikely to be unchanged by the experience.

Pain Disorders

A duration of 6 months or longer is required to meet the clinical criteria for a DSM-IV diagnosis of ***pain disorder***.

DSM-IV Criteria for Pain Disorder (APA, 1994)

1. Pain in one or more anatomical sites is the predominant focus of the clinical presentation and is of sufficient severity to warrant clinical attention
2. The pain causes clinically significant distress or impairment in social, occupational, or other important areas of functioning
3. Psychological factors are judged to have an important role in the onset, severity, exacerbation, or maintenance of the pain
4. The symptom or defect is not intentionally produced or feigned (as in factitious disorder or malingering)
5. The pain is not better accounted for by a mood, anxiety, or psychotic disorder and does not meet the criteria for dyspareunia

Pain Disorder Associated with Psychological Factors

Psychological factors are judged to have the major role in the onset, severity, exacerbation, or maintenance of the pain. (If a general medical condition is present, it does not have the major role in the onset, severity, exacerbation, or maintenance of the pain.) This diagnosis is not made if criteria are also met for somatization disorder. Acute is a duration of less than 6 months and chronic is a duration of 6 months or longer.

Pain Disorder Associated with Both Psychological Factors and a General Medical Condition

Psychological factors and a general medical condition are judged to have important roles in the onset, severity, exacerbation, or maintenance of the pain. The associated general medical condition or anatomical site of the pain is coded on Axis III. A pain diagnosis is determined following a medical history and physical findings. The practitioner can determine if pain is nociceptive or neuropathic and what psychological contributions may be involved. In some patients, organic pain is present, but the far greater dysfunction comes from psychological issues.

Hypochondriasis, Malingering, Factitious Disorder, and Somatization Disorder

The most difficult types of expressed physical pain disorders for practitioners are defined by Eisendrath (1995) as hypochondriasis, malingering, factitious disorder, and somatization disorder. ***Hypochondriasis*** pain is associated with an individual's psychological preoccupation with a fear of having a serious disease. ***Malingering*** is the expression of physical pain that is motivated by hoped-for secondary gains. Eisendrath points out that if observers had full information regarding the malingerer's true circumstances, the individual's motivation for malingering would be obvious. Therefore individuals who are malingering are highly motivated to withhold information.

Factitious pain disorder differs from malingering in that the individual is seeking both primary and secondary gain. In factitious pain disorder the individual expresses physical pain to achieve a psychological purpose that is both unconscious and primary. This purpose is almost always to obtain care and attention by being hospitalized. This disorder is extremely troubling to health care providers because some individuals will go to extraordinary lengths to achieve hospitalization, including life-threatening self-harm.

Eisendrath (1995) offers the following clues to the assessment of factitious disorder: the individual's symptoms can be shown to be exaggerated; any symptom improvement is always followed by relapse; symptoms appear to be made worse by self-manipulation; the individual is very willing to submit to highly invasive procedures; the individual seems able to forecast exacerbations; the individual resists allowing open communication with previous health care providers; the individual or a family member is employed in a health care setting; there is strong resistance to psychiatric consultation; the individual has a long history of treatment with little or no continuity of care. Specialists work with such people with the goal of helping them reduce the psychological need for hospitalization. In severe cases, however, the individual is completely unconscious of the psychological drive for hospitalization and may continue to do whatever is necessary to obtain admission.

Somatization disorder differs from factitious disorder or malingering in that the individual is not intentionally pretending or producing symptoms. Specific DSM-IV criteria must be satisfied in order to warrant this diagnosis. The individual must have a minimum of four different types of pain (e.g., head, back, menstrual, joint), at least two gastrointestinal symptoms other than pain (e.g., nausea), one sexual symptom (e.g., lack of sexual arousal), and one pseudoneurological symptom (e.g., paralysis, weakness, double vision). These symptoms must be present, and either they cannot be fully explained by any known illness or condition or substance abuse or, if a health condition is diagnosed, the individual's symptoms clearly exceed what would be expected. Eisendrath recommends that practitioners arrange for the individual to see one provider rather than the usual different provider for each symptom, avoid invasive procedures, and schedule regular visits so that the individual need not use symptoms as a way of maintaining a relationship with the practitioner.

Gender, Culture, and Pain

Gender Issues

When pain is not associated with a physical condition or a mental disorder, other factors may be considered. Regardless of the actual experience of pain, the expression of pain is influenced by many psychosocial factors. Two of the most important are gender and culture. There has been extensive research and social debate on the observed differences in practitioners' responses to the expression of pain by men versus women. Consistently, male expressions of pain are taken more seriously than female expressions of pain (Vallerand, 1995).

According to Vallerand, women's reports of physical pain are more likely to be suspected and treated less aggressively, so much so that being a woman is a predictor of poor pain management. Regardless of the type of pain being expressed or the individual variations in female tolerance for and expression of physical pain, a primary assumption of Western culture is that women do not tolerate pain as well as men do, and therefore a man's expression of pain signals a higher level of more intense pain and is thus more important and valid. This cultural bias is so strong that even in studies of cancer pain, female expressions of pain are not taken as seriously as male expressions of pain. It should also be noted that men who experience pain are more likely than women to become angry, hostile, or aggressive, and these behaviors can contribute to the cultural bias of responding more to male expressions of physical pain (Fernandez and Turk, 1995).

Cultural Issues

The experience and expression of physical pain is also subject to cultural norms and biases. Traditional expressions of physical pain vary across ethnic groups so that, just as with any other learned behavior, differences can be expected. In their study of more than 350 Caucasian, Hispanic, Irish, Italian, Polish, and French-Canadian adults with chronic pain, Bates et al, (1993) found that ethnic identity predicted locus of control style (internal or external) and that locus of control style and age predicted reports of pain intensity. The researchers concluded that individuals followed their cultural norms in their expression of pain and in their response to pain. Ethnic differences in the meaning or importance of physical pain were also observed.

Because support is also culturally defined and the type of support that is available will vary across ethnic groups, it is reasonable to assume that an individual's request for support in coping with pain may be highly appropriate within one's cultural group. For example, if an individual has learned to request sympathy from others when experiencing pain, that individual's expression of pain will match the desired support resource, in this case sympathy, as defined within that cultural group. Both the desired resource (sympathy) and the expression of pain as a request for that resource are learned cultural norms. However, outside of the individual's cultural group, the very same expression of pain that is intended to solicit sympathy might produce just the opposite response. Ethnic and cultural minorities who seek health care in settings that are culturally incompetent may find that their expressions of pain are not recognized, understood, or responded to, and, like women, their expressions of pain may be suspected.

Mood and Pain

Pain and Anger

Anger has been studied in relation to pain, as a complicating factor in both the experience and the expression of pain. Fernandez and Turk (1995) recommend that anger be viewed as one of the three emotional components of chronic pain, the other two being depression and anxiety. They define anger, a phenomenon that is separate from hostility or aggression, as negative consequences for the self that can be attributed to or blamed on external factors (e.g., an auto accident). Aside from anger related to the experience of physical pain, the researchers point out, the individual's basic anger style, established before the development of chronic pain, is an often overlooked but important influence. Individuals with state versus trait anger, suppressed versus expressed anger, or passive-aggressive anger may differ significantly in their expressions of pain-related anger. These variations notwithstanding, anger is a common experience of chronic pain patients, and it can have severe negative effects on the individual's psychosocial functioning and well-being.

Fernandez and Turk's (1995) review of recent pain-related anger research led them to conclude that anger may be a response to negative stimuli of which the individual may not always be consciously aware. This conclusion was based on the findings of studies of noxious physiological stimuli and anger responses, such as inclement weather, foul odors, or snoring. In their model of anger and pain, Fernandez and Turk view the regulation of pain as vital to restoring biopsychosocial functioning. Expressed anger related to chronic pain can have a negative impact on interpersonal interactions, including those with health care providers, and it is correlated with poor health habits (e.g., alcohol abuse) and poor treatment compliance. Suppressed anger, on the other hand, may create physiological responses that in turn exacerbate pain, leading to yet more anger and increasing the risk of severe depression and physical illness (e.g., hypertension).

Pain and Depression

Most individuals living with chronic pain experience depressed mood, and a significant proportion may develop a depression disorder, such as adjustment disorder, or depressive symptoms that are secondary to chronic pain (Estlander, Takala, Verkasalo, 1995). Many individuals with depression related to chronic pain may express anger as a primary symptom or they may strive to deny all emotional components of their pain (Cassem, 1991). In theory, the relationship between pain and depression seems to be self-reinforcing. Cairns et al,(1996) conducted a study of pain and depression in patients with acute traumatic spinal cord injury and concluded that changes in pain predicted changes in depression over time. A reduction in pain had a greater effect on reducing depression than vice versa. However, moderate to high depression symptom levels can interfere with the expression of and relief from pain. When an individual experiences both pain and depression, improvement in mood often follows rehabilitation treatment for pain. This improvement may be the result of pain management, improved functioning, or both. When pain persists, depression may deepen, with increasing risk of hopelessness and spiritual distress.

Pain and Anxiety

Anxiety occurs in 30% of patients with chronic pain and is usually manifested as generalized anxiety or panic anxiety, whereas 60% have comorbid psychiatric disorders, most commonly depression, alcohol abuse, or substance abuse (Cassem, 1991). Anxiety is usually the result of disruption in important relationships, bodily functions, or sense of self. Fernandez and Turk (1995) found that mild pain was associated with both anger and anxiety, but extreme pain was associated with anxiety only. Stressful life events that ordinarily cause anxious feelings can reduce or compromise the individual's capacity to tolerate pain (Craig, 1994). Major negative life events, such as the death of a loved one, or loss of position, and daily hassles are associated with higher levels of pain.

Anxiety may be closely related to the experience of physical pain due to the interaction between the physiology of anxiety and the physiology of pain. In some cases anxiety can produce pain.

The prolonged muscle tension associated with anxiety may trigger other points of pain and induce vasoconstriction that can intensify pain. Relaxation training has been used to demonstrate the importance and benefit of interrupting the feedback loop between anxiety and physical pain.

Pain and Relationship Conflict

Chronic pain implies that the individual must adjust to living with the experience of physical pain. When this is the case, those around the individual must also adjust. Without an absolute diagnosis, and with interpersonal differences in pain tolerance or in the expression of pain, chronic pain can quickly become a major source of conflict within important interpersonal relationships. Spiritual distress and a loss of faith and trust in health care providers and significant others can lead to anxiety and depression that further taxes the relationship. At the same time, family members and other loved ones may feel helpless and manipulated when there is no improvement in the ability to regulate pain.

New coping skills may be needed if the relationship or the family is to grow and maintain itself, and the family will look to the practitioner for assistance in this area (Rowat, Jeans and LeFort, 1994). Within close family groups, members may be hypersensitive to expressions of both positive and negative moods, so that expressions of pain may be misinterpreted as signals related to other feelings or problems within the relationship or family, such as longstanding feelings of helplessness or fears of abandonment. Living with a person who has chronic pain can mean being forced to give up enjoyable activities or change the routines and structure in one's life in order to accommodate the needs of the individual with pain, quickly paving the way for both expressed and suppressed anger, hostility, and aggression.

When normal and pleasant activities are set aside and the individual's pain becomes the center of the family or the focus of every interaction, then avoidance, rejection, regression, and blame can begin to define the family group or relationship. Under these circumstances the family or relationship is not an effective resource for anyone, either the individual with pain or the significant others. The family or relationship may be divided by accusations of manipulation and abandonment. Individuals who must give up important social roles due to chronic pain can place a considerable strain on others. For example, the adult who no longer works may need more assistance and thus be looked upon as an unfair source of problems for others. Relationships, households, and families that were in distress prior to the individual developing a chronic pain condition are particularly vulnerable to the negative interpersonal effects of chronic pain.

Chronic Pain in Children

In children chronic pain, such as severe headaches or recurrent abdominal pain, is generally seen after the age of 5 (Goldberg and Gabriel, 1991). Three episodes of incapacitating pain over not less than 3 months indicate a need for aggressive intervention. The prognosis improves significantly if treatment produces improvement within 6 months. Children who are at risk are those with a genetic predisposition or hypersensitivity to pain stimuli, those who live in an environment in which physical symptoms are used to expressed distress, and those whose emotions are disallowed and must be suppressed.

Recurrent abdominal pain is a classic childhood physical reaction to emotional stress that typically turns out to be an established pattern in the child's household. Children with chronic pain may have a parent or a sibling who has a severe mental illness (SMI) or chronic disorder, the most common of which are parental depression or alcohol abuse. A number of family problems have been associated with children's chronic pain. These problems include parental conflict or violence, parental preoccupation with physical illness, parental absence, school problems, inconsistent or ineffective responses to the child's expression of aggressive, hostile, or sexual feelings, and negative parent-child relationships.

Pain and HIV Disease

Pain management protocols for providing comfort have been well defined and, in other than critical cases, are highly effective (Storey, 1996). Hospice organizations have been very successful in offering both physical and emotional pain management. Meeting the complex pain management, emotional support, and psychosocial needs of individuals with HIV and AIDS has become the focus of a great deal of research. Breitbart (1996) states that "pain in AIDS is highly prevalent, dramatically undertreated, and has a significant impact on functioning and quality of life (p. 20)."

Although there are many parallels between the needs of individuals with cancer and those with HIV and AIDS, the former group is not subject to the same stigma and painful social rejection. When the meaning of pain associated with HIV and AIDS is assumed to be somehow different from another life-threatening condition, the individual can be vulnerable to significant depression, anxiety, and spiritual distress. Those who view their pain as a signal of the disease's progression report more severe pain than those who do not view it this way (Breitbart, 1996). More pain is associated with more depression, which in turn can lead to more perceived pain. This feedback between pain and depression can increase the risk of substance abuse and other self-harm behaviors. Individuals who are most vulnerable to these negative cumulative effects are women, individuals with less education, and injection drug abusers.

Individuals with HIV or AIDS are vulnerable to undertreatment of their pain as a result of wishing to avoid negative encounters with health care providers. Women with children may be concerned that a visit to a health care setting will lead to someone questioning whether they are able to provide a safe home for their children. Practitioner barriers to adequate pain management can be identified for any number of patient population groups, but individuals with HIV or AIDS may be more vulnerable and more sensitive to prejudice and concerns about rejection. Adequate pain management should be viewed as necessary treatment, particularly for the long-term benefits in protecting the individual from depression, anxiety, and anger.

Management of Psychosocial Problems Related to Pain

1. Chronic pain should not be referred to as psychological pain. Although psychological factors may play a role, this does not diminish either the quality or the quantity

of pain that patient endures. Active measures to decrease pain are required.

2. In addition to medications, management should include relaxation techniques and education. Alternative techniques, such as transcutaneous nerve stimulation and massage, should also be considered.
3. The goal of pain management may not be immediate improvement or full relief; therefore a long-term approach is required, with reassurances that the individual will not be abandoned or rejected if he or she "fails" to become pain free.
4. Practitioners, as well as the individual in treatment, should strive to maintain hope.

Counseling

The two counseling skills needed for working with individuals with pain are talking and listening. Individuals with severe psychological symptomatology or extremely poor interpersonal skills may require specialized counseling. However, the individual who is very angry or anxious as a result of unmanaged pain may not need specialized care but instead may need reassurance and more time to talk. Individuals with chronic pain will more than likely have suffered a great deal of damage to their self-esteem and may have developed spiritual distress. Initially the practitioner may be a target of rage, but usually when the individual's fears of rejection are not realized, the anger dissipates. It is always helpful to encourage the individual to talk about difficult interpersonal problems related to the pain and to learn how these interactions correlate with the individual's experience of pain.

Individuals who reveal fantasies of unrealistic expectations of being rescued should be encouraged to adopt a more realistic attitude toward their pain and toward their health care. Some individuals, for cultural or gender reasons, may have ways of expressing their experience of pain that are not helpful and, without giving the impression that the individual has done something wrong, an agreement on more suitable expressions should be made. It is also important to allow the individual to engage in expressions of anger and anxiety that are appropriate for the setting.

High levels of self-awareness can be very helpful as the individual begins to learn to manage the pain. This single goal can make a great deal of difference in the long-term effectiveness of pain management counseling. Individuals who are unaware of changes in their thoughts, feelings, and behaviors are more likely to act after the fact, or after pain has become so intolerable that a great deal of effort is required to regain a measure of pain control. Individuals must be fully aware of their role in the management of their pain and, without exception, this must be as active a role as possible.

In cases where family strain has developed as a result of being unable to effectively cope with the individual's needs, the family should be referred for family therapy. Family therapy will be needed, rather than family counseling, because longstanding interpersonal conflicts are likely to be revealed and will require more time than is normally available in primary care.

Finally, direct communication of pain, rather than changes in mood or behavior that hint at changes in pain, should be established as a fundamental expectation of treatment. Individuals may require assistance in coming up with a system for describing the nature, intensity, and duration of their pain that accurately conveys their experiences. Self-recording of daily activities allows the patient to set realistic daily goals that incorporate the steps of pain management.

References

Bates M, Edwards W, Anderson K: Ethnocultural influences on variation in chronic pain perception, *Pain* 52:101, 1993.

Benoliel J: Multiple meanings of pain and complexities of pain management, *Nursing Clinics of North Am* 30(4):583, 1995.

Breitbart W: Pain management and psychosocial issues in HIV and AIDS, *Am J of Hospice and Palliative Care* 1:20, 1996.

Cairns D, Adkins R, Scott MD: Pain and depression in acute traumatic spinal cord injuring: origins of chronic problematic pain, *Arch Physical Med Rehab* 77(4):329, 1996.

Cassem N: *Massachusetts General Hospital Handbook of General Hospital Psychiatry,* 3rd Edition, St. Louis, 1991, Mosby.

Craig KD: Emotional aspects of pain. In Wall P, Melzack R (editors): *Textbook of Pain,* 3rd Edition, London, 1994, Churchill Livingstone.

Eisendrath S: Psychiatric aspects of chronic pain, *Neurology* 45(12 suppl 9):S26, 1995.

Estlander A, Takala E, Verkasalo M: Assessment of depression in chronic musculoskeletal pain patients, *Clin J of Pain* 11(3):194, 1995.

Fernandez E, Turk D: The scope and significance of anger in the experience of chronic pain, *Pain* 61(2):165, 1995.

Goldberg IS, Gabriel HP: Recurrent nonorganic abdominal pain: current concepts. In Lewis M (editor): *Child and adolescent psychiatry*, Baltimore, 1991, Williams and Wilkins.

Goldman H: *Review of General Psychiatry,* 4th Edition, East Norwalk, 1995, Appleton and Lange.

Portenoy RK: Chronic pain management. In Stoudemire A, Fogel B (editors): *Psychiatric care of the medical patient*, New York, 1993, Oxford University Press.

Rowat KM, Jeans, ME, LeFort SM: A collaborative model of care: patients, family, and health professional. In Wall P, Melzack R (editors): *Textbook of Pain,* 3rd Edition, London, 1994, Church Livingstone.

Storey P: The vision of hospice and total pain relief, *Am J of Hospice and Palliative Care* 1:40, 1996.

Wall P, Melzack R (editors): *Textbook of Pain,* 3rd Edition, London, 1994, Church Livingstone.

Vallerand A: Gender differences in pain, *Image: J of Nursing Scholarship* 27(3):235, 1995.

Psychosocial Problems Related to Spirituality 13

This chapter presents some of the current thinking on spirituality, health, and the practitioner's role in helping individuals who are in spiritual distress. When science became the source of answers to many questions that had long troubled society, it also became easier to focus on the body and the mind than the soul or the spirit. The body's anatomy and physiology could be scientifically observed and tested, and the workings of the mind, like the anatomy and physiology of the brain, continue to be discovered. But the soul, once considered a person's most valuable possession, does not submit easily to the rules of laboratory science; it therefore has been all but ignored in the science and practice of health care. The intention here is to discuss aspects of spirituality that practitioners may find useful to consider when they encounter a person who is experiencing the common and disabling condition once known as "soul sickness," or in modern terms, a person with a broken spirit.

Spirituality

In everyday life, spirituality is hope that is attached or anchored to a positive force and is thus a source of support. The *Diagnostic and Statistical Manual of Mental Disorders, fourth edition* (DSM-IV), includes a diagnosis of religious or spiritual problem as a category of focus of clinical attention unrelated to mental disorder (Lukoff et al, 1995). Most expert definitions of spirituality distinguish it from religion and identify potential psychosocial problems related to spiritual distress. ***Spirituality*** has been defined as a transcendent relationship between a person and a higher being that goes beyond religious affiliation; it is a universal experience rather than a universal theology (Turner et al, 1995).

These researchers define ***religion*** as an adherence to the beliefs and practices of an organized church or institution.

Many experts cite dictionary definitions of spirituality, such as attitudes, beliefs, and practices that animate people's lives and give dimension to the human experiences of identity, purpose, and meaning (Gelo, 1995). Gelo expands this definition of spirituality to include spiritual growth as a development process, with the view that individuals must strive to reach emotional, psychological, and spiritual maturity. Experts who do not distinguish spirituality from religion define religion as an aspect of spirituality. For example, Mickley and Carson (1995) define spirituality as a belief in and a relationship with a higher power and an aspect of life that gives purpose, meaning, and direction, with religion considered a part of this.

The most comprehensive definition of spirituality is the definition most commonly used in relation to health and health care. Citing Rentzky (1979), Ross (1994) defines spirituality as a need to find meaning, purpose, and fulfillment in life, suffering, and death; a need for the hope and will to live; and a need to believe in and have faith in oneself, others, and God or a positive force. As suggested by these definitions, spirituality is an important resource that impacts all aspects of an individual's health, well-being, and psychosocial functioning.

When an individual experiences spiritual distress, it can be said that the basis of his or her hope has somehow been shaken or threatened and therefore does not provide needed support. Health care providers routinely assess and intervene to help individuals who are experiencing spiritual distress. When a formal religion is the basis of the individual's spirituality, suitable arrangements can be made to accommodate that individual's religious requirements, thereby supporting his or her need for meaning, purpose, and fulfillment. When religion is not the basis of the individual's spirituality, or when the individual's spirituality cannot be excluded from his or her illness (e.g., cancer) or health care experience (e.g., surgery), practitioner support is invaluable.

Experts in the study of religious and spiritual problems draw clear distinctions between the two experiences. ***Religious problems*** directly correspond to a specific aspect of the individual's religious beliefs or practices. Common religious problems are a change in church membership or conversion to a new religion, intensification of religious beliefs and practices, loss of or questioning one's religious faith, guilt caused by failure to keep prescribed religious tenets, and membership in a destructive cult (Turner et al, 1995). ***Spiritual problems*** are related to universal experiences, including health and illness.

For example Turner et al, (1995) defines a spiritual problem as one that causes a person to question that which had been accepted and valued. Widely accepted spiritual problems are mystical experiences, near-death experiences, spiritual transformation experiences, negative meditation experiences, separation from a spiritual teacher, serious or terminal illness, and addiction (Lukoff et al, 1995; Turner et al, 1995). In short, psychosocial problems and illness impact the mind, the body, and the spirit, and for some individuals, healing results from health care that addresses each of these spheres.

Assessment of Problems

This section is a brief review of some of the universal pathways to spiritual distress. Many factors determine whether or not an individual who is faced with one or more of these problems will actually experience spiritual distress. Those who do experience distress will differ in the nature of their distress and their need for spiritual comfort or spiritual care. Each of the following problem experiences share a single basic characteristic: each negates that which the individual had accepted as positive or true and which therefore served as a basis for meaning, purpose, and fulfillment in that individual's life. When faced with such problems, effective coping may mean that the individual must redefine his or her spirituality, a process that may force the individual to search for new meaning, purpose, or fulfillment, thereby precipitating spiritual distress (Carr, 1995).

Loss

Although a tenet of common wisdom states that there are no possessions that one can have that cannot be lost (including life), loss is one of the most shocking and disturbing life events that can lead to spiritual distress. ***Actual loss*** implies that the individual was once in possession of what was lost, whereas ***perceived loss*** does not. Common losses include loved ones (due to death or separation), possessions, important social roles, and a hoped-for future. Individuals gain a great deal of meaning and fulfillment from life by surrounding themselves with people and things that define who they are and what their lives are about. To suddenly be without one's partner, home, or job, or to no longer be able to look forward to graduating from college, for example, are losses that can be spiritually weakening.

Although it is a fact of life that good things happen to bad people and bad things happen to good people, the initial reaction to loss is to question its fairness or rightness. Most people have a gut reaction of "Why me?" Perhaps as a long-term effect of childhood, it is not uncommon for an individual to react to a painful loss by asserting that he or she has done nothing to deserve this. These reactions suggest that the individual feels compelled to make sense out of the event, as if by making sense of the loss the individual will feel less vulnerable. This cause-and-effect premise to coping with loss is very culture-bound, for many of the world's ancient cultures do not subscribe to the belief that humans are capable of explaining life.

Nevertheless, most people are able to find a way to understand the loss and incorporate that experience into their reality. Those who are unable to do so can become highly distressed and begin to question their values, or they may devalue important relationships and possessions in fearful anticipation of future loss. Individuals who have suffered a loss need time to talk about it. They will need to continue talking about it until they are able to assign meaning and purpose to the loss and then incorporate this information into their personal reality.

Disruption

Even the most disorganized life can be disrupted. People build structure into their everyday lives, and this structure literally supports their day-to-day functioning. Events that disrupt or remove the structure from a person's life, such as a change in residence or employment, can be unsettling. ***Disruption*** suggests that the individual is able to reorganize, unlike loss, which assumes that the individual cannot regain what was lost. Disruption does not imply destruction, an experience that would most likely include loss.

Individual coping style and character are large determinants of how distressed an individual will become when his or her life is disrupted. Those who are intolerant of change will be more distressed than those who are more accustomed to change.

Crisis in Beliefs or Values

Individuals rely a great deal on their beliefs and values, although many people may be only semiaware of them or of their need for them. ***Crisis*** implies that the individual has developed painful doubt. The more important the belief or value that is now doubted, the more distress the individual is likely to experience. The source of the doubt is also important. For example, an individual who believes in and values fidelity learns that his or her partner has broken this commitment. This experience could cause the person who placed great value on the commitment to have an extreme crisis in belief.

Meaningless Destruction

At first glance ***meaningless destruction*** seems to be an odd concept, implying that destruction can or should be meaningful. Humans react to overwhelming destruction, usually the result of disasters such as fire or flood, by trying to assign meaning to the event. Destructive human acts, such as arson or a bomb explosion, immediately cause people to wonder why. Most of the people who ask this question will assume that there was something mentally or morally wrong with the individual who committed the act. The more difficult task is to try to understand the disaster and all of its consequences, including loss. It is not so much a matter of actually coming up with an accurate explanation of destruction, but more a matter of trying to classify the experience within one's understanding of reality. Was it bad luck, revenge, punishment? How the individual answers this question can determine how vulnerable one feels under the circumstances and thus the level of distress that will be experienced.

Loss of Self-Esteem

It is difficult if not impossible to believe in or value much of anything if one does not believe in or value oneself. Maintaining adequate levels of self-esteem can often be extremely difficult. Any event or experience can trigger anger at oneself that may lead to a lowered opinion of oneself. Low self-esteem has been associated with numerous self-harm behaviors, including substance abuse and violence. Low self-esteem is one of the most powerful loss events in life. Children like themselves and enjoy being who they are. Painful life experiences, such as prejudice or poverty, can lead to a child's first major loss, the loss of self-esteem. Adults routinely struggle to maintain their self-esteem within their work, academic, and social relationships. Because loss of self-esteem is such a powerful experience, it is often viewed as a symptom of a disorder, such as depression.

Victimization

Being assaulted or in any way harmed by another person is always shocking. Some victims have this reaction instantly, whereas others may not feel the shock for months. Being victimized can also seem to be a failure, and many individuals become totally focused on what they could have done to have avoided the painful experience. When they find that there is nothing they could have done—or worse yet, if they think they could have acted to prevent being victimized—feelings of guilt and self-hate can develop. In effect, an individual can become a victim of oneself by attacking one's own actions. Thoughts and feelings such as these are painful enough, but often the individual begins to view the world differently than before, such as seeing it as a dangerous place and spending a great deal of energy preparing oneself for the "next time."

Isolation

Isolation is disorienting because external stimulation from interaction with others or within other environments shapes and influences how the individual views oneself and the world. Always being alone with one's thoughts and feelings, having to meet one's own needs, and similar experiences can undermine both self-concept and self-esteem. At some point, if not routinely, the individual who is isolated tries to make sense of this experience, and the more isolated an individual is, the more important social relationships seem to become. It is not uncommon for individuals who have been isolated for long periods of time to become hypersensitive to interpersonal interactions. Although it is a temporary response, the individual may misinterpret this reaction as proof that he or she is isolated for legitimate reasons. Although the individual is not always likely to come to this conclusion, the psychological experience of long-term isolation is to feel forsaken or abandoned.

Fear or Uncertainty

Psychological survival requires that individuals maintain little or no awareness of their fears in order to go about their daily life with feelings of certainty about events yet to unfold. Passengers on a plane or in a car concentrate on their plans at their destination, which effectively reduces the awareness of their fears of being in a fatal accident. Awareness of severe fear or uncertainty can impair functioning, but equally important, fear and uncertainty interfere with the ability to experience the little joys that give meaning to life.

Lack of Faith or Trust in Health Care

Faith and trust are two vital elements of good health care. In just a few decades society has shifted from having high levels of faith and trust in doctors and hospitals to an almost adversarial patient-provider relationship. Corporate health care, like any other industry, is highly concerned with product management, and being a successful health care consumer requires a great deal of individual effort. The results of this transformation include complex consent forms that are designed to protect providers, increasingly high malpractice insurance rates, and a growing number of lawyers who specialize in health-related malpractice litigation. Most people still have faith and trust in their health care providers, but their faith and trust tends to be more easily shaken. Some people have opted to place all their faith and trust in health care technology, so that simple health care procedures are suspect. This is just the opposite of what people believed decades ago, when "less" was thought to be better. The benefit of the current trend is that it is not unusual, for example, for patients seeing a provider to have highly technical information about their condition. The negative aspect is that health care is still an interpersonal interaction, and the depersonalization of providers or patients undermines faith and trust.

Severe or Life-Threatening Illness

Severe or life-threatening illness takes away or changes the meaning of everything. A beloved garden, a favorite sweater, and a good friend all have value to the individual, but illness can change the value of life and of all of the experiences that define the meaning of one's life. In a very real sense illness takes away one's life by forcing the individual to focus on survival. For example, a family with a seriously ill child may have to decide whether to put every resource at their command toward finding health care that may save the child. To struggle for survival changes the meaning and definition of life. Most important, the individual is forced into a full awareness of thoughts and feelings that are normally set aside, such as questions about the value and purpose of one's life.These are extremely difficult questions to ask or to answer. Those who found purpose in their lives while healthy are not necessarily better able to deal with these very upsetting questions.

Assessment of Spirituality

The beneficial interpersonal interactions of listening, compassion, and empathy form the ideal context for the assessment of spirituality and potential spirituality problems. Practitioners must provide this context for the individual, since as a result of spiritual distress the individual is likely to seem unmotivated, disappointed, uninterested, angry, scared, or worried and may directly or indirectly express strong feelings of hopelessness to the practitioner (Younger, 1995). An individual in this state of distress may challenge the practitioner's interpersonal skills or question his or her sincerity. Practitioners should keep in mind that an individual in spiritual distress who challenges and questions a practitioner may only be projecting his or her own internal spiritual challenges and questions. In asking such individuals if the challenges and questions being expressed are those that they themselves are experiencing, the answer obtained is often "yes."

Fleischman (1993) states that the healing spirit has immediate value to health care in that it facilitates listening to, understanding, and empathizing with individuals of diverse cultural backgrounds. In effect, by supporting the individual's need for spiritual comfort and strength, the practitioner promotes healing by empowering the healing nexus of mind-body-spirit (McSherry, 1996; Mornhinwig and Voigner, 1996; Wooten, 1996). The practitioner helps the individual to utilize his or her personal resources, which include people, particularly confidants, and reading materials that can lend strength to an individual in need. In so doing, practitioners can help individuals to take more control over their coping efforts and to search for meaning, purpose, and fulfillment in life regardless of actual health status.

Valuing the quality of one's life does not negate the basic human desire for a long life, but spiritual comfort comes from the value that one gives to life rather than the amount of time that one lives. This form of comfort is directly challenged by the painful losses that are associated with any serious illness, whether acute or chronic, physical or mental. Although no one can truly share the suffering of another, lonely suffering is unbearable and undermines the individual's search for meaning (Carr, 1995).

Maugans' (1996) spiritual history is a brief, uncomplicated approach to assessment that can provide practitioners with a clear understanding of a given individual's interest in and need for spiritual care or comfort. This assessment assumes that spirituality is the individual's system of beliefs regarding that which is intangible but which gives meaning to life events. The assessment identifies five topics that practitioners can invite the individual to discuss:

1. Spiritual belief system
2. Personal spirituality
3. Integration with a spiritual community

4. Ritualized practices and restrictions
   Implications for health care
5. Terminal events planning

In this assessment, spiritual belief system and personal spirituality refer to the individual's formal and personal spiritual and/or religious affiliations, practices, and beliefs. For example, an individual may identify as a Christian and may have developed a personal system of Christian practices and beliefs. Integration with a spiritual community refers to membership within a formal religious group, church, or spiritual family. Ritualized practices and restrictions are proscribed or personal activities that can be said to be the practice of one's spirituality or religion, such as prayer, meditation, or song. Implications for health care are any and all spiritual or religious beliefs and practices that are significant for the individual's health, health care, or death; for example, an individual who for spiritual/religious reasons does not wish to receive or donate body organs, who follows strict dietary rules, or who receives a visit from a member of the clergy immediately before and after surgery.

Health-related spiritual and religious practices have been incorporated in many health care settings for some time, and terminal planning, such as whether the individual wishes to use life support technology, is also an established practice. The content of the spiritual history is not complicated or excessive and may be accomplished in a single interview or over a period of time. However, the process of the assessment can become a very important spiritual intervention when, as a result, the individual is successful in formulating and expressing his or her spiritual needs, and those needs are validated by the health care provider.

Spiritual Care and Spiritual Comfort

Spiritual care and spiritual comfort should focus on the health condition, illness, or psychosocial problem with which the individual is striving to cope. Practitioners are not expected to replace spiritual or religious specialists who address the individual's general spiritual needs. The terms ***care*** and ***comfort*** are used here to suggest a meaningful clinical distinction between the two levels of intervention. In essence, many patients may be better able to cope with a health condition, illness, or psychosocial problem when they are provided with basic spiritual comfort or they have their spirits lifted. Those who are in severe spiritual distress may need spiritual care aimed at helping them to achieve spiritual healing or relief from spiritual distress. Spiritual care becomes important when the individual's spiritual distress has had a negative impact on one's ability to cope.

The impact of spirituality on health is in partly determined by the individual's spiritual orientation, most commonly defined as either extrinsic or intrinsic (Mickley et al, 1995). ***Extrinsic*** orientation implies that spirituality is a means to an end, such as safety, status, or power. ***Intrinsic*** orientation implies a constitutional spirituality. These researchers note that the negative connotation of extrinsic orientation has led to a debate about the value of making such a distinction. The distinction is helpful as long as practitioners refrain from judging a person's spiritual orientation and view the individual's spirituality as a positive source of support for him or her. Understanding the individual's orientation can help practitioners to understand the individual's spiritual distress as a first step of spiritual care.

Citing Pargament (1988), and Mickley et al, (1995) summarize three basic ways in which a positive spiritual force or God can influence individual coping style: self-directed, deferring, and collaborative. The ***self-directed*** individual views coping as a personal responsibility that requires personal action, which is in turn supported by a spiritual force. The ***deferring*** individual relies on a spiritual force as a coping solution without the requirement of personal responsibility or personal action. The individual who has a ***collaborative*** coping style shares responsibility and action with a spiritual force. When personal responsibility and personal action are vital elements of effective coping with a health condition, illness, or psychosocial problem, the deferring individual may be more vulnerable to distress than a person with a more active spiritual coping style.

The process of providing spiritual care for individuals who are coping with an illness follows the same process of all health interventions: assessment and identification of the individual's spiritual needs, planning, implementation, and outcome evaluation (Ross, 1994). In a study of nurses' perceptions of patients' spiritual needs, Ross found that the top three patient needs identified by nurses were (1) the need for belief and faith, (2) the need for peace and comfort, and (3) the need to give and receive love and forgiveness. The researcher identified four factors that significantly influenced the provision of spiritual care: the patient, other professionals, the environment, and the nurse. In this study, patients who had trouble communicating or who could not communicate at all were less likely to receive spiritual care; if spiritual or religious specialists were not available, nurses were less likely to attempt spiritual care. If the work environment was extremely stressful, understaffed, dominated by physical care practices, or without an available quiet and private area, providing spiritual care was extremely difficult. Perhaps the most revealing finding of the study was that nurses who had themselves experienced a crisis that became a force for personal growth were more likely to address the spiritual well-being of their patients than nurses who had not had such an experience.

Individuals who have themselves experienced spiritual distress may be more likely to recognize this condition and therefore more likely to intervene. The practice of spiritual care, as with any health care practice, is clearly a matter of experience, resources, time, space, and patient need.

References

Carr W: Spiritual pain and healing in the hospice, *America* 8(12):26, 1995.

Fleischman P: *Spiritual aspects of psychiatric practice*, Cleveland, SC, 1993, Bonne Chance Press.

Gelo F: Spirituality: a vital component of health counseling, *J Am College Health* 44(1):38, 1995.

Lukoff D, Lu F, Turner R: Cultural considerations in the assessment and treatment of religious and spiritual problems, *The Psychiatric Clinics of N Am* 18(3): 467, 1995.

McSherry W: Raising the spirits, *Nursing Practice* 92(3):48, 1996.

Maugans TA: The SPIRITual history, *Arch of Fam Med* 5(1):11, 1996.

Mickley JR, Carson V, Soeken KL: Religion and adult mental health: state of the science in nursing, *Issues in Mental Health Nurs* 16(4):345, 1995.

Mornhinweg GC, Voignier RR: Rest, *Holist Nurs Pract* 10(4):54, 1996.

Pargament K, Kennell J, Hathaway W, Grevengoed N, Newman J, Jones W: Religion and the problem-solving process: three styles of coping, *J for the Scientific Study of Religion*, 27(1):90, 1988.

Renetzky L: The fourth dimension: applications to the social services. In Moberg D (editor) *Spiritual well-being: sociological perspectives*, Washington, 1979, University Press of America.

Ross LA: Spiritual aspects of nursing, *J of Advanced Nursing* 19(3):345, 1994.

Turner RP, Lukoff D, Barnhouse RT, Lu FG: Religious or spiritual problem: a culturally sensitive diagnostic category in the DSM-IV, *J of Nervous and Mental Disease* 183(7):435, 1995.

Wooten P: Humor: an antidote for stress, *Holist Nurs Pract* 10(2):49, 1996.

Younger JB: The alienation of the sufferer, *Adv Nursing Sci* 17(4):53, 1995.

Part IV

Special Populations and Problems

Children 14

The *Diagnostic and Statistical Manual of Mental Disorders, fourth edition*, (DSM-IV) distinguishes between disorders or problems that are first diagnosed in infancy, childhood, or adolescence and disorders that begin in adulthood. However, the trend is to use the same diagnostic criteria for all age groups, with age as a special assessment consideration. This chapter presents basic assessment information for children with attention deficit disorder, separation anxiety, obsessive-compulsive disorder, and mood disorder. Issues related to learning disabilities, difficult temperaments, psychosocial problems, and family dynamics are also discussed. The essential difference between the assessment of children and adults is that the assessment of children requires a great deal of collaboration among practitioners, specialists, parents, and teachers. In addition, because of their young age and dependence on the family, children require counseling and preventive health care aimed at meeting the needs of both the child and the child's family.

Assessment

As noted by Long, Starfield, and Kelleher (1995), childhood mental disorders and psychosocial problems are often not assessed or diagnosed in primary care. Practitioners may instead focus on physical conditions, to the exclusion of mental health and psychosocial concerns, partly because of the complexity of symptom assessment and partly because of some practitioner's lack of confidence in the efficacy of childhood mental health treatments. When practitioners encounter evidence of both mental and physical problems they may, with good reason, focus on the child's physical problem as the mandatory primary care problem; the mental problem may be viewed as secondary. Mental health problems are also less likely to be assessed in children in primary care if the language of assessment does not seem useful, is too general, or seems to require detailed information that is not readily available. Despite these practice problems, the importance of psychiatric primary care assessment and counseling for children cannot be overstated (Schneider, 1996). In their community study of the prevalence and incidence of childhood mental health problems, Riley and Wissow (1995) found that 18% to 20% of the children that were seen had a diagnosable mental disorder, and about 11% of the children had symptoms severe enough to warrant treatment. Unrecognized and untreated mental health problems place children at immediate risk for acute problems and also increase the risk of adolescent and adult onset disorders and problems. Practitioners play a vital role in the early detection and timely treatment of childhood disorders.

As children develop physically, cognitively, socially, and emotionally, changes in their moods, attitudes, and behaviors occur, and these changes can be rapid and extreme. Therefore the mental health assessment of children must be within the limited context of the child's current stage of development, relative to other children of the same age. An apparently standard approach to assessment can sometimes backfire when the comparison group selection is not obvious or realistic or when the child's symptoms are highly unusual. Similarly, practitioners must employ age-appropriate assessment methods (e.g., play, draw) or methods that are appropriate for the child's current behavioral and cognitive functioning. Neurodevelopmental status is also a complicating factor in assessing children. Neurodevelopmental status in a school-age child can account for a broad range of assessment observations regarding the neurologic and cognitive capacities at the time. Neurologic and cognitive development is critical to a child's developing sense of mastery and competency as the child strives to meet new challenges and acquire new skills. Assessment must take into account each child's unique neurodevelopmental status in terms of strengths, weaknesses, and meeting important developmental expectations (e.g., expressive communication skills) and challenges.

Mental disorders and psychosocial problems that develop in childhood are by nature multifactorial, and they may best be revealed by cognitive and developmental testing to assess the child's strengths and possible areas of impairment, loss, or delayed functioning. Dependent children are highly vulnerable to external environmental and psychosocial factors as well as to internal neurodevelopmental changes. Tanner (1995) explains the importance of neurodevelopmental changes as the core of the complaints of parents of children who have experienced neurological trauma or impairment. Physical problems typically associated with neurodevelopmental trauma or impairment in school-age children include congenital disorders, metabolic disorders, toxic intrauterine exposure, neurologic insult, and postnatal toxic exposures. As a result of the trauma or impairment the child may be at risk for developing hearing impairments, seizure disorder, or speech and language delays. These conditions can lead to yet another set of behavioral problems, such as medication side effects from anticonvulsant medications.

Because of the multiple variables involved, primary care practitioners are well positioned to effectively bridge the gap between neurodevelopmental concerns and behavioral or performance problems that may suggest a mental disorder or a psychosocial problem. This approach ensures full consideration of all possible causes of behavioral and developmental problems, from temper outbursts at school to idiosyncratic response to physical illness. Along with neurodevelopmental factors, general health, temperament, family, socioeconomic, cultural, and community factors may all affect a child's behaviors and performance. Without making assessment so complex that the findings reveal little useful information, the aim is to ensure that multiple factors are considered. It is unlikely that any single factor can account for symptoms observed in children, but unless multiple factors are given their full importance, such a conclusion is not uncommon. For example, parental alcoholism is often viewed as a single explanation for a child's separation anxiety. A basic neurodevelopmental assessment includes sensory and motor capacities, speech and language, visual/spatial responses, memory, higher cognitive functioning, social awareness, and behavioral patterns.

Learning Disabilities

Learning disabilities, which are particularly threatening to childhood developmental mastery, are associated with school failure, inadequate personal and social adaptation, impaired adult occupational functioning, and adult low self-esteem. Working with parents and teachers, practitioners can monitor a child's learning progress across a range of cognitive, psychological, and social criteria, with the main objective being the comprehensive assessment of the needs of the child found to be at risk.

Kaplan and Sadock (1995) offer a three-step approach to neurodevelopmental screening and assessment. The first step is a broad overview of what is known about the child in a variety of environments, how the child responds during the assessment, and any neurodevelopmental risk factors that were noted in previous routine health care visits, including problems observed during the assessment. Helpful screening questions for children include: How is school going? What do you like about school? Dislike about school? Do you have a favorite friend? What kind of things do you like to do? Do you play sports or games? Are you a member of team/group activities? Helpful follow-up questions for parents are: Are you satisfied with your child's progress in school, at home, and with same-age friends? How are your child's school grades,—any Ds or Fs? Have you observed any signs of unhappiness, worry, or frustration? How much school has your child missed? Does your child have problems with sleep or appetite? During the assessment, the child can be asked to demonstrate specific learning tasks, such as reading a funny poem or completing an interesting spelling, math, or writing puzzle. More advanced assessments include copying simple geometric forms and drawing a person. Draw-a-person assessment is a powerful method of revealing a great deal of cognitive, visual-spatial, and fine motor abilities as well as offering important clues to any psychosocial stressors with which the child may be coping. Interpretation of a draw-a-person assessment should be performed by a specialist in this area. Evidence of problems in any of these assessment areas indicates a need to continue with the second step of the assessment.

The second step is to talk to the child's teacher or have the teacher complete an assessment questionnaire. Teacher assessment information should be regarded as extremely important, but in cases where neurodevelopmental deficits or a mental disorder is suspected, teacher assessment information is required. Teachers may have records of previous assessment findings, academic performance measures such as grades and class-administered achievement tests, and child evaluations completed by school staff. The objective is to obtain whatever information has previously been collected and to ensure that teachers contribute to the current assessment. When there is little or no previous information or history available, standardized assessment questionnaires for teachers can make this step convenient and easy. Pediatric specialists or specialist school staff will be able to recommend assessment questionnaires that may be suitable.

The third step, if necessary, is to obtain a specialized assessment. Any number of childhood specialists can be of assistance, but in most cases consultation with a child psychologist will be most helpful. Otherwise a specialized assessment can be obtained from a child educational specialist, a child speech and language specialist, a physical or an occupational child therapist, or a child psychotherapist (e.g., nurse clinical specialist, social worker specialist, child psychiatrist). Both the child and the parents should be well informed about what to expect and why the practitioner thinks this additional assessment will be helpful to the child. Among the many types of specialized assessments for children, the most common are assessments for possible abuse or neglect, family violence (adult-adult, adult-child), or severe mental illness (SMI). Many schools now employ or contract with child-assessment specialists in order to comply with public laws that mandate that schools will take the necessary steps to determine if a child requires and is therefore eligible for special education services due to a learning disability.

Difficult Temperament

Children, like adults, have innate character traits that can complicate the already demanding and difficult tasks of child rearing. In terms of SMI and mental disorders, children with difficult temperaments are considered normal but difficult to manage because of their characteristic manner of approaching tasks (e.g., getting dressed). Specialists may refer to a child's temperament as the child's developmental style (Novak, 1996). Temperament is largely constitutional in origin and is affected by a broad range of factors, including genetic make-up, pregnancy and delivery complications, childhood allergies, chronic ear infections, and uneven language and learning skills development. The fact that these conditions are significantly related to difficult temperament suggests that there are important, biological elements of temperament. The following difficult temperament styles, from infancy to childhood, are common (Parker and Zuckerman, 1995).

High activity level: very active, restless, fidgety; easily over-stimulated; impulsive, aggressive, hates confinement.

Distractible: trouble with concentration unless interested; inattentive, tunes out, daydreams, forgets instructions.

High intensity: loud and forceful expression of emotions.

Irregular or unpredictable: uncooperative when tired or hungry; conflicts over meals and bedtime; waking up during the night; changeable or unpredictable moods; good or bad days with no obvious explanation for either.

Negative persistence: becomes stubborn; continues nagging, whining, or trying to negotiate for something; is relentless, will not give up, becomes locked into prolonged tantrums.

Low sensory tolerance: reacts to color, light, sights, textures, noise/sounds, smells, taste, heat, or cold; may have strident and unusual preferences; may be fussy about getting dressed; does not like certain foods because of their appearance, smell, or taste.

Initial shyness: acts reserved with new people; withdraws in new situations; holds back; protests by crying or clinging; may have a tantrum if forced to engage; trouble adapting to any changes in routine.

Negative mood: serious or cranky; doesn't show pleasure openly; does not have a sunny disposition.

Truly difficult children can be hard to understand. Their behavior confuses and upsets even the most experienced parent or teacher, since the normally effective child rearing methods seem to have no impact. Parental discipline usually becomes very inconsistent, with frequent power struggles between parent and child. Excessive punishment and overindulgence of the child are both common. The child can literally dominate the family and household, leaving everyone bewildered, overinvolved, or exhausted. Irrational parental feelings of guilt or of somehow being victimized by the child may develop, because the parents cannot understand why nothing seems to works. At this point parents can become extremely critical of each other, adding to the already high levels of stress and strain in the marriage and the family. Susceptible adults can develop depression, anxiety, or substance disorders in response to the stress. This adds yet another complicating factor to the family dynamics when that parent isolates, avoids, or withdraws, thereby becoming unavailable to the family. Siblings of the child with a difficult temperament can feel neglected when everything always revolves around the difficult child (Kaplan and Sadock, 1995).

The most difficult children consistently have trouble with transition and change and can be extremely strong willed and stubborn. The DSM-IV does not identify difficult temperament as a mental disorder; it only includes difficult temperament as a feature of mental disorder symptomatology. When a child does not meet the DSM-IV diagnostic criteria for a mental disorder and does not appear to have a difficult temperament, the child's behavior can be described in terms of strengths, weaknesses, vulnerabilities, and the impact of these characteristics on the parent-child relationship and the child's family.

Psychosocial Problems

Psychosocial assessment of children covers the range of emotional, behavioral, and psychological problems associated with impaired functioning that do not meet DSM-IV diagnostic criteria for a mental disorder or victim of abuse (Riley and Wissow, 1995). These include the severe psychosocial problems of family violence, family dysfunction, community violence, and poverty. The aim here is to identify children who may be at risk for abuse, neglect, exploitation, or violence. The children who are most at risk are generally young children who live in poverty, have absent or emotionally unavailable parents, or are in transition from elementary to middle school. Children are devastated by family violence whether they are targets or witnesses of it. Sexual and physical abuse, neglect, and exploitation of children are difficult for many adults to understand and cope with, but the impact on children is even greater. Children react to these horrors, but they also struggle to try to answer their own questions about their experiences of humiliation, pain, and fear (Monteleone, 1994). Because children's psychological universe is so much smaller than that of adults, their experience of abuse can take on global proportions, and they can come to believe that they must change in order to survive in such a hostile and dangerous universe. Children may not have full awareness of their coping responses or answers to their own questions, but how they cope (cognitively, psychologically, and behaviorally) can become a significant predictor of long-term adult psychosocial problems and mental disorders. Practitioners may not be in the position to assess a child for abuse. The DSM-IV has a special code for victims of abuse, without giving the child a mental disorder diagnosis per se. When evidence of abuse is observed, a specialist should assess the child immediately. Practitioners should take note of the following psychosocial characteristics as possible indicators that a child has suffered abuse and that an assessment by a specialist is warranted (Monteleone, 1994).

1. Lack of or low trust
2. Low self-esteem
3. Must guess about what is and is not normal
4. Poor interpersonal communication skills
5. Does not enjoy life
6. Aggressive and hyperactive or withdrawn, passive, and overly compliant
7. Apathetic and unresponsive
8. Developmentally delayed
9. Poor decision-making skills
10. Self-defeating with risk of self-injurious behaviors
11. Substance abuse
12. Excessively manipulative
13. Poor self-control and feelings of powerlessness

There continues to be rigorous social debate about when and how to assess children who have suffered abuse. Unfortunately, at the heart of the debate is the question of when adults should believe and act on a child's report of abuse. Standard primary care practice should include some form of screening for maltreatment with all children. Specific child responses to maltreatment include vague but persistent somatic complaints, including abdominal pain and headache, fatigue or weakness, anorexia, and suicidal thoughts (Riley and Wissow, 1995). Aggressive or violent behavior in children can be a response to maltreatment.

Family Issues

Parents and caretakers can provide helpful information about a child's background, including medical history; family history;

prenatal, neonatal, and developmental history; adult perspectives on apparent problems; and a current history of present problems. These adults can provide information on psychosocial stressors with which the family is currently coping, sibling information (including ages and sibling responses to family stressors), and their own responses to the child who is being assessed. Family information should include social-cultural values and behavioral norms. Any and all violence in the family should be noted, including violence among extended family members, adult partners, sibling violence, and other children who may be targets of maltreatment. When both parents are present, family assessment information includes the practitioner's direct observations of the couple's interactions during the assessment.

Family dynamics worth noting include relationship issues, how conflict is handled within the family and between the family and outsiders, and how frustration is expressed and resolved. Families can be assessed in terms of how open, warm, giving, and safe they appear to be. Families that are closed, cold, withholding, and less than safe for children create enormous stress for the child who is dependent on that family. Indicators of potential adult emotional or psychological problems should be noted, particularly in the child's primary caretaker.

A depressed parent is a tremendous psychosocial burden for a child, but this is easy to overlook if the practitioner views the child as the single focus of assessment. What may at first appear to be a child's symptoms of a mental disorder may prove to be the child's response to a depressed caretaker parent or the child's efforts to cope with the caretaker's symptoms, such as negative thinking. Adult conflicts that cause the child to fear being abandoned by the adults involved represents a severe threat to the child. In some cases such children may behave in ways that they believe will protect the adult upon whom they depend.

Family chaos or disorganization that threatens the survival of the family is a critical assessment concern when the child's needs become secondary to the family's struggle for survival. Parents can become so involved in adult problems that they may misinterpret a child's need for reassurance and security as troublemaking. Highly stressed parents can also become truly unaware of their children's feelings, such as anxiety, sadness, anger, or fear. Just the opposite can also occur when highly stressed parents minimize their own problems and maximize the child's problems. Finally, any and all adult substance use should be considered. Adult substance abuse—in terms of money and time spent, physical and mental health losses, unpredictable changes in behavior, and safety dangers—is a major stressor for children. Children can themselves be at increased risk for adolescent and adult substance abuse from observing the substance abuse of important adults. Children can be at immediate risk when the adult becomes impaired as a result of acute intoxication or chronic substance abuse. A depressed or substance-abusing parent can become self-absorbed to the point where the child's needs and responses go unnoticed at home but are apparent to teachers, relatives, and practitioners.

Abusive parents may greatly exaggerate what they believe to be the child's provocative nature. This exaggeration is most apparent when the abusive parent is rationalizing his or her harsh treatment of the child. Usually the same child will have a teacher or child care worker who describes the child as interpersonally engaging but very needy. Conflicting and inconsistent adult reports can actually be helpful in the assessment of children. When the child seems to interact differently in different environments, it may be possible to determine which psychosocial environments are supportive and which are nonsupportive in meeting the child's needs. The assessment of children clearly takes a great deal of time, and no two assessments will be alike in content or process, but assessments based on inadequate information are not helpful and can misrepresent a child's mental health status.

Mental Disorders in Children

Attention Deficit/Hyperactivity Disorder (ADD or ADHD)

Attention deficit disorder (ADD) is actually a group of behavioral symptoms observed in children, adolescents, and adults. The essential symptoms of ADD are short attention span, difficulty sustaining attention, and poor impulse control. Some children with ADD are highly distractible, but some are impulsive rather than distractible. These symptoms can cause mild, moderate, or severe impairment in functioning with significant learning problems. Coleman (1993) describes four major elements of ADD: altered attention, attention span, distractibility and impulse control.

Altered Attention. Attention is the ability to increase concentration while simultaneously disregarding or minimizing unnecessary or unrelated information. Interest and motivation can influence attention. The ability to increase concentration can be improved by external factors, such as individual attention and encouragement from others that fuels interest and motivation. Internal factors, such as personal commitment and determination, can also lead to increased concentration ability. The personal-interest value of an activity is important, since individuals are more likely to pay attention to something that is interesting to them.

Not being able to increase one's attention can be a major turn-off or discouraging after one has tried to focus on something of potential or actual interest. Children with learning disabilities or ADD generally start out interested and motivated to learn, but they lose their interest and motivation when they find they are unable to bring their attention to the task at hand. The combination of experiences is a source of tremendous frustration for the child, family, and teachers. Confusion, failure, and unpredictable results accelerate the process, leading to still greater discouragement and frustration. Children with ADD have trouble filtering information, both internal and external, so that sounds in a room or ideas that suddenly come to mind may take over their attention. They might not be able to attend to the cues to which they are supposed to respond, and they can have problems absorbing and remembering important information. Attention requires vigilance that allows the individual to renew one's concentration when distractions occur.

Attention Span. Attention span is an individual's ability to intentionally sustain attention for significant periods of time across a range of situations and various amounts and types of material content. Impairment implies that the individual is susceptible to distraction or is unable to place one's full attention or prolonged attention on an activity. The exception appears to be activities that constantly provide new information that re-establishes the individual's attention (e.g., computer games).

Distractibility. The type or amount of alternative stimulation that is needed to draw an individual's attention away from one focus and on to another is the individual's level of distractibility. Someone who is highly distractible has little to no ability to concentrate on a focus when faced with alternative or additional information. Individuals who are distractible can also have difficulty bringing their attention to focus on a single activity that has many elements, such as a complex set of instructions.

Impulse Control. Impulses can be viewed as ever-present urges to act that individuals learn to control or delay so that they do not act automatically or on impulse. Poor impulse control therefore implies that the individual tends to act on impulse or act automatically. Since acting without forethought implies that the consequences of the act are not fully considered in advance, unanticipated consequences usually follow impulsive acts. The individual may end up in one unexpected situation after another and be clueless as to how to next proceed. When asked to explain the behavior, the individual may be unable to do so. Being unable to explain or understand one's actions, tends to be the first consequence of acting on impulse, for children as well as adults. The more primitive the impulse, the more extraordinary the behavior and its consequences tend to be—for example, aggressive or sexual impulses.

Hyperactivity

Hyperactive children have trouble regulating their activity levels and engage in a great deal of aimless, purposeless, nonstop actions. Because hyperactivity is not always present with ADD, the diagnosis for this condition is specifically stated as attention deficit-hyperactivity disorder (ADHD). Children can outgrow hyperactivity symptoms but may continue to experience attention deficits well into adolescence and adulthood.

Parents, teachers, and providers who work with a child who has ADHD may find it difficult to understand that the symptoms of this disorder occur every day, every week, and every year and invade multiple areas of functioning, with longstanding effects on the child's sense of well-being and development. Those who deal with a child with ADHD are soon worn out and become unable to continue to interact effectively with the child or keep to the exact routines and schedules that the child needs. Any significant changes in environment may intensify ADHD symptoms, but there is little that seems to improve these symptoms. The child is difficult to discipline, does not follow directions, seems to dawdle over simple tasks, leaves projects and chores incomplete, forgets homework assignments or, if the classwork is done, forgets to turn it in. Children with ADHD may impulsively touch or bump other children or dash into the street, and they do not like to wait for their turn in a game. Sitting still is an unrealistic request to the child, who continues to fidget, squirm, and move about within whatever space is available. Relationship problems with peers and family members, poor school achievement, and low self-esteem are predictable stressors for the child. Unlike many disorders, ADHD is usually diagnosed early.

The diagnosis of ADD or ADHD requires that symptoms be present before age 7, but diagnosis may be delayed until the child enters school or day care since these environments require controlled, directed, purposeful behavior and adequate attention span. As more young children are being placed in similar settings, the age of first diagnosis may begin to decrease, with much younger children being diagnosed with and treated for ADD and ADHD. Despite the dramatic symptom profiles of ADD and ADHD, some parents will strongly resist the idea that their child may have the disorder and insist that their child will grow out of the problem behavior. Although parents may resist or deny their child's ADD or ADHD diagnosis, the diagnosis is still made based on a parent's or family's description of the child's behavior, school reports, teacher observations, specialized testing, and the practitioner's assessment.

ADD and ADHD symptoms may wax and wane or vary in content and style, so that continual assessment is often necessary. Individual differences in personality traits and coexisting psychosocial problems can also make diagnosis more difficult. The line between normal misbehavior and symptoms of a disorder is sometimes difficult to ascertain when, for example, impulsive behavior is not uncommon within the family or community. In these circumstances the practitioner will need to collaborate with specialists to determine the relative importance of possible contributing factors before diagnosis and treatment can be considered. Positive behavioral responses to stimulant medication are not unique to children with neurologically based attention deficits, so a successful trial of medication should not be used as proof of ADD or ADHD.

ADD and ADHD is more common in boys than girls but occurs across all socioeconomic groups. Concurrent psychosocial and behavioral problems are common with approximately two thirds of children with ADD and ADHD, such as conduct disorder, learning disability, perceptual motor skills delay, expressive language problems, impaired organizational skills, oppositional defiant disorder, and mood disorder. As is evident by the range of disorders listed here, the actual etiology of ADD and ADHD is not clear. Evidence of genetic or family risk is indicated by the high incidence of the disorders in first-degree relatives. Additional possible causative factors include prenatal or perinatal insult, prenatal drug and alcohol exposure, and lead poisoning (Coleman, 1993; Kaplan and Sadock, 1995).

ADD and ADHD Treatments

Psychopharmacological treatment with psychostimulants (methylphenidate, dextroamphetamine, and pemoline) is effective with most children diagnosed with ADD. When helpful, these medications can improve attention, increase attention span, and decrease distractibility to age-appropriate levels. Antidepressants (imipramine, desipramine, bupropion, and clonidine) have also been effective with some children (DeVane and Sallee, 1996; Fisher and Fisher, 1996). When medications are prescribed as treatment for ADD or ADHD, specific hoped-for benefits should be identified before starting the medication. Close consistent monitoring of medication effects at home, school, and day care is mandatory. The adults involved must be made aware that medication alone is rarely sufficient to produce major improvements in behavior. Long-term counseling and parent training in the management of ADD behaviors will be necessary. Contingent reinforcement (e.g., rewards), time-outs, and daily school behavior reports can help parents meet the child's needs for structure and consistency. Parents will always need new strategies to direct and maintain the child's attention and to organize each day.

Children need counseling aimed at protecting and promoting their self-esteem, positive peer relationships, and coping with setbacks and failures. It was once assumed that children with ADD outgrew their symptoms when they entered adolescence, making it possible to discontinue medication at that time. ADD and ADHD have been diagnosed in adolescents and adults, however, thereby making this assumption questionable. Some children will improve as they age, but adults who are known to have had untreated childhood ADD have been observed to have poor impulse control, poor attention, and difficult-to-treat disorders, such as antisocial personality disorder and substance disorder (Kaplan and Sadock, 1995).

The day-to-day frustrations of parenting a child with ADD or ADHD cannot be avoided or overstated. Parents will be subject to intense caretaker burdens. Referral to a specialist for assessment and diagnosis is indicated when these are made difficult by the child's young age (e.g., preschool), with newly diagnosed adolescents, or when assessment and diagnosis are complicated by comorbid disorders. Children who do not respond to medication and consistent behavior management may require long-term specialized care. Children who experience unacceptable medication side effects, who are developmentally disabled, or who are severely hyperactive may also require specialized care (Barbaresi, 1996).

Separation Anxiety

The essential feature of separation anxiety is excessive and developmentally inappropriate symptoms of anxiety that is aroused by real or anticipated separation from home or primary attachments (caretaker/parents) and begins before age 18. All children experience a stage of separation anxiety sometime between infancy and 4 or 5 years of age. A 1 year old's protest at separations from his or her parents is a normal expression of attachment, but most children gradually become comfortable with being temporarily separated from their home, family, and parents. ***Separation anxiety disorder*** is the persistent or recurrent fear of separation that occurs well after a child is expected to have become comfortable with separation. Anxiety symptoms must be present for at least 4 weeks and should be distinguished from brief periods of the anxious dysphoria that is associated with going away to camp or the first few days of school.

A better prognosis is indicated when separation anxiety symptoms occur in very young children who are closer to an age at which separation worries are expected. Separation anxiety disorder in older children or adolescent onset indicate a more severe condition. The anxious child or adolescent may stay close to home or a parent, will not join with peers in "sleep-overs" away from home, may have poor school attendance, and may have fierce tantrums to resist being forced to separate from home or parents against his or her will. Anxiety may be associated with a fear of harm coming to the parent, of becoming lost, or of being abducted if away from home. Sleep onset problems, refusing to sleep in a room alone, and recurrent nightmares may also occur. Physical anxiety symptoms such as headaches, stomach aches, rapid heart rate, and dizziness occur at times of actual or anticipated separation. Physical symptoms and school refusal are more common symptoms with adolescents. School refusal may become related to anxiety about poor academic performance, being teased or bullied by peers, or fearful reactions to teachers. Depression is a common comorbid condition with separation anxiety disorder.

Children with posttraumatic stress disorder may feel unable to leave home. Anxiety disorders are the most common mental disorders in children and adolescents, and separation anxiety disorder in prepubertal children is particularly common in both males and females. A family history of anxiety disorder, agoraphobia, panic disorder, depression, or alcoholism is common. Separation anxiety can develop as a maladaptive response to a severe negative life event or a crisis within the family, such as serious illness, moving away from the community, or divorce.

When assessing a child with separation anxiety, it is important to try to define the fear or worry that fuels the child's anxiety. The child's concerns about attending school or being away from home and parents should be identified precisely and, where possible, resolved. If school refusal appears to be a phobic anxiety—that is, anxiety develops in response to being in school rather than away from home, or as an excessive response to minor illness, learning disability, physical disability, or defiance—specialized intervention is indicated. A diagnosis of severe depression or SMI should be ruled out as a possible explanation for the child's behavior.

When school-related separation anxiety disorder is diagnosed, the family should be actively involved in the plan to help the child return to school as soon as possible. Any evidence that would suggest that the child's anxiety is actually the mother's anxiety about being separated from her child should be evaluated by a specialist. When school refusal is related to actual physical illness, parent education in meeting the health needs of the child may make it less difficult for the child to attend school. In this case family therapy or parental-couples therapy may be required. As with adult anxiety disorders, behavioral therapy, cognitive therapy, desensitization therapy, and antidepressants may be helpful for some children (Kaplan and Sadock, 1995).

Obsessive-Compulsive Disorder

Obsessive-compulsive disorder (OCD) is diagnosed in children, adolescents, and adults, but children are more likely to be underdiagnosed or to not receive treatment (March et al, 1995). The disorder is characterized by intrusive thoughts, followed by anxiety and compulsive behavior rituals intended to relieve the anxiety. The need to diagnose OCD in children is indicated by the fact that approximately one third of adults who are diagnosed with OCD actually developed the disorder in childhood or adolescence. OCD in children may be biologically related to conditions such as Tourette's syndrome, Sydenham's chorea, an autoimmune inflammation of the basal ganglia triggered by bacterial infection, and beta-hemolytic streptococcus. A child with a dramatic onset of OCD symptoms, exacerbation of mild OCD symptoms or tics may need to be evaluated for group A beta-hemolytic strep infection.

There can be left-sided soft signs on neurological examination, with poor visual-spatial processing. Selective serotonin reuptake inhibitor (SSRI) antidepressants can be effective in some cases, but in most cases psychostimulants will exacerbate OCD symptoms. Males with OCD tend to be shorter and to have a flatter growth curve, suggesting neuroendocrine dysfunctions. Males are more likely than females to have prepubertal onset of OCD and tics. Females are more likely to have OCD symptom onset at puberty. Because of the amount of time and energy that is spent engaged in OCD rituals, children with this disorder can have significant problems with school performance but may also have a learning disability as a comorbid disorder.

Anxiety and OCD Treatment

Clomipramine has been approved for treatment of OCD in children and adolescents 10 years of age and older. SSRI antidepressants such as fluoxetine have been effective with adults, but only at extremely high doses. Cognitive-behavioral therapy is the treatment of choice for children and adolescents with separation anxiety or OCD. The goal of treatment is to extinguish anxious responses through repeated exposure to the source of anxiety and through the use of behavior modification. This specialized treatment follows a gradual course of exposing the child to the feared experience without the fear response or the feared consequences. Parent education about the child's disorder is critical to successful treatment outcomes. Without this education parents may find it difficult to refrain from "saving" their child when he or she becomes distressed, rather than allow the child to improve. Parents may need to participate in support groups, self-help groups, or psychotherapy to helping them reduce their feelings of frustration and to prevent treatment burnout.

Mood Disorders

The prevalence rate of mood disorders in school-age children is 9% (Laraia, 1996). Incidence rates for mood disorders in children living in developed countries suggest dramatic increases in depression, mania, and suicide in recent generations. Children can experience negative moods that have major effects on their behavior and functioning. As with adults, children can have severe episodes of many types of negative moods, such as sadness, guilt, and anger, with concurrent negative changes in their daily routine and habits, including changes in sleep, appetite, appearance, and energy. DSM-IV criteria for major depression, bipolar disorder, and dysthymic disorders also apply to children and adolescents. Children differ somewhat in that mood disorder symptoms are more likely to be somatic with significant irritability, isolation and withdrawal, academic problems, school refusal, extremely negative attitudes, aggression, and antisocial behavior. Symptoms such as motor retardation, hypersomnia, and delusions, which are observed in severely depressed adults, are uncommon in children. Childhood depression occurs in males and females at about the same rate. Common concurrent problems or disorders with depression are conduct disorder, ADD, and anxiety disorders.

Depression symptoms in children include overreacting to events, fear of leaving or being without parents or primary caretakers, being moody with periods of extreme anger and sadness, restlessness or not being able to settle down, poor concentration, difficulty making decisions, changes in weight that may be associated with vomiting or binge eating, and compulsive behaviors. When depressed, children may refuse to go to school or may develop phobic anxiety about school. Although more rare, dangerous behaviors such as setting fires or attempting suicide are associated with depression in highly distressed children (Coleman, 1993).

The depressed preschool and school-age child looks sad. The child may complain of headaches or stomach aches, have problems sleeping, and develop separation anxiety. Depressed children may begin to do poorly in school and may experience psychomotor agitation with impaired concentration. These last two symptoms should be distinguished from the hyperactivity and attention symptoms of ADD and ADHD. As with adults, depressed children may have very low self-esteem and may call themselves stupid, ugly, or bad. The child with depression related low self-esteem can become unwilling to attempt tasks such as reading, drawing, or participating in performance activities (e.g., playing ball). Their negative thinking is typically expressed with flat statements of "I can't."

The limited language and cognitive skills of children make it all the more difficult for them to describe their feelings of sadness, worthlessness, guilt, or thoughts they may have about death or suicide. Parents may be unwilling or unable to acknowledge the depths of their child's despair but may be able and willing to acknowledge their child's unhappiness. Children's suicidal thoughts and behaviors may be associated with depression but may also be associated with conduct disorder, substance disorder, and impaired impulse control.

A study of 8- to 13-year-old patients being treated in a child psychiatry outpatient department found that 58% of the children had suicidal thoughts and 9% had actually attempted suicide. In that study 39% of children who did not have a mood disorder had suicidal thoughts. The most common methods of attempted suicide were substance overdose, stabbing or cutting, running in front of a moving car, jumping from a building, asphyxiation by hanging or gas fumes, and gunshot wounds. As with many mental disorders, depression strikes families, so a depressed child typically has a family history of depression. Earlier-age onset, or childhood depression, suggests that the incidence of depression within the family may be very high (Puig-Antich et al, 1989). A high rate of depression relapse and a 20% incidence of bipolar disorder have also been associated with childhood depression (Gellar, Fox and Fletcher, 1994; Kovacs, Feinberg and Crouse-Novak, 1984).

Management of Mental Disorders in Children

➢ Counseling

Children with psychosocial problems, learning disabilities, difficult temperaments, or mental disorders may seek primary health care for reasons unrelated to these conditions (e.g., an immunization). Routine assessment for potential long-term problems makes early intervention and prevention possible. With children, delayed psychiatric primary care counseling or specialized psychiatric care can delay psychological growth and development, compounding what may already be a difficult time for the child and the family and increasing the risk for adolescent or adult onset disorders.

Early recognition of psychosocial problems and mental disorders requires parents to be fully aware of the child's multiple environments (e.g., home, school, peers) and day-to-day stressors. Without this information it is extremely unlikely that environments or stressors with which the child is having trouble coping, or family biopsychosocial risk factors that put the child at risk for disorder, can be identified. Advocacy is the most important intervention for very young children, in primary or specialized care. But to advocate effectively on behalf of a young child, the practitioner must be able to enlist the participation of the child's family and teachers.

Just as child assessment requires the active participation of those who are directly involved with the child every day, counseling requires the assistance of many caring adults. One of the most important roles that the practitioner can play is to ensure that the family and teachers have the resources they need to meet the child's needs. When the family and teachers do not fully understand the child's needs or have excessive personal needs of their own, the child may not have the psychosocial resources that are necessary to prevent long-term problems or to effectively resolve normal developmental crises.

Family counseling can be effective in mobilizing participation and developing a plan that will address the child's immediate, short-term, and long-term needs. Practitioners can provide much-needed guidance, support, and reassurance to the child and the adults involved, since the group must work together to the child's benefit. This may involve establishing new partnerships among the adults and building an interpersonal structure of relationships and resources that are effective. With adults, and perhaps even more so with children, meaningful goals (e.g., behavioral goals) must be clearly stated and used as a point of reference for intervention. In most cases these goals will target the child's social skills, behaviors, activity level, cognition functioning, and self-esteem (and the parent's self-esteem as well).

Within age-appropriate expectations, children and their parents can be encouraged to pay more attention to the child's negative thoughts and the relationship between the child's thoughts and behaviors. The child should be encouraged and expected to take appropriate responsibility for his or her behavior, but this responsibility must be age appropriate. Regardless of age, unacceptable behavior should be clearly and consistently defined and responded to by adults. At the same time, the child should be provided with numerous opportunities to participate in pleasurable activities, to be successful, and to learn basic social and communication skills. When improvement in self-control is a goal, the child must be given realistic self-control expectations so that success is always within reach. Like adults, children may be defensive or resist changes. When this is the case, change will take longer, but goals for improvement need not be reduced.

However, hoped-for changes in behavior require a high level of cooperation and participation by all the involved adults and the child. When the parents rather than the child become defensive or resist changes, they may need more psychosocial support and resources to improve their ability to effectively participate in their child's health care.

Parents benefit from helpful information about their child and his or her needs. This information should be in a form that the adults can use when at home, at work, or in public settings. Many excellent commercial materials are available (e.g., books, videos) on a wide range of child mental health and well-being topics, but parents and teachers should have specific information about the particular child and his or her treatment plan. General information is always useful, but it is a well-informed plan for the particular child that will determine the outcome. General information can be difficult to apply or may be misunderstood. It can also be extremely negative and a source of gloomy defeat for parents. Parents need information that acknowledges the difficulty they may have accepting their child's diagnosis or problem, but a parent's hope for improvement should be supported at all times.

Parents who do not resist or deny their child's needs may still require a fair amount of time and support as they try to absorb a great deal of information. Parents may have a kind of delayed or slow reaction to any diagnosis or problem,—from depression to ADD to substance abuse—and they need time to adjust to the idea that their child needs professional help. Community resources and self-help groups for parents are important and helpful, although initially parents may be more concerned with immediate problems than with the long-term needs that such groups can meet.

Parent's needs in response to their child's needs can become complicated when the parent has poor coping, communication, or parenting skills. Individuals who are rigid and controlling or blaming and demanding can feel threatened by their child's problems and may become hostile and aggressive towards the child. At some point all parents feel overwhelmed. Parents who have severe negative reactions to their child's needs should be strongly encouraged to seek individual or parental therapy for as long as it takes to come to terms with what is likely to be a very different life from what was expected. When a child's needs are acute and the family is in crisis, all members of the family may have needs that must be addressed before they can begin to effectively mobilize to meet the needs of the child. When family members feel powerless, there is a greater possibility that their reaction will be to blame the child or accuse the child of intentional misbehavior, rather than accepting that the child has different needs. They may add to the child's problems by trying to force the child to change his or her behavior by using unpredictable and severe punishment or lavish gifts. Even worse, the family may abandon the child and create a more comfortable family subgroup that excludes the child with special needs.

The potential for family tension and conflict is obvious. Children who feel abandoned or rejected by their family will react to their perception of rejection, which only increases the risk of establishing a pattern of parent-child conflict that is extremely difficult to change and very painful to everyone involved. If the child is depressed or acting out, it is not likely that his or her mood or behavior will improve in a family environment that is bounded by conflict. Family conflict, stress, and tension negatively affect everyone in the household, but the effects for the child with a disorder can be immeasurable. It is not helpful to take the perspective that any single individual or family subgroup is at fault for the family's struggles. To do so is to invite that individual or subgroup to defend itself by blaming or accusing someone else, including the practitioner. Practitioners can greatly aid the child and the family by helping them to understand that everyone's feelings count. No one's feelings are more important or less important than another's feelings. The practitioner must include everyone in the work.

Finally, the child's ongoing developmental needs must continue to be met. Growth and development needs cannot be set aside until a later time, especially learning and social skill development. Many communities have reestablished local support programs for families who live in areas with limited resources and opportunities. Programs such as Family Enhancement in Madison, Wisconsin benefit children by addressing the needs of the entire family, and they are an excellent referral resource.

References

Barbaresi W: Primary care approach to the diagnosis and management of attention-deficit hyperactivity disorder, *Mayo Clin Proc* 71:463, 1996.

Biederman J, Faraone S, Milberger S, Guite J, Mick E, Chen L, Mennin D, Marrs A, Quellett C, Moore P, Spencer T, Norman D, Wilens T, Kraus I, Perrin J: A prospective 4-year follow-up study of attention-deficit hyperactivity and related disorders, *Arch Gen Psychiatry* 53(5):437, 1996.

Coleman W: *Attention Deficit Disorders, Hyperactivity, and Associated Disorders*, Madison, 1993, Calliope.

DeVane CL, Sallee FR: Serotonin selective reuptake inhibitors in child and adolescent psychopharmacology: a review of published experience, *J Clin Psychiatry* 57(2):55, 1996.

Fisher RL, Fisher S: Antidepressants for children, is scientific support necessary? *J of Nervous and Mental Disease* 184(2):99, 1996.

Gellar B, Fox I, Fletcher M: Effect of tricyclic antidepressants on switching to mania and on the onset of bipolarity in depressed 6 to 12 year olds with major depressive disorder, *J of Am Aca of Child and Adoles Psychiatry* 32:43, 1994.

Kaplan HI, Sadock BL (editors): *Comprehensive Textbook of Psychiatry VI*, Baltimore, 1995, Williams & Wilkins.

Kovacs M, Feinberg TL, Crouse-Novak MA: Depressive disorders in childhood: a longitudinal prospective study of characteristics and recovery, *Arch of Gen Psychiatry* 41:229, 1984.

Laraia MT: Current approaches to the psychopharmacologic treatment of depression in children and adolescents, *JCAPN* 9(1): 15, 1996.

Long N, Starfield B, Kelleher K: Co-occurrence of medical and mental disorders in pediatric primary care. In Miranda J, Hohmann A, Attkisson C, Larson D (editors) *Mental Disorders in Primary Care*, San Francisco, 1995, Jossey-Bass Publishers.

March JS, Leonard HL, Swedo SE: Neuropsychiatry of obsessive-compulsive disorder in children and adolescents, *Comprehensive Therapy* 21(9):507, 1995.

Monteleone J: *Recognition of Child Abuse*, St Louis, 1994, Mosby.

Novak LL: Childhood behavior problems, *Am Fam Physician* 53(1):257, 1996.

Parker S, Zuckerman B (editors): *Behavioral and Developmental Pediatrics: a handbook for primary care*, Boston, 1995, Little, Brown, and Company.

Puig-Antich P, Goetz D, Davies M: A controlled family history study of prepubertal major depression disorders, *Arch of Gen Psychiatry* 46:406, 1989.

Riley AW, Wissow LS: Recognition of emotional and behavioral problems and family violence in pediatric primary care. In Miranda J, Hohman A, Attkisson C, Larson D (editors): *Mental Disorders in Primary Care*, San Francisco, 1995, Jossey-Bass Publishers.

Schneider D: Meeting provider health care objectives for children and adolescents by the year 2000, *Children's Health Care*, 25(1):1, 1996.

Tanner JL: Neurodevelopmental variation in school-age children, *Comprehensive Therapy* 21(9):499, 1995.

Adolescents 15

American norms allow individuals who are 18 years old to develop the healthy physical, psychological, and social characteristics needed for effective adult psychosocial functioning and to set forth on the path of a meaningful life. From ages 11 to 18 adolescents feel the pressure of meeting these long-term adult goals, but at the same time they are faced with some of the most difficult and important immediate choices they will ever have to make. To adolescents, the concept of positive adult psychosocial functioning can seem relatively unimportant compared to immediate problems, such as deciding whether to talk to or listen to adults, smoke tobacco, drink alcohol, use marijuana, study and learn, refrain from sexual intercourse or use condoms and contraceptives, exercise, eat healthily, drive safely, choose friends wisely, and believe in a difference between right and wrong. Adolescents with good physical health, good mental health, positive social resources, and the ability to successfully navigate the high seas of adolescent choices are more likely than their counterparts to be able to look forward to the many opportunities of healthy adult life. This chapter describes three of the many threats to positive adolescent growth and development: acting out and conduct disorder, violence, and substance abuse.

Adolescence

In biopsychosocial terms, a great deal of an adolescent's day-to-day life is devoted to coping with powerful internal and external demands, using what may be relatively untested and unreliable coping skills (e.g., confrontation) and social resources (e.g., peers). Effective coping skills and adequate social resources can reduce the perceived demands of adolescence, thereby increasing the probability of positive adolescent growth and development and preparation for adult life. For as many reasons as there are adolescents, some adolescents arrive at this critical stage of development unprepared (Korenblum et al, 1990). Many of these adolescents are unprepared and at increased risk for mental disorders (e.g., depression), severe psychosocial problems (e.g., academic failure), or negative growth and development, because the single most important and most overlooked adolescent risk factor is the period of childhood that precedes adolescence.

The findings of a study of adolescent development (Allen, Aber and Leadbeater, 1990) led the researchers to conclude that adolescents are challenged by four severe, perplexing problems: adolescent crime, school dropout, substance abuse, and pregnancy. For adolescents and society in general, the full financial, social, and psychological impact of these problems is difficult to calculate due to the cumulative interaction effects of their negative consequences. With problems like these in mind, it comes as no surprise to practitioners that increasingly higher numbers of adolescents are at risk for mental disorders and severe psychosocial problems.

The fundamental barriers to adolescent health care service utilization are cost and lack of health insurance, lack of parental consent, lack of skilled providers, ethnicity as a cultural barrier, and poverty (US Office of Technology Assessment, 1991). Adolescents need positive support, guidance, and reassurance from their parents. Many families have little time together, with the net result that everyone goes his or her own way. These highly individualized households can be a lonely place for a 14 year old. Family violence is also a national concern and a serious problem for children and adolescents. When home is not the primary source of support, adolescents look elsewhere. Peers become an easy, though less than reliable, substitute for family. An important psychological cost to adolescents who depend on their peers to meet their needs for support is that they become more vulnerable to the painful interpersonal rejection that follows when adolescents fail to conform to a group's ever-changing membership rules. Even positive peer groups can be difficult for adolescents to manage if the group becomes extremely powerful.

According to Millstein (1989), most adolescent deaths are related to preventable causes, such as motor vehicle accidents, suicide, family violence, and gang violence. Because of the severity of these problems, preventive measures alone are now viewed as insufficient (Kazdin, 1993). Active promotion of adolescent health and well-being is required (American College of Physicians, 1989). This means that adolescence should be viewed as a critical stage of growth and development and not simply as a period of transition between childhood and adulthood. For example, a study of four school-based adolescent clinics demonstrated that although adolescents did seek out health care, the reasons for their clinic visits were often masked or not fully disclosed to practitioners. The concerns that adolescents may find most difficult to disclose are often those with the greatest health and well-being consequences. For example, adolescents who are victims of emotional abuse at home or who have serious academic problems may choose to seek emotional support from peer sexual relationships rather than seek help to address the experience of abuse and academic problems. There are many risks in adolescent sexual relationships, including pregnancy, partner violence and academic problems (Harold and Harold, 1993; Spitz et al, 1996).

Data from Riggs and Cheng's (1988) study of adolescent health care visits indicated that 28% of the adolescents seen were seriously depressed, and 12% reported having attempted suicide. Studies of depression and suicidal thoughts such as these indicate that most adolescents are doing well, but a significant proportion are having serious problems and are highly distressed. A similar study of 104 adolescents seen in a teen primary care clinic found that about half of the adolescents came with a problem that was psychological only. Half of that number were depressed and one quarter had serious thoughts of suicide (Cappelli et al, 1995). In this study 60% percent of the adolescents who complained of both physical and psychological symptoms were seriously depressed. These findings clearly indicate that distressed adolescents may seek health care but may not easily disclose the problems that are most troubling to them.

Distressed adolescents may be more likely to engage in high-risk behaviors; therefore, adolescent health promotion services now specifically target adolescent needs rather than waiting for problems to develop. For example, the American Medical Association's Guidelines for Adolescent Preventive Services (Blum and Beuhring, 1995) recommends five categories of routine adolescent health and well-being screening: biomedical, physical health, psychosocial health, substance use, and sexual behavior. Annual adolescent health care visits are recommended, with a focus on adolescent developmental concerns, sociocultural concerns, confidentiality concerns, health guidance and teaching needs, health checkups, and immunization checks.

Adolescent sexuality is of concern to adults, to adolescents who have chosen to be sexually active, and to adolescents who have chosen to not engage in sexual activity. Sexuality is a correlate of adolescent psychological health and well-being and a major test of adolescent psychological and social coping skills. The pressure on adolescents to be sexually active is relentless. In the 1950s, an adolescent could be considered attractive by peers, an extremely important adolescent psychological need, without being sexually active. Today, in many schools sexual attraction that is not acted on is less common, but social rejection continues to be as painful today as it was in the '50s, when adolescents had more societal support and faced fewer sexual demands.

Higher numbers of sexually active adolescents can mean an increased adolescent risk of being the target of sexual victimization by adults or peers (Spitz et al, 1996). Large numbers of adolescents spend more than half a day away from school and home, either working or "hanging out" with peers. Burkhart and Sherry (1993) suggest that although biopsychosocial sexual development is a necessary developmental task of adolescence, overconfidence, depression, anger, intoxication, and inexperience make adolescents highly vulnerable targets for sexual victimization. The immediate short-term, and long-term consequences of adolescent sexual victimization, such as mood disorder, substance disorder, and academic failure, cannot be overstated. Adolescents who have been victimized may not report what happened to them, may blame themselves, or may develop a negative view of the world to match the negative experience, which can lead to negative or antisocial behavior.

Adolescents who are ethnic minorities or who grow up in severe poverty can be at increased risk for depression and multiple psychosocial problems when minority social status or poverty effectively decreases the availability of positive support resources (e.g., good schools) or increases the adolescent's exposure to painful psychosocial stressors (e.g., discrimination). The majority of the studies of psychosocial problems experienced by minority adolescents who live in poverty indicate that poverty increases adolescent vulnerability to substance abuse, violence, and pregnancy. For example, the findings of a study of over 3000 African-

American, Asian-American, Caucasian, and Mexican-American adolescents ages 13 to 17, who received outpatient treatment within the Los Angeles county mental health system, indicate that poverty is perhaps the most important but most overlooked factor of minority mental health problems (Bui and Takeuchi, 1992). In that study, African-American adolescents had more mental health treatment contacts than Caucasian adolescents, but no significant racial differences were observed in treatment dropout rates or length of treatment, two factors that are significantly related to positive treatment outcomes. The researchers concluded that poverty predicted a higher number of treatment contacts, a higher rate of treatment dropout, and a shorter length of treatment. In this study, 90% of the African-American adolescents lived in poverty.

In summary, adolescents are vulnerable to depression and substance disorders and complex psychosocial problems related to family, school, violence, and sexuality. To be an effective resource for adolescents, practitioners must routinely screen adolescent patients for potential disorders and problems, with the assumption that an adolescent may be more likely to disclose important information when invited to do so (Faigel, 1996).

Adolescent Psychosocial Assessment

The psychosocial assessment of adolescents varies from the assessment of adults, primarily in terms of the unique developm-
tal milestones, psychosocial contexts, and pote-
associated with these stages of development
are significant individual variation
personal attitudes, beliefs
sonal and social st
coping skills (
assessment of a
adolescence are
be helpful. Some
style, such as facia
suggestive clothing
adults, which all incr
behaviors mean that
unnoticed but in most ca

social demands, such as graduating from high school or looking forward to the future. Most adolescents experience brief episodes of what they and their families may refer to as "difficult times," but these times almost always occur as well-defined crises, such as the ending or beginning of an important peer relationship or adolescent struggles with self-esteem.

The findings of a large self-image survey of adolescents (Offer et al, 1990) indicate that the following are important areas of adolescent assessment.

Impulse Control

Adolescents with poor impulse control may appear to be disorganized, have a low tolerance for frustration, and act on impulse. An adolescent with age-appropriate impulse control is able to delay gratification, think through important choices, and is not highly susceptible to peer impulses.

Emotional Patterns

Adolescents should experience a balanced range of emotions without excessive extremes in mood. Moods by definition change, but an adolescent who seems, for example, to always be angry without significant periods of a relaxed mood or a positive mood can be said to have a ***restricted mood range***. Another example of restricted mood range is an adolescent who becomes excessively distressed with a loss of control or difficulty regaining emotional balance. Adolescents should be able to exercise normal vels of control over their emotions rather than being dominated heir feelings.

Image

e refers to psychological adjustment to one's body.
range of socially acceptable male and female ado-
es is significantly greater today than in the past,
truggle with positive body image. Hair contin-
important, followed by facial features, com-
t, and secondary sex characteristics. How
rmal changes in their bodies depends in
s occur. Physical changes that occur

much earlier or later for them than for their peers can be a source of distress. Adolescent peer groups always have physical standards of "normal," which determine those who will be treated as different. Being different is no longer an automatic social deficit, but it can require greater social skill.

Social Relationships

What are an adolescent's primary relationships? Ideally adolescents have relationships with a variety of friends and relatives, and these relationships do not follow rigid or negative patterns, such as interpersonal dominance, fear, or demands for absolute loyalty, or self-destructive behaviors, such as binge drinking. The absence of meaningful peer relationships can indicate that an adolescent finds such relationships to be too demanding or unrewarding, but an adolescent should participate in positive interactions with others that can provide companionship and support.

Conscience

What has traditionally been referred to as the superego or moral development can more easily be understood as conscience or the experience of discomfort as a result of wrongful thoughts, feelings, or behavior. Adolescents should not have excessive feelings of guilt or self-hate, but neither should they be free of self-judgment, such as an individual who is not discomforted by a wrongful act towards another, believing instead that the end always justifies the means or that it is the other person's responsibility to avoid being harmed. The classic example of this is males who manipulate females for the purpose of sexual conquest.

Sexuality

What are an adolescent's sexual attitudes, beliefs, thoughts, feelings, behaviors, experiences, and worries? Adolescents often have one set of sexual attitudes for other people and another set for themselves and their close friends. Although most adolescents may feel comfortable talking about sex, it can still be difficult to talk about their personal sexuality. A major assessment concern with sexually active adolescents is that they may find themselves in sexual relationships that they don't want, but they continue with them because they find it easier to remain in such relationships than to end them. Finally, traditional sexual double standards for males and females hold that adolescent boys have the option of having sexual intercourse as a game that boys win and girls lose. The pressure to "score" negatively affects both boys and girls.

Family Relationships

This refers to the adolescent's feelings for and relationships (positive and negative) with all members of the family and his or her need for such relationships. Adolescents should be able to take their parent's and sibling's feelings into consideration without being dominated by the fear of saying or doing something that might upset the family. Fear may suggest conditional family support, in which the adolescent can enjoy good family relationships only under the condition that he or she meets family expectations.

Vocational/Educational Goals

Adolescents should have future plans that are of personal importance or value. These plans should give the adolescent a sense of personal responsibility and purpose and should not be unrealistic or harmful—for example, an adolescent who refuses to attend school because his or her goal is to become a rich ball player or model. Perhaps more than in any other generation, vocational and educational anxiety and ambivalence are troubling concerns for many adolescents. Anxiety and ambivalence about future goals should be distinguished from apathy.

Psychological Well-Being

Are there symptoms of severe distress, a mental disorder, or psychosocial problems? The adolescent's interpersonal style can increase the difficulty of this assessment. For example, some adolescents may adopt a hostile interpersonal style or may prefer a great deal of interpersonal distance and therefore adopt an odd interpersonal style to maintain this distance. Adolescent well-being tends to be fluid however it is assessed, but the first rule of assessment is to distinguish style from substance.

Adjustment

How is the adolescent coping with or adjusting to the various demands she or he is facing, including the demands of adolescence as a stage of development? Does the adolescent seem challenged or overwhelmed? Is the adolescent marking time until he or she reaches age 18, or is the adolescent enjoying this stage of life? A well-adjusted adolescent has more hope than despair, more interest than apathy, and looks forward to the future. The well-adjusted adolescent is not trouble-free, but there should be evidence of basic problem-solving skills, age-appropriate functioning most of the time, and a capacity for moral judgment.

Acting Out and Conduct Disorder

Acting out is often impulsive or thoughtless behavior, but it can also be the indirect expression of important thoughts and feelings. Individuals may act out important thoughts and feelings when direct verbal expression is difficult (e.g., the individual is uncertain), impossible (e.g., the individual is confused), dangerous (e.g., the individual fears, abuse, violence, or punishment), or unacceptable (e.g., the individual is negative). Acting out a message to others also makes it possible to avoid feedback, consequences, or to disown the message if necessary. With adolescents, acting out can also be a way to express feelings of low self-esteem.

Children and mature adults may act out important thoughts and feelings, but adolescents seem to be particularly adept at this form of communication. Acting out seems to be more common with adolescents who believe that others will not take their thoughts and feelings seriously if they are expressed directly, or in some cases it is the adolescent who does not take his or her own thoughts and feelings seriously. Adolescents may also act out impulsively even when they have the option to express themselves in a more direct and less dramatic manner. Adolescent acting out will appear to be a deliberate attempt to manipulate others when it consists of a lot of behavior with little or no message. Examples of this are adolescents who stay out all night but do nothing, or those who take the family car without permission but go nowhere. To many well-meaning adults, this type of acting out is assumed to be the adolescent's request for adult attention. If asking adults for attention is difficult, or the adolescent feels threatened by what he or she perceives as inadequate adult attention, acting out may indeed be a request for attention.

When adolescent acting out is not impulsive, potentially dangerous to the adolescent (e.g., sexual acting out) or to others (e.g., violent acting out) and is not a symptom of a mental disorder, it is generally viewed as a phase of growth and development. When acting out signals occupational, academic, or social relationship problems that are important to the adolescent, those problems, rather than the acting out, should be the focus of attention.

Adolescent conduct disorder is a *Diagnostic and Statistical Manual of Mental Disorders, fourth edition*, (DSM-IV), disorder with behaviors that exceed acting out or normal misbehavior. Conduct disorder consists of predelinquent or delinquent behaviors that violate social norms, rules, and laws, interfere with the basic rights of others, and are repetitive and persistent. Adults with antisocial personality disorder typically have a history of adolescent conduct disorder. Antisocial personality disorder requires evidence of antisocial behaviors during adolescence. DSM-IV conduct disorder criteria include physical fighting, physically threatening others, stealing or destroying property, setting fires, forcing others to submit to sexual contact, chronic lying, conning people, running away, staying out overnight, truancy, and breaking and entering (APA, 1994). A conduct disorder diagnosis is defined by the severity of the behavior and symptom onset in early or late adolescence.

Adolescents who are diagnosed with conduct disorder are at risk for other mental disorders, including substance abuse, depression, and impulsive suicide attempts. Adolescents with conduct disorder often have a family or community environment that is characterized by neglect, abuse, deprivation, adult social deviance, or parental psychopathology, including parental substance abuse and parental antisocial personality disorder. The adolescent and his or her parents or caretakers may blame society or deny the adolescent's conduct disorder by taking the position that he or she has not been treated fairly or has been misunderstood. Both the parents and the adolescent may believe that the world is a negative and hostile environment and that the adolescent's conduct is therefore appropriate, necessary, justified, or acceptable.

Adolescents who are victims of abuse, neglect, or deprivation are significantly more likely to view the world as a hostile place. Adolescents who blame the world for their conduct can be provocative, aggressive, or hostile towards everyone, including practitioners, thereby soliciting the negative social responses that in turn validate their hostile world view. Adolescents with a conduct disorder diagnosis may engage in bravado and go to great lengths to outsmart or hustle authority figures. This interpersonal style is also an excellent psychological defense against feelings of guilt and wrongdoing; therefore, it is not likely that such an adolescent would easily give up his or her "style." Interactions with these adolescents can feel superficial and staged, as though the practitioner has been reduced to playing a part in the adolescent's psychological theater. However provocative the adolescent's conduct may be, interpersonal isolation and rejection is a very high cost to pay, a cost that few adolescents can easily afford.

Conduct disorder is more common in boys than girls. Adolescents with this diagnosis quickly come to the attention of the court system, at which time counseling is usually court-mandated. Before a conduct disorder is diagnosed, seizure disorder, head trauma, and severe mental illness (SMI) should be considered first; if any of these is diagnosed, it should be treated with the hope that the treatment will lead to an improvement in the adolescent's conduct. Educational testing and intervention should be included to reduce long term learning disability and to help the adolescent with conduct disorder to increase his or her feelings of self-esteem. Social intervention, such as out-of-home placement, is used when the adolescent's conduct is harmful or potentially dangerous or when the family environment contributes to the adolescent's conduct disorder. When the family environment is able and willing to provide positive support, long-term family therapy will be required for improvement to be a realistic goal. Community support groups and therapy groups for adolescents can provide valuable opportunities for learning new social skills and new verbal communication skills.

Violence

Adolescent violence is not a new phenomenon. However, with the advent of relatively easy access to firearms, drugs, alcohol, and gangs organized for the purpose of making money by stealing and selling firearms and drugs, adolescent violence has become unpredictable and deadly. The majority of the victims of adolescent violence are themselves adolescents. Fear of violent peers can be the basis for school refusal and academic failure in nonviolent adolescents. Communities and school districts have been required to fund high-profile security measures, and legislation has been necessary to establish drug- and firearm-free zones around schools.

Deadly adolescent violence is a news staple, but other more common forms of adolescent violence have received far less public attention, especially sexual and physical assaults on peers and adolescent assaultive behavior in the home. Assessment of violent adolescents who do not yet have a long history of violence should first determine whether the adolescent has a mental disorder (including substance abuse), represents a danger to oneself and/or others, has used or has access to firearms, has targeted a particular individual (e.g., a homosexual student) or a group of individuals (e.g., girls), or is a member of an organized hate group (e.g., Skinheads, gang bangers).

Mental Disorder

Psychosis is not a cause of violence, but individuals who have an altered state of reality as a result of intoxication, head injury, bipolar disorder, or thought disorder can become violent. Use of alcohol, crack cocaine, and stimulants is highly correlated with violent behavior. Violence is also indirectly related to substance buying and selling and to retribution for acts committed when intoxicated. Sadistic violence may occur, unrelated to a formal mental disorder, although there continues to be a great deal of social pressure to view all violent behavior as a symptom of a mental disorder. Most important, adolescent violence may be an indication of family violence that would otherwise go undetected.

Danger to Oneself and/or Others

Adolescents can become a danger to themselves or suicidal when they are disorganized, confused, impulsive, humiliated, or enraged. Adolescent threats of harm or injury to oneself, adults, peers, or groups should be acted on accordingly, and named targets should be notified. Local authorities should be notified if the adolescent has access to weapons but refuses to reveal their location. Adolescents who are recent victims of violence are significantly more likely to themselves become violent toward others. Any adolescent who has suffered a major loss, such as the end of an important peer relationship or the death of a loved one, can behave on impulsive in very aggressive or dangerous ways, such as reckless driving.

Firearms

A weapon turns a violent impulse into a life-threatening event (Stringham, 1995). Recently in Madison, Wisconsin two adolescent boys decided to steal a car. The owner saw the boys and did not try to stop them, but one of the boys had a gun and shot the owner in the head at close range. After months of intensive care the owner of the car survived; the boys were convicted and will spend their adult lives in prison. The car owner had the opportunity to ask the boy why he used the gun. The boy's sincere response was, "I don't know." In the opinion of many people, he shot the owner because he had a gun in his hand and fired the weapon on impulse, an image that many adolescents have watched (on television, in movies, and video games) for entertainment purposes for most of their lives. There are adolescents who, for any number of reasons, have divided the world into winners and losers, with winners defined as the people with the better weapons. Some adolescents base their entire identities and self-esteem on the fact that they have firearms and are willing to use them. Any adolescent who has access to firearms or who in the past has used firearms has a significant potential for unpredictable violence.

Hate Groups

There are two basic types of adolescent hate groups: those who rationalize their violence with the belief that they are biologically, morally, socially, culturally, or politically superior to others, and those who rationalize their violence with the belief that the end (e.g., status, power, profit) justifies the means (violence). Ironically, well-organized hate groups have strict rules of conduct for all members, with no tolerance of nonconformity, but these groups view all nonmembers as legitimate targets for their hate. Adolescent alienation, once manifested in the introspective, adolescent loner, is an important psychological criteria for hate-group membership. Adolescent hate groups wear many colors, such as the easy-to-recognize black boots of neo-Nazis, the "colors" of urban gang bangers, and the less-than-obvious jeans and T-shirts of gay-bashers.

Level of Risk for Violence

Adolescent risk of violent behavior can be assessed as minimal, moderate, or major (Stringham, 1995). ***Minimal risk*** of violence is assessed when the adolescent has a previous history of fighting with no current episodes of fighting, and the adolescent's parent or caretaker denies any concern about actual or potential violent behavior in the home. There should be no history of serious threats of violence or weapon possession. ***Moderate risk*** of violence is assessed when the adolescent has a recent history of fighting without inflicting or receiving major injuries. Neither adults nor children in the adolescent's household should feel unsafe with the adolescent in the home. There should be no criminal behavior, the adolescent is not a member of a hate group (or pretending to be in manner or dress), and does not have access to or possession of a firearm. These adolescents are often described as boys or girls who like to fight. ***Major risk*** of violence is assessed when the adolescent and/or the victims have suffered major injuries, when others are afraid of the adolescent, or when the adolescent possesses or has access to firearms, makes verbal threats to adults and peers, has a long history of fighting, enjoys fighting, and makes statements such as, "I would never walk away from a fight."

Substance Abuse

Adolescent substance abuse does not differ from adult substance abuse, but the substance's effects can be less predictable or more severe in adolescents. Adolescent substance abuse can create serious problems quickly (Kandel and Davis, 1996; Shaffer et al, 1996). For example, adolescents with family conflict over their substance abuse may run away from home and try to support themselves by living on the street. The primary health care goal for adolescent substance abuse is prevention. Over the previous decades a great deal has been learned about some of the factors that can predict adolescent substance use, including those that contribute to its start and those that contribute to its progression.

Specific psychosocial risk factors for adolescent substance disorders were identified in a study of more than 1500 randomly selected high school students ages 14 through 18 (Lewinsohn, Gotlib, and Seeley, 1995). ***General risk factors*** were defined as increasing the adolescent's risk for a range of disorders, and ***specific risk factors*** were defined as increasing the adolescent's risk for depression or substance abuse. Adolescent substance abuse was generally predicted by poor academic performance and prior episodes of substance abuse. Specific risk factors for substance abuse were (1) previous tobacco use, (2) current tobacco use, (3) days missed at school, (4) days late for school, (5) parental dissatisfaction with grades, and (6) past substance disorder diagnosis. The researchers concluded that a high number of risk factors reliably predicted substance abuse. In this study 3.2% of the adolescents with two risk factors, compared to 23.8% of adolescents with four or more risk factors, were diagnosed with a substance disorder.

There is little doubt that academic functioning problems and tobacco use are related to substance disorders, but, as is frequently the case with such powerful outcome predictors, it is difficult to determine the relationship, if any, between academic problems and tobacco use. Academic problems can have the same painful psychological impact on adolescents that employment problems have on adults. Troubled 14-year-old smokers can be quite clear about the positive nicotine mood effects they seek and obtain from tobacco, and that for them these benefits outweigh the health risks.

These observations indicate that adolescent personality characteristics are important substance abuse risk factors.

Researchers have hypothesized that childhood personality factors are associated with adolescent personality factors, which in turn are associated with young adult substance abuse (Brook et al, 1995). More than 700 students ages 11 to 27 participated in the study. This longitudinal study began following these children at the age of 5.The study's measures of personality were conventional or unconventional (e.g., noncompliance, rebelliousness, sensation seeking, church attendance), control of emotions (e.g., temper tantrums, anger, impulsiveness), intrapsychic functioning (e.g., ego integration, guilt), and interpersonal relating (e.g., fearlessness, aggression against siblings and peers). In this study the students who were fearless, who had trouble controlling their emotions, and who were unconventional were at higher stages of substance use as young adults than their counterparts. The researchers concluded that childhood personality risk factors predicted adolescent substance use by affecting the way the adolescent interacted within important environments (occupational, academic, social), and that these interactions in turn reinforced substance abuse.

Finally, ethnicity is indirectly related to adolescent substance abuse. In a study of more than 6000 African-American, Caucasian, Cuban, and other Hispanic sixth- to eigth-grade boys, researchers hypothesized that substance use was a basic coping mechanism and would be related to a higher number of risk factors (Vega et al, 1993). Ten risk factors were measured in relation to the use of alcohol, tobacco, inhalants, marijuana, cocaine (crack and powder), PCP, barbiturates, amphetamines, and tranquilizers. These risk factors were low family pride, family substance abuse, parental smoking, low self-esteem, depression, suicide-attempt history, perceptions of high peer substance use, perception of peer approval of substance use, willingness to engage in nonnormative behavior, and delinquent behavior. All the risk factors were important, but different risk factors were important for different ethnic groups. African-Americans and Hispanics were vulnerable to depressed mood and low self-esteem; Cubans and Caucasians were most likely to believe their friends used drugs; Caucasians reported the lowest levels of family pride. The African-American group had the highest group average number of risk factors, and the Caucasians were significantly more likely to have seven or more risk factors.

These findings highlight the point that adolescent substance abuse is a significant problem that is related to every aspect of the adolescent's life, including temperament; ethnicity; parent and peer substance use; family, community, and school problems; socioeconomic status; and type of substance (Lowery et al, 1996). These findings also suggest that adolescents who begin to smoke and drink may have several longstanding psychosocial problems that will need to be addressed before their risk of lifetime substance abuse can be decreased.

References

Allen P, Aber LJ, Leadbeater BJ: Adolescent problem behaviors: the influence of attachment and autonomy, *Psychiatric Clinics of N Am* 13(3):455, 1990.

American College of Physicians: Health care needs of the adolescent, *Ann of Internal Med* 110:130, 1989.

Blum R, Beuhring T: Guidelines for adolescent preventive services: addressing youths' risky behaviors, *Minnesota Med*, 78:29, 1995.

Brooks JS, Whiteman M, Cohen P, Shapiro J, Balka E: Longitudinally predicting late adolescent and young adult drug use: childhood and adolescent precursors, *J Am Acad Child Adolesc Psychiatry* 34(9):1230, 1995.

Bui K, Takeuchi D: Ethnic minority adolescents and the use of community mental health care services, *Am J Community Psychology* 20(4):403, 1992.

Burkhart B, Sherry A: Sexual victimization in adolescents, *Advances in Med Psychotherapy* 6:171, 1993.

Cappelli M, Clulow M, Goodman J, Davidson S, Feder S, Baron P, Manion MP: Identifying depressed and suicidal adolescents in a teen health clinic, *J Adoles Health* 16(1):64, 1995.

Erickson SJ, Feldman S, Steiner H: Defense mechanism and adjustment in normal adolescents, *Am J Psychiatry* 153(6):826, 1996.

Faigel HC: Primary care of the adolescent patient, *Hospital Prac* 31(4):127, 1996.

Harold R, Harold N: School based clinics: a response to the physical and mental health needs of adolescents, *Health and Social Work* 18:65, 1993.

Ho M: *Minority children and adolescents in therapy*, Newbury Park, CA, 1992, Sage.

Kandel DB, Davies M: High school students who use crack and other drugs, *Arch Gen Psychiatry* 53(1):71, 1996.

Kazdin A: Adolescent mental health: prevention and treatment programs, *Am Psychologist* 48:127, 1993.

Korenblum M, Marton P, Golomek H, Stein B: Personality status: changes through adolescence, *Psychiatric Clin of N Am* 13(3):389, 1990.

Lewinsohn P, Gotlib I, Seeley J: Adolescent psychopathology: IV. Specificity of psychosocial risk factors for depression and substance abuse in older adolescents, *J Am Acad Child Adolesc Psychiatry* 34(9):1221, 1995.

Lowry R, Kann L, Collins JL, Kolbe LJ: The effect of socioeconomic status on chronic disease risk behaviors among U.S. adolescents, *JAMA* 276(10):792, 1966.

Millstein S: Challenges for behavioral scientist, *Am Psychologist* 44:837, 1989.

Offer D, Ostrov E, Howard K, Atkinson R: Normality and adolescence, *Psychiatric Clin of N Am* 13(3):377, 1990.

Riggs S, Cheng T: Adolescents' willingness to use a school-based clinic in view of expressed health concerns, *J Adoles Health Care* 9:208, 1988.

Shaffer D, Gould MS, Fisher P, Trautman P, Moreau D, Kleinman M, Flory M: Psychiatric diagnosis in child and adolescent suicide, *Arch Gen Psychiatry* 53(4):339, 1996.

Spitz AM, Velebil P, Koonin LM, Strauss LT, Goodman KA, Wingo P, Wilson JB, Morris L, Marks JS: Pregnancy, abortion, and birth rates among U.S. adolescents- 1980, 1985, and 1990 *JAMA* 275(13):989, 1996.

Stringham P: Violent youth. In Parker S, Zuckerman B (editors): *Behavioral and development pediatrics: a handbook for primary care*, Boston, 1995, Little, Brown, and Company.

U.S. Office of Technology Assessment: *U.S. Adolescents face barriers to appropriate health care*, Washington DC, 1991, Government Printing Office.

Vega V, Zimmerman R, Warheir G, Apospori I, Gil A: Risk factors for early adolescent drug use in four ethnic and racial groups, *Am J Public Health* 83(2):185, 1993.

Elders 16

In anticipation of the first generation of adults over 65 to sit at the head of America's social table, society has had to redefine the aging individual as an American elder. This generation of American elders will differ little from previous generations its biopsychosocial needs, but it will differ significantly in the ability to command the necessary resources, including highly skilled primary care services (Cornman and Kingson, 1996).

By the year 2020 a significant portion of American elders in their seventh decade will have just retired or will be starting a third or fourth career. Many will enjoy highly independent lifestyles, with active and satisfying peer relationships. These elders will expect to participate in life fully and will seek those services that can best help them to protect their health, well-being, and way of life. Skilled practitioners will be looked upon as resources that can help elders continue to meet important life goals, rather than as professionals who manage the loss of health and well-being that occurs at the end of life. This chapter covers delirium, depression, anxiety, and alcohol and substance abuse, four common conditions experienced by elders of any age.

Aging

Age is no longer an accurate reflection of aging (Young, 1996). An individual who begins the process of normal biological and psychological aging experiences tremendous internal and external demands. Successful aging requires that the individual copes effectively with the stressors of aging, adapt adequately to the biopsychosocial changes of aging, and continue to put forth the necessary effort to meet one's personal needs for comfort and spiritual resolution (Spar and LaRue, 1990; Strawbridge et al, 1996). Large families were once organized in such a way that meeting the complex physical, psychological, social, and spiritual needs of aging family elders was a normal part of everyday life. Today's smaller families, typically a two-income married couple and their children, are still able to meet the needs of their aging elders, but in the absence of plentiful human resources the small family may have to expend considerable time and money to care for a loved one. Many couples are struggling to meet the needs of both their parents and their children. Although the strain for these couples has been great, it is anticipated that when this baby-boom generation ages, these elders will have even smaller family groups to care for them, and so the strain will be even greater.

However gradual or sudden the onset, or whatever the age of onset, aging is primarily the loss of biological capacities that in turn diminish functioning (Reichel, 1995). Most individuals feel anxious and a little sad when they anticipate their aging, particularly when they think about experiencing a serious loss of functioning or even suffering, and if they will be alone—the two great unknowns of aging. Everyone thinks about aging, and the thoughts are realistic if the individual has both positive and negative expectations. Individuals who have an imbalanced appraisal of aging, whether too positive or too negative, may have more anxiety about aging or may be less able to protect themselves from anxiety. When individuals reach the stage of aging, they may experience a sharp increase in anxiety, sadness in reaction to feelings of extreme stress related to physical, psychological, and social vulnerability, or they may react to ordinary stressors that they would have once disregarded. To others, this individual may seem to have undergone a total change in character or to have developed a mental disorder rather than extreme stress. Stress has traditionally been viewed as a fact of life for working adults and is only now being widely accepted as a problem for children, adolescents, and elders (Ensel et al, 1996). In short, aging is usually a very stressful experience. Some people will cope better than others, but almost everyone has some level of anticipatory anxiety about the problems and changes with which they will have to deal (Kalayam and Shamoian, 1990).

Elders require highly skilled care to prevent the poor physical and mental health conditions that can be avoided. Prevention requires the active participation of the aging individual with the practitioner. Practitioners can expect that more people will seek primary health care for the purpose of maintaining their health and personal life-styles well beyond what used to be the age of retirement. Elders will look to practitioners to perform routine screening, health promotion and illness prevention assessment, and to have a positive attitude and approach to meeting their health care needs. These expectations are particularly important in providing effective psychiatric primary care aimed at reducing the stress of normal aging. The assessment and management of common mental disorders and psychosocial problems are presented below. Prescribing medication for an elder who needs it requires a great deal of expertise, and the practitioner should consult with the appropriate primary care or psychiatric specialist.

Delirium

A recent symposium on delirium in elders generated the following information and recommendations (Rummans et al, 1995). Delirium is an alteration of the mental state to one of acute confusion. The condition is somewhat common but frequently unrecognized or misdiagnosed. Family and friends, as well as practitioners, may fail to recognize delirium thinking instead that the individual has become mean or lazy, or worse yet, they may simply assume that delirium is a normal consequence of aging. Delirium is a reversible state of confusion that impairs conscious awareness of important information. The individual is unable to focus, sustain, or change one's attention. The experience of delirium is frightening for the individual as well as for family and friends, and can precipitate a state of crisis that adds to what is already a very stressful situation. The prevalence rate for delirium among elders who are hospitalized is as high as 50%, with a preadmission rate of up to 24% (National Center for Health Statistics, 1992).

Delirium symptoms are cognitive, perceptual, and emotional. ***Cognitive symptoms*** include disorientation, language difficulties, or impairments in absorbing (learning) and retaining (memory) information. The individual may not know or may be uncertain of the time, a place, or a person; he or she may be unable to use words effectively or to express ideas and feelings clearly and may seem unwilling or uncooperative. Severe ***perceptual symptoms*** include illusions, delusions, and hallucinations. Illusions are misperceptions of actual experiences, delusions are false beliefs, and hallucinations are false perceptions. Each of these experiences is devastating to the individual and to his or her loved ones. Illusions can be more difficult to assess than delusions and hallucinations because, the latter two experiences are based entirely on false information, whereas illusions may include factual information. For example, an individual may feel hungry but may have illusions about this sensation, thinking instead that part of the gastrointestinal system is separating or dissolving. The individual is having a true experience (hunger), but due to delirium he or she is having frightening misperceptions about that experience. ***Emotional symptoms*** of delirium can be prominent, intermittent, or unpredictable. Common emotional symptoms are anger, sadness, extreme irritability, or euphoria.

The onset of delirium is usually related to physical illness, substance intoxication, medication or substance abuse side effects, or medication or substance withdrawal effects, but a vast range of conditions or separate factors can precipitate delirium in elders (Cole and Primeau, 1993). Onset tends to be rapid, occurring over a few hours or a few days, but symptoms may be mild, moderate, or intermittent, making assessment and diagnosis difficult. The individual may literally seem to be going in and coming out of a state of confusion, or, as is unfortunately all too often the case, the individual's symptoms may be seen as intentional or manipulative. Rapid changes in mental state significantly increase the difficulty of assessment. Within the span of minutes, an individual can cycle from a state of drowsiness to hypervigilance to normal wakefulness, then to agitation. The individual may also cycle through the same mental states over a period of days, which increases the probability of the symptoms being overlooked or misdiagnosed. Rummans et al (1995), note that delirium remains undetected in up to half of the individuals who have it.

Delirium may be classified in terms of the individual's level of psychomotor activity. ***Hyperactive delirium*** is the most common of the delirium diagnoses, mostly because this condition is obvious even to the casual observer. It is often associated with adverse medication effects from anticholinergic drugs or substance intoxication or withdrawal. Individuals with hyperactive delirium become agitated and may experience psychosis (full loss of contact with reality) or rapid changes in mood; they may become uncooperative or belligerent and may engage in highly disruptive behaviors, such as shouting for help or being physically aggressive. In this state the individual is at significant risk for injury due to falling, combativeness, or removing treatment catheters or intravascular lines. Unless otherwise prohibited, sedation is usually required. If the individual is experiencing psychosis, illusions, delusions, or hallucinations, treatment is generally the smallest effective dose of antipsychotic medication.

Hypoactive delirium is characterized by decreased psychomotor activity. Hypoactive delirium is also frequently unrecognized or dismissed as a temporary problem that is not highly significant. Metabolic conditions, such as hepatic or renal encephalopathy, are frequently associated with hypoactive delirium, but there are many other common causes of this condition. The individual with hypoactive delirium appears lethargic as well as confused. The absence of disruptive, bizarre, or injurious behaviors makes this condition more difficult to recognize. The quiet state of withdrawal, apathy, and clouded inattention that defines hypoactive delirium can be difficult to distinguish from drowsiness. The two conditions differ in that the individual who is merely dozing or sleeping can be aroused with a mild stimulus and will stay awake. With hypoactive delirium, a strong, vigorous stimulus, such as shaking or shouting, is required to increase the individual's level of alertness, an increase that will never-the-less be incomplete and temporary.

A combination of hypoactive and hyperactive delirium symptoms is not unusual, and about 40% of individuals will experience illusions, delusions, or hallucinations regardless of their level of psychomotor activity. Delirium can produce a range of somatic symptoms, including incontinence, impaired gait, and tremor. Symptoms of receptive and expressive aphasia are not unusual. Impaired information processing or impaired memory is thought to be an inability to receive and register information due to impaired attention. This impairment can affect recall of information in both short-term and long-term memory. Higher-order cognitive functions are impaired in much the same way. The individual has a great deal of difficulty making plans, solving tasks, or following a set of instructions. These symptoms increase in intensity and impact with fatigue, a process that is referred to as ***sundowning***. With delirium, the risk of severe injury from falling is so great that specific measures to prevent falls are necessary. Individuals with this disorder sleep poorly and are not likely to feel rested even if they have been able to sleep. Many individuals develop a pattern of daytime napping and nighttime wakefulness.

Individual variations in the course of delirium are considerable. Onset tends to be abrupt, with brief periods of symptom relief, but overall the course of delirium fluctuates, with acute symptom episodes that persist for a few days to a few weeks at a time. Between acute episodes the individual can become totally lucid, and in fact a cycle of increasing, decreasing, and absent symptoms clarifies a diagnosis of delirium. However, these brief periods of full awareness are extremely distressing and upsetting to the individual, who may, for example, become lucid only to find that he or she has been physically restrained. It is impossible to overstate the embarrassment, hopelessness, and grief that individuals may experience. Statements of suicidal intent are not unusual, because few people would not become fearful of living with such a condition (Devons, 1996).

Treatment of delirium begins with treatment of the condition for which the delirium may be a symptom (e.g., stroke, alcoholism). Treatment outcomes are uncertain. Many people will have full recovery or will continue to experience mild to moderate symptoms. Fragile individuals may be unable to withstand the biopsychosocial stress of delirium, thereby increasing the risk of death. Delirium may also be the reason for long hospital stays or institutionalized care that can also be stressful.

It was once thought that delirium predicted dependence, decline, and death. This observation seems to be related more to persistent than to brief episodes of delirium. A study of 125 hospitalized elders diagnosed with delirium found that only 4% had recovered completely by the time of discharge (Cole and Primeau, 1993). At 3 and 6 months after discharge, 21% and 18%, respectively, had fully recovered. In this study, individuals with subclinical symptom levels tended to have a similar course of illness, with prolonged hospital stays, persistent symptoms, and decreased independence, though with lesser acuity. Such research findings indicate that delirium is a serious condition, but many people can improve or recover with treatment.

Delirium can develop as a secondary condition related to dementia, a stable and progressive illness of deterioration. Individuals who are treated for delirium should be reassessed 3 to 6 months after recovery before a diagnosis of dementia is considered. The Folstein mini-mental exam is a well-standardized measure of cognitive capacity that can be useful in distinguishing delirium from dementia (Folstein, Folstein, and McHugh, 1975). Fluctuations in mini-mental exam scores occur with delirium, but scores remain below 23 with dementia. Individuals with mild delirium in which poor concentration is the main symptom will have dramatic improvement in their mini-mental exam scores with successful treatment of delirium symptoms. Unrelated conditions, such as physical fatigue, dehydration, medication, pain, infection, metabolic disorder, or less-than-eighth-grade reading level will also have a negative impact on the individual's mini-mental exam scores.

Pathophysiology of Delirium

Delirium is considered a nonspecific, neuropsychiatric disorder of cerebral metabolism and neurohormone transmission. Alterations in neurotransmitter activity are believed to account for symptoms of delirium, including alterations in acetylcholine, dopamine, and gamma-aminobutyric (GABA) along cortical, subcortical, and central nervous system pathways. Delirium may be caused by medications, drug abuse, alcohol abuse, or toxins that act upon vital neurotransmitter systems and produce periods of confusion rather than a global disturbance in cerebral function.

Abnormalities in cholinergic neurotransmission, such as those seen with anticholinergic drugs, can produce symptoms of delirium. Memory-related symptoms and changes in level of consciousness that occur with delirium appear to be associated with cholinergic pathways. Anticholinergic delirium is characterized by agitation, psychosis, memory loss, disorientation, confusion, and in severe cases coma. Severe dry mouth and dry skin can be early signs of anticholinergic reactions, indicating the need for a significant decrease in the amount of medication being taken, or even a complete discontinuation of the medication, in order to decrease the risk of delirium reaction to anticholinergic drugs.

Excessive dopamine activity has also been implicated in the onset of delirium and may explain why medications that block dopamine, such as the antipsychotic medication haloperidol, can provide delirium symptom relief despite their anticholinergic properties. Dopamine-specific antipsychotic medication, at the lowest effective dose, can also be effective in remitting hallucinations and decreasing the illusions and delusions of delirium.

GABA, the predominant inhibitory central nervous system (CNS) neurotransmitter related to anxiety, has also been found to be related to hepatic encephalopathy. Increased serum ammonia levels associated with the condition may contribute to increased glutamate and glutamine levels, which in turn increase GABA levels. Study findings suggest that an endogenous, benzodiazepine-like toxin is produced as an effect of liver failure, and this toxin contributes to the development of encephalopathy by binding to hypothalamus benzodiazepine receptors. Overstimulation at these receptor sites produces somnolence, a symptom normally observed in individuals with hepatic encephalopathy. Individuals who have abused benzodiazepines, barbiturates, or alcohol and are undergoing withdrawal can experience a sudden understimulation at these receptor sites, resulting in hyperactive delirium. Serotonin (the neurotransmitter related to depression) histamines, opioids, and glucocorticoids have also been implicated as pathophysiological factors in the onset of delirium.

The aging body has a lower lean-to-fat body-mass ratio and decreased rates of glomerular filtration and creatinine clearance. Total plasma protein levels, particularly albumin levels, tend to be lower. The combined effect of these biological changes can account for excessively high plasma medication levels and increased risk of toxicity in elders who are taking normal doses of otherwise safe medications. Given the biological implications of normal aging, fat-soluble medications that require renal clearance tend to have a longer half-life, and water-soluble medications tend to have a much smaller volume of distribution, which also increases plasma medication levels and the risk of medication toxicity.

With most medications, a dose that would otherwise be considered therapeutic could easily be excessively high for an elder. Most medications that are metabolized within the hepatic or renal systems, such as medications to control pain and improve sleep, can precipitate the onset of delirium. Similarly, the abrupt discontinuation of a prescribed medication can predispose the individual to delirium onset. As more and more prescribed medications become available over-the-counter (OTC), these OTC medications must also be considered as factors in the sudden onset of delirium. Finally, decreases in cortical brain cells, acetylcholine storage, and muscarinic receptor plasticity associated with normal aging can lead to lower neurotransmitter reserves and activity levels, thereby increasing the risk of delirium in elders who are taking anticholinergic medications.

Perceptual disturbances that are associated with delirium in patients with a history of schizophrenia, depression, or mania should be distinguished from psychotic symptoms that are associated with these disorders. Elders with baseline cognitive impairment, depression, alcoholism, or poor physical health may also be at increased risk for delirium. Specific physiological risk factors for delirium include male gender, age greater than 70 years, poor premorbid functioning, and impaired vision. Illnesses that have been related to the onset of delirium include Alzheimer's dementia, Parkinson's disease, cerebrovascular disease, stroke, fracture on hospital admission, symptomatic infection, total knee arthroplasties, cardiac and noncardiac thoracic surgical procedures, and surgical repair of aortic aneurysms.

Depression

At a time when the individual as a whole is less resilient, elders are having to cope with major changes in health, well-being, and physical and psychosocial functioning. How an individual appraises these changes or the meaning of these changes is important to one's ability to cope and therefore one's risk of depression. The series of losses and the many disruptions that can occur at this stage of life, particularly the loss of important attachments, are a source of pain and stress to those who are already facing the many challenges of aging (Johnston and Walker, 1996). Retirement once served as a clear social milestone or signal of the changes and challenges that define aging, but this event is less likely to serve such a purpose for coming generations of elders.

Depression in elders is usually classified as early or late onset. The age of 60 has traditionally been used to distinguish early from late onset, but as people live longer this age is not quite as useful for this purpose. However, the age at which depression onset occurs is extremely important, both for the course of the illness and for treatment reasons. Clinically, ***early onset depression*** is major depression without age-related complications, whereas ***late onset depression*** includes the age-related symptoms of early morning insomnia, hypochondriasis or somatizing, agitation, and a markedly higher incidence of delusions.

Depression is sometimes said to be *masked* or to exist behind presenting somatic and cognitive complaints. With masked depression, the individual does not seem to have emotional distress or complaints. In many cases this is due to the fact that the individual is unaware of his or her sadness, stress, or anxiety or is semiaware of these negative mood states but attributes them to a physical illness. Masked depression is further complicated by the problem of ***polypharmacy***: when elders are taking a lot of medications with possible direct and interactive depressive side effects, depression itself is not easy to recognize due to these effects.

Cimetidine, antipsychotics, benzodiazepines, barbiturates, narcotics, and digitalis can also cause masked depression. Antihypertensive medications (e.g., reserpine, clonidine, and propranolol), antiparkinsonian medications (e.g., L-dopa), hormonal medications (e.g., progesterone and prednisone), and antineoplastic medications (e.g., vincristine) are possible causes of depression in elders.

Many physical illness conditions can cause stress-related depression due to the severity of the illness, related biological changes, or depression as a complicated grief response to the illness. Severe physical conditions such as postmyocardial infarction, renal failure, seizure disorder, Alzheimer's disease, and Parkinson's disease can be also be viewed as stressors associated with depression. And depression as a symptom of an illness condition, such as hypothyroidism, is more common in this population of individuals, who are more likely to have such illnesses. Any physical condition that involves a great deal of physical and social changes, such as menopause or recovery from cardiac arrest, can be related to the onset of depression in individuals who find change difficult.

Traditionally depression, like delirium, was viewed as a normal part of aging rather than as a disorder likely to be experienced by elders. It was once assumed that men who no longer worked and women who no longer had children in the home would have no other interests in life and would think of these events as the close of the most meaningful chapters of their lives. The social expectation was that people would grieve and mourn the loss of a meaningful life and become depressed. Bereavement due to the loss of a lifemate continues to be the major depression-related stressor for elders , but retirement, whether from employment or homemaking, is much less likely to be viewed as the end of a meaningful life. Nevertheless grief, bereavement, stress, and anxiety related to aging are important threats to the emotional health and well-being of elders.

Loss of a child or a partner can directly increase the risk of early or late onset depression or of somatic complaints with masked depression, with a resulting decrease in functioning that can lead to such a decline that it was once assumed to be a normal part of the aging process (Kane, Ouslander and Abrass, 1994). The loss of loved ones is a stressful but unavoidable fact of aging, so emphasis must be put on the individual's ability to cope with these stressors. This, and the early identification of a distressed elder, are important determinants of short-term and long-term depression risk. Women and caretaker spouses (male or female) are at increased risk for stress-related depression. Caretaker spouses are especially susceptible to depression if they have cared for an ill partner for a prolonged period of time and have been physically and emotionally drained by the experience. The sudden unexpected loss of a partner can be a significant depression risk factor, since the loss occurs so quickly or under such circumstances that the individual is susceptible to a state of crisis, which may in turn interfere with the process of grief and mourning.

For treatment, most elders tolerate serotonin selective reuptake inhibitor (SSRI) antidepressants better than tricyclic antidepressants. This makes prescribing medication for depression safer and more likely to be effective. The SSRIs are significantly less anticholinergic than tricyclics, which contributes to the safety and increased prescribing options with these medications. However, SSRIs are expensive and, as is the case for all age groups, the expense of medication as a potential source of financial stress must be considered.

Delusion depression, seen more often in elders than other age groups is difficult to treat with antidepressant medication or with a combination of antidepressant and antipsychotic medications.

At the same time, delusion depression can be a very dangerous condition, including the increased risk of behavior that is potentially harmful to oneself or others. Electroconvulsive treatment of delusional depression in elders is extremely effective and is a sound alternative when the risk of medication side effects or prolonged depression with loss of function indicate the need for alternative treatment. Negative social attitudes toward electroconvulsive treatment for depression and the fact that the precise mode of treatment effect has yet to be discovered make this treatment unacceptable for many people. When these barriers are not a factor, all too often the high cost of electroconvulsive treatment is prohibitive.

In conclusion, depression in elders is not a fact of aging, but there are normal life events that occur in this stage of life that represent profound loss, and loss is one of the most important depression risk factors.

Anxiety

The prevalence rate of anxiety disorders among elders does not differ greatly from the rate among the general population; however, phobic anxiety disorders tend to be more common. A diagnosis of anxiety disorder can be more difficult with this population because most of the symptoms of anxiety disorders are physical—and no different from the physical symptoms of physical illnesses (Alexopoulos, 1990). Diagnosis can also be complicated when the individual has both a physical illness and an anxiety disorder. Some of the health conditions commonly associated with anxiety in elders are major depression, adjustment disorder, dementia, late onset psychosis, personality disorders, alcoholism, benzodiazepine abuse and dependence, chronic pain syndrome, crisis, and physical illness (e.g., cardiovascular, chronic respiratory, or Parkinson's disease).

Common symptoms of anxiety are dysphoric apprehension, trembling, shakiness, aches, restlessness, easily fatigued, shortness of breath or smothering sensations, tachycardia, palpitations, sweating, dry mouth, dizziness, nausea, diarrhea, flushes or chills, frequent urination, trouble swallowing or hypervigilance, exaggerated startle response, difficulty concentrating, trouble falling asleep, and irritability. Symptoms of anxiety can be very distressing to the individual and difficult to distinguish from physical illness conditions. How the individual ***reacts*** to the anxiety symptoms is also a factor, but the interaction here may be difficult to determine. Individuals can have reactions to their physical symptoms of anxiety that are less than helpful or that can make assessment more difficult. For example, some individuals become mistrustful and accusing if their physical symptoms of anxiety are not treated with a full cardiac evaluation, even though laboratory findings have clearly ruled this out.

Physical symptoms of anxiety are extremely unpleasant but not usually life threatening. Anxiety symptoms can be relieved by emotional support, antianxiety medication, or both, depending on whether the basis of the anxiety is an event or a chronic condition. Prescribing antianxiety medications for elders is made difficult by the fact that these medications are sedating and can create obvious hazards such as falls or delirium, and the few nonsedating antianxiety medications available are not helpful for some people. On the other hand, some individuals with more generalized anxiety symptoms may improve with SSRIs. Transient anxiety associated with stress, loss, or change seldom improves with medication, or the individual who receives medication may complain that it is not providing the desired effects.

Emotional support with structure and reassurance is a very effective intervention for mild to moderate symptoms of anxiety, but both interventions require time and effort that may not always be available. Individuals who experience very specific symptoms of anxiety, such as muscle weakness in the arms, legs, and back, can improve with stress management and relaxation training, but both interventions require a considerable amount of individual motivation and energy—certainly more effort than is required for treatment with a prescribed medication.

It is not uncommon for family and friends to take the position that an elder should not be refused easy comforts or expected to learn new coping skills when medication will do. This logic contributes to the problem of polypharmacy treatment with elders. If an individual's age is used to determine how much effort should be made to reduce anxiety, medication will always be the treatment of choice. This approach seems less than rational since relaxation training can be effective and allows elders to remain in control and use effective self-care practices that can support their self-esteem. When persistent symptoms of anxiety occur with frustration or interpersonal conflict, for example, these events should be addressed directly as a means of reducing the basis for the individual's anxiety. Cognitive impairment or severe physical illness can make interventions such as relaxation impossible. In such cases medication may be the only suitable treatment.

The most common treatment for anxiety continues to be antianxiety medication, but benzodiazepines used for the treatment of anxiety expose the individual to significant health hazards, including dependence, delirium, and falls. Because the half-life of most medications, including benzodiazepines, may be substantially longer with elders, their use requires routine monitoring to decrease the risk of toxicity. When anxiety symptoms greatly interfere with day-to-day functioning or activities, and symptom relief produces normal functioning, the individual may be quite clear about the decision to use benzodiazepine medications. The problem with this plan is that tolerance may be associated with decreased effectiveness, so that an individual must take more medication, which can lead to more health risks but not necessarily any improvement in anxiety. Evidence of a history of substance abuse or dependence prohibits the use of benzodiazepines.

Diazepam, chlordiazepoxide and clonazepam are frequently used. Long-acting benzodiazepines are usually taken twice a day for a limited period of time. Short-acting bezodiazepines have several advantages over drugs with longer half-lives. These medications tend to have very rapid onset, usually within minutes, which means they can be useful with episodes of acute anxiety. They also have shorter half-lives, with lower levels of active metabolites, which means less risk of cumulative effects. The primary disadvantage of short-acting antianxiety medications is that they are not useful for long-term management of anxiety.

Lorazepam is one of the most commonly prescribed antianxiety medications, primarily because it has a short predictable half-life and can be prescribed in small doses. Its short half-life makes it useful in the treatment of situational anxiety. Buspirone hydrochloride, an atypical, nonsedating antianxiety agent, has proved useful in the long-term treatment of chronic generalized anxiety disorder, but it is less helpful with acute anxiety or panic.

Alcohol and Substance Abuse

Estimates of alcoholism rates are substantially higher among clinical populations regardless of age since these individuals are more likely to use health care services. The approximate rate of alcoholism for clinic, hospital, and nursing home populations is between 15% and 58 % (Closser and Blow, 1993).

Alcohol abuse is often underdiagnosed and untreated in elders because their substance abuse tends to be out of public view. Unless observed by family members or close friends who are not drinking companions, alcohol abuse may develop and continue for years, until the individual's health begins to fail. At the same time, elders who abuse alcohol can avoid detection by avoiding interactions with others. They may insist on being alone or that they are too ill or too tired to spend time with friends and family. Often loneliness, anxiety, depression, and fear maintain alcohol abuse among elders.

When the alcohol abuse of an elder does not create immediate hazards to that individual or to others, many believe that there is no harm in it. Compared to an adolescent boy who abuses alcohol, drives while intoxicated, gets into physical fights, or is sexually aggressive, an elder who quietly drinks alcohol every day seems much less of a problem.

This social attitude toward alcohol abuse is related to the fact that problems at work, school, or within important relationships are viewed as symptoms of the condition. In fact, the hazards of alcohol abuse to elders are not less serious than with younger-age problem drinkers, and in some respects the problems are worse. Elders may be able to drink alone without being observed, but they are not unaffected by the drug. Elders who abuse alcohol can become emotionally unavailable to family and friends as well as interpersonally aggressive, hurting people with words. They represent a serious hazard to others in terms of home fires started by falling asleep with a lighted cigarette, leaving lighted cigarettes unattended, or attempting to cook a meal while intoxicated. Intoxicated elders may also drive under the influence if they have access to a car. Low-income elders who abuse alcohol may also be considered a hazard to others when they combine their assets with underage adolescents to obtain alcohol. Adolescents have the money to buy alcohol, and elders who buy large amounts of alcohol are not likely to be questioned.

When none of these problems is a factor, the health hazards of alcohol abuse become the primary concern. Because elders as a group do not have a high social status, there continues to be the assumption that their alcohol abuse is somehow more acceptable or should be viewed differently. Some argue that it would be more of a hazard to try to treat the elder's drinking problem than to allow him or her to continue to abuse alcohol. The negative physical and mental health effects of alcohol abuse for elders are so great that just the opposite assumption should be made: Without alcohol abuse this individual would probably have a dramatic improvement in physical health, mental status, and social relationships. Instead, it can be all too easy to take the view that an elder's drinking is not harmful but is simply enjoyable.

The health risk of alcohol abuse for elders can be significantly greater than the risk to adolescents and adults, because of age and decreased physical ability to metabolize the drug. Alcohol abuse may be hazardous enough in many cases to be considered dangerous behavior to oneself, such as when the elder is taking OTC or prescribed medications. The risk of interactive effects cannot be overstated. However, nearly every experienced practitioner has encountered elders who take a dozen prescribed medications every day and abuse alcohol. These individuals have multiple physical and mental health problems that seem resistant to treatment, such as congestive heart failure and anxiety. All too often yet another medication is tried, rather than attempting to help the elder stop the alcohol abuse.

Denial is a major treatment problem because elders are no more likely than any other age group to easily admit to an alcohol problem. In fact, it may be easier for elders to seek health care for physical symptoms that are related to their alcohol abuse without disclosing their drinking problem (Closser and Blow, 1993). It is unreasonable to assume that an elder who abuses alcohol would be unable to benefit significantly from alcohol abuse treatment or to tolerate alcohol detoxification and withdrawal.

Many elders take benzodiazepines daily and have become physically dependent on them. This is another important substance abuse problem in this population. However, when the individual does not increase the daily dosage or take single doses large enough to produce intoxication, substance dependence is not likely to become a focus of health care attention; just the opposite is true with adolescents and adults who are dependent on benzodiazepines. Aging can be a stressful experience, rife with unpredictable and unpleasant events, but these events do not define aging, and alternative support resources are becoming more and more available. Treatment programs for elders with substance abuse must become more accessible and available and offered with formats that are socially acceptable to this population group. Elders can and do benefit from treatment for alcohol abuse, but it must address the stressors related to aging with which the elder is trying to cope. Elders who have had a lifetime of alcohol abuse and who have extremely fragile health status as a result can present some of the most difficult challenges for practitioners and specialists. Those who ***begin*** to abuse alcohol as an elder, perhaps in response to a painful loss, should be treated with a goal of alcohol abuse remission (Blazer, 1996).

Assessment of elders should include substance use questions, and when substance abuse is suspected, a full assessment of risks and needs should be performed. This should address the individual's changes in mood, thoughts, and behavior, as with all mental disorder assessments, past diagnosis and treatment for mental disorders, and current physical or mental health concerns. Psychosocial problem assessment should focus on aging but not to the exclusion of other common concerns. For example, there is an increasing number of elders who are the primary caretakers of their grandchildren because the parents are unable or unwilling to care for the children. There are also many elders with adult children who have returned home, and this arrangement can be the source of painful relationship conflicts or other problems that may have little to do with aging. Assessment should place a great deal of attention on what resources are available to the elder. Inadequate resources (e.g., financial, social, health care, transportation) are second only to poor health as a major concern and problem for elders. Because the potential of physical abuse always exists, assessment of an individual's alcohol abuse and physical safety around others should be clarified, and evidence of harmful or poor coping skills or suicidal thoughts should be fully addressed (Devons, 1996; Groc, 1993).

Management of Mental Disorders Common among Elders

➤ Counseling

Psychiatric primary care counseling should support the individual's needs for self-esteem and well-being as important elements of routine care. Important friends and relatives may be involved, but these individuals do not speak for the elder. Any evidence of unrecognized cognitive impairment should first be evaluated as a potential medication side effect or as a symptom of a physical illness before a diagnosis of mental disorder is even considered. Exercise, physical safety, and nutritional assessment and counseling should be routine.

Individual brief therapy can be helpful for elders who have lost loved ones, but support groups are more useful for caregiver lifemates and for elders who need more social interaction opportunities. Counseling does not have to be totally problem focused; elders have concerns and interests other than aging, such as politics, social change, and local community issues. Aging is always considered, but aging is not the total life experience of an individual over 70. Interpersonal support is always important and should be discussed. Some individuals may be reluctant to enter into new social settings to meet new people, but in most cases their reluctance has more to do with not knowing what to expect than not wishing to meet people.

Families may want to help their elder relatives but may not know how, or they may feel that they have little to offer. Family counseling can help the family to determine what is needed and to make plans to be together with the elder. Families often need a great deal of education about how to help, how to know when "help" is not helping, and how to handle an emergency. A particular source of stress for some families is an elder who insists on being totally independent when in fact the individual needs their help. Practitioners can help the family to find a compromise that does not demean the elder or the family's good intentions. Elders who rely on their families may have feelings they would like to talk about or problems they would like to address, without implying that they are dissatisfied or anything other than grateful. They may look to the practitioner as a resource for this need.

Elders who are clearly in a state of confusion that could indicate delirium will require hospitalization for severe symptoms and immediate treatment for moderate or mild symptoms.

Finally, a unique form of counseling with elders is reminiscence, with the focus on remote memory. Photos and other retrieval cues can be used to stimulate reminiscing, which is a very comfortable format for counseling (Rentz, 1995). The individual is often better able to interact and may feel less out of place. The more comfortable an individual is, the more comfortable and effective counseling becomes. It can also be informative to talk with elders when they are on comfortable ground, so to speak, and to compare their moods and comfort levels then to when the topic of conversation is something with which they are less comfortable.

References

Alexopoulos GS: Anxiety-depression syndromes in old age, *Int J Geriatric Psychiatry* 5:351, 1990.

Blazer DG: Alcohol and drug problems. In Busse EW, Blazer DG (editors): *Textbook of Geriatric Psychiatry,* 2nd Edition, Washington DC, 1996, American Psychiatric Press.

Closser MH, Blow FC: Special populations women, ethnic minorities, and the elderly, *Psychiatric Clin of N Am* 16(1):199, 1993.

Cole MG, Primeau FJ: Prognosis of delirium in elderly hospital patients, *Can Med Assoc J* 149:41, 1993.

Cornman JM, Kingson ER: Trends, issues, perspectives, and values for the aging of the baby boom cohorts, *The Gerontologist* 36(1):15, 1996.

Devons CA: Suicide in the elderly: how to identify and treat patients at risk, *Geriatrics* 51(3):67, 1996.

Ensel WM, Peek MK, Lin N, Lai G: Stress in the life course, *J of Aging and Health* 8(3):389, 1996.

Folstein MF, Folstein SE, McHugh PR: Mini-mental state: a practical method for grading the cognitive state of patients for clinicians, *J Psychiatr Res* 12:189, 1975.

Groc S: *The thirst for wholeness: addiction, attachment, and the spiritual path*, New York, 1993, Harper Collins.

Johnston M, Walker M: Suicide in the elderly recognizing the signs, *Gen Hosp Psychiatry* 18(4):257, 1996.

Kane RL, Ouslander JG, Abrass IB: *Essentials of Clinical Geriatrics*, New York, 1994, McGraw Hill Company.

Kalayam B, Shamoian CA: Geriatric psychiatry: an update, *J Clin Psychiatry* 51(5):177, 1990.

National Center for Health Statistics: Current estimates from the national health survey 1991, *Vital and Health Statistics Series 10, No. 184*, 1992.

Reichel W (editor): *Care of the elderly,* 4th Edition, Baltimore, 1995, William & Wilkins.

Rentz C: Reminiscence: a supportive intervention for the person with alzheimer's disease, *J of Psychosocial Nursing and Mental Health Services* 33(11):15, 1995.

Rummans RA, Evans JM, Krahn LE, Fleming KC: Delirium in elderly patients: evaluation and management, *Mayo Clinic Proc* 70:989, 1995.

Spar JE, LaRue A: *Geriatric Psychiatry*, Washington DC, 1990, American Psychiatric Press.

Strawbridge WJ, Cohen RD, Shema SJ, Kaplan GA: Successful aging: predictors and associated activities, *Am J ofEpidemiology* 144(2):135, 1996.

Young K: Health, health promotion and the elderly, *J of Clin Nursing* 5(4):241, 1996.

Survivors of Trauma 17

Rhonda Michele Kutil

When individuals are confronted with life-threatening events that are beyond their control, they experience high levels of physical and psychological stress. High levels of stress can cause individuals to react abnormally, becoming dazed, stunned, disorganized, or aggressive, or crying and screaming for help. When the human body is confronted with extremely high levels of stress, there is a strong "fight or flight" crisis response (Southwick et al, 1994). In an acute crisis, this response is adaptive and may be critical for survival, but the response can also be maladaptive, leading to psychological crisis and long-term psychological problems (Van der Kolk, 1996). Individuals who experience traumatic events, such as sexual assault, war, disaster, catastrophic illness, or accidents, are at risk for immediate psychological crises and long-term psychological problems. Immediate and appropriate health care can reduce the risk of both by altering the short- and long-term effects of the traumatic event that produced the crisis response. This chapter reviews the effects of traumatic events on survivors as well as treatment strategies for survivors.

Post-traumatic Stress Disorder (PTSD)

The psychological effects of severe trauma were first examined in soldiers. During the Civil War, physicians noted symptoms of generalized weakness, heart palpitations, and chest pain among traumatized soldiers. During World War I many soldiers complained of fatigue, exhaustion, and anxiety, but it wasn't until the Vietnam War that the formal diagnosis of post-traumatic stress disorder (PTSD) was developed and then documented in veterans. Since the introduction of the PTSD diagnosis, its appropriate use has been broadened to include individuals who have experienced assault, crime, torture, disaster, accident, and abuse (Tomb, 1994). The *Diagnostic and Statistical Manual of Mental Disorders, fourth edition*, defines four diagnostic criteria for PTSD

(American Psychiatric Association [APA], 1994). The individual has witnessed, been confronted with, or experienced a traumatic event that involves actual or potential death or serious injury, and the individual's response to the event is

1. Fear, helplessness, or horror
2. Intrusive psychological reexperiencing of the event
3. Avoidance
4. Increased stress arousal (APA, 1994)

Reexperiencing means that the individual keeps reliving the traumatic event in the form of intrusive thoughts and feelings, nightmares, or flashbacks. ***Flashbacks*** are a full sensory reexperience of the traumatic event, as though it were actually occurring again. Reliving experiences can be triggered by cues that, to the individual, have come to symbolize or be similar to the original traumatic event. For example, a women who was sexually assaulted in a public park may relive the assault when she is again in a public park. Weather (e.g., rain) and seasons (e.g., New Year's Eve) can also trigger a reliving experience.

Avoidance symptoms are conscious or subconscious avoidance of thoughts of the trauma. Avoidance symptoms include amnesia, dissociation, emotional numbing, and distancing. ***Amnesia*** of the traumatic event is a prominent feature of PTSD, associated particularly with severe trauma. ***Dissociation*** refers to episodes of acting automatically, without conscious self-awareness. An everyday example of dissociation is driving a familiar route home and then not remembering the drive after you have arrived. ***Emotional numbing*** can manifest as emotional detachment from friends and family, loss of interest in people and events, and an inability to feel or experience most normal emotions (e.g., happiness). Avoidance may also manifest as a sense of a foreshortened future, or the belief that one will not survive into the future.

Increased arousal as a symptom of PTSD requires at least two of the following symptoms: sleep difficulties, irritability, concentration difficulties, hypervigilance, or exaggerated startle response. ***Sleep difficulties*** are often due to nightmares that wake the individual up during the night or recurrent nightmares that cause the individual to wish to avoid sleep. ***Irritability*** may manifest as outbursts of anger and may be triggered by a reminder of the traumatic event. ***Concentration difficulties*** can be related to intrusive thoughts and avoidance symptoms. ***Hypervigilance*** is excessive monitoring for possible sources of dangers even when one is in relative safety.

A diagnosis of PTSD requires that all four symptom criteria be present for at least 1 month. The DSM-IV distinguishes between ***acute PTSD*** (1 to 3 months) and ***chronic PTSD*** (more than 3 months). ***Delayed-onset PTSD*** is diagnosed when symptom onset occurs 6 months or longer after the traumatic event.

There is considerable comorbidity associated with PTSD. The most common mental disorders associated with PTSD are anxiety disorder, major depression or dysthymia, and substance disorders. Disorders that occur less frequently with PTSD are phobias, personality disorders, and somatoform disorders. The most important symptom criterion for distinguishing PTSD from these other disorders is the history of a traumatic event. Because amnesia of the traumatic event is a symptom of PTSD, the diagnosis cannot be ruled out without a complete patient history. PTSD symptoms in children and adolescents may differ significantly from adult symptoms. The type of symptoms found in children depend on the child's age and cognitive development at the time of the traumatic event (Eth and Pynoos, 1985).

PTSD symptoms in infants include excessive crying, eating, sleeping, overstimulated states, and failure to thrive. Symptoms in preschool children include sleep disorders, repetitive play associated with the traumatic event, hyperalertness, regressive behaviors, fear, sadness, and shame. Symptoms in school-age children include sleep disorders, anxiety, depression, hyperalertness, retelling the event, return of old fears or the onset of new fears, and loss of interests. Adolescents have many of the PTSD symptoms experienced by adults, with the addition of acting-out behaviors such as suicidal gestures, hypersexuality, substance abuse, truancy, and minor self-injury. Although trauma is presented here as a criterion for the diagnosis of PTSD, trauma during childhood and adolescence can also precede adult substance abuse, personality disorders, depression, anxiety disorders, and eating disorders.

Treatment of PTSD

The majority of individuals who experience severe trauma do not develop PTSD. It is estimated that about 30% of those individuals who are exposed to severe trauma (war, rape, and disasters) will develop PTSD (Tomb, 1994), and these individuals need extensive specialized care. Referral to a specialist is indicated when the individual meets all four of the DSM-IV criteria for PTSD. This means that the individual is fearful and has reexperiencing, avoidance, and stress-arousal symptoms for at least 1 month. If the individual is experiencing only one or two PTSD symptoms, then information, emotional support, and crisis intervention may be adequate. If there are more than two PTSD symptoms that persist of intensify, referral to specialized care is necessary. Referral may also be necessary if there is significant comorbidity, such as an anxiety disorder or major depression in addition to PTSD symptoms.

Treatment of PTSD usually requires a combination of treatment approaches (McFarlane, 1994), including individual psychotherapy, group therapy, family therapy, and medication. Cognitive-behavioral therapy is very helpful because individuals can learn to identify internal and external PTSD symptom triggers. Individuals can continue to work through the personal meaning of the traumatic event, with the goal of increasing control over intrusive thoughts and feelings. Cognitive-behavioral therapy also helps the individual to begin to realistically assess the amount of danger at the time of the trauma and presently. With this process individuals are able to confront their PTSD symptoms of hypervigilance and stress arousal by learning to focus on current safety rather than past traumas.

Group therapy can be very helpful for a number of reasons. First, group members have the opportunity to talk about their traumatic events, which allows for emotional catharsis. Second, group members are able to see that other individuals have experienced the same or a similar trauma, which can decrease negative feelings of uniqueness and isolation. Third, group members can talk about how they cope with their PTSD symptoms, and this sharing allows group members to learn new coping methods as well as strengthen their effective coping skills. Finally, group therapy can serve as a support network. Because PTSD symptoms include emotional numbing and interpersonal distancing, PTSD survivors can become alienated from close friends and family. Group members who build connections with each other may find it easier to rebuild their relationships with their significant others. Family therapy may be necessary when the individual becomes alienated from family members due to severe avoidance symptoms.

The most common type of medications given for PTSD are antidepressants (Southwick et al, 1994). Tricyclic and selective serotonin reuptake inhibitor (SSRI) antidepressants have been found to decrease the reexperiencing and avoidant symptoms of PTSD. Other medications that have been used for PTSD include benzodiazepins, lithium, carbamazepine, and propranolol, to treat specific symptoms rather than PTSD as a whole (Sutherland and Davidson, 1994). Benzodiazepines have been used to treat anxiety and sleep disorders, and lithium and carbamazepine have been used to treat impulsivity and mood lability. Propranolol has been used to treat hyperstress arousal and hypervigilance.

Two final points must be made about the treatment of PTSD. First, practitioners who treat individuals who have experienced a severe trauma need to be aware that some individuals are more at risk for developing PTSD than others and therefore should be followed up closely. These groups are: (1) survivors with psychiatric disorders, (2) close relatives of traumatically deceased individuals, (3) children, especially if they have been separated from their parents, and (4) individuals who are more dependent upon stability, such as elders and the disabled (Lundin, 1994). Second, practitioners who treat PTSD survivors may also experience psychological stress as a result of being exposed to traumatized individuals and their suffering (McFarlane, 1994). Health care professionals (practitioners and specialists) can become overwhelmed and may withdraw emotionally, becoming numb or avoidant of their own emotional responses and the emotional responses of others. The number of PTSD survivors seen by one provider should be limited.

Acute Stress Disorder

Acute stress disorder can be a precursor to PTSD (APA, 1994). Symptoms of acute stress disorder occur within 4 weeks of a traumatic event and last a minimum of 2 days and a maximum of 4 weeks. Those individuals who demonstrate an immediate, severe stress response at the time of a traumatic event may be more likely to develop long-term effects than those who do not. The criteria for acute stress disorder are very similar to the criteria for PTSD. The individual must have experienced a traumatic event that caused fear, helplessness, or horror and must also be reexperiencing the trauma, and manifesting avoidance and increased stress arousal. The difference between the two is that in acute stress disorder, avoidance must occur in the form of dissociative symptoms, whereas in PTSD the dissociative symptoms are one of several types of avoidance symptoms. Early identification and treatment of acute stress disorder may decrease the risk of PTSD (Lundin, 1994).

Treatment of Acute Traumatic Stress

Psychological treatment of acute trauma can begin at the scene of the trauma, in an emergency room, in a primary care setting, or in the individual's home shortly after the traumatic event occurs. The first step in treating an individual who has experienced a traumatic event is assessment. The two most important areas of assessment are (1) the type of traumatic event experienced and (2) the individual's response to that event. The assessment should help to determine the type and amount of intervention needed. Some individuals may experience relatively little psychological distress in response to a traumatic event, while others will become highly distressed in response to a seemingly minor event. Different types of trauma require different types of treatment strategies. Individuals who have survived a flood or an earthquake will require different types of support than an individual who has been assaulted. After the initial assessment, the practitioner may decide that no immediate interventions are needed, that support and counseling are needed, or that immediate specialized care is needed. Specialized care may be needed on an emergency basis when the individual has severe dissociative symptoms, such as catatonia, or when the individual becomes suicidal.

The majority of cases of acute trauma can be effectively treated with information, emotional support, and crisis intervention (Lundin, 1994). However, acute stress symptoms can be very frightening and cause the individual to believe that he or she is going crazy or is about to lose control. It can be a great relief to learn that this is a normal response to an abnormal situation. Helpful ***information*** about the many aspects of trauma is important, both for the survivor and for his or her family, who may have become frightened by the survivor's reactions. The survivor and the family need to be informed that acute symptoms are temporary. Information about self-help and support groups for survivors who have experienced the same or a similar trauma can be useful. In cases of persistent symptomatology, specialized care should be considered.

Support involves listening and encouraging the individual to actively cope. It is important for individuals to be able to talk about a traumatic event following the experience. Individuals may need to tell the story of what happened to them over and over again. Telling the story allows the individuals to begin to make sense of what happened and to find personal meaning in the event (Weinrich, Hardin, and Johnson, 1990). Emotional catharsis may accompany the telling of the story and is a way of coping with the stress arousal that was experienced. Other adaptive coping strategies used by survivors include a focus on survival, humor, religion, altruism, crying, and resting. Negative coping strategies used by survivors include substance abuse, aggression, and overeating. Support includes helping survivors connect with their normal support resources (e.g., supportive relationships). Survivors should be encouraged to spend time with helpful friends and family members who will listen and provide emotional support. Practitioners can in turn support family members by providing information on the effects of trauma and adaptive coping methods as well as by listening to their concerns. ***The family should not be overlooked.*** Family members may experience extreme distress when a loved one has survived a traumatic event and may need help.

Finally, the usual treatment of acute trauma is ***crisis intervention.*** This involves short-term, problem-solving counseling. Crisis intervention, which is based on crisis theory (Aguilera, 1994), assumes certain universal human reactions to crisis or trauma, such as anxiety and depression. It also assumes that individuals go through stages of emotional reactions in response to traumatic events and that most individuals eventually recover. The purpose of crisis intervention is to support individuals as they proceed through the stages of a crisis response.

Hoff (1989) developed a four-step approach to help individuals in crisis: assessment, planning, intervention, and follow-up. ***Assessment*** involves evaluating the origins of the crisis, the individual's personal resources (including past coping behaviors), and social and family resources. ***Planning*** involves the identification of immediate problems and a plan to deal with them. Hoff (1989) identifies specific principles for setting up a plan: it should be developed with the individual; it should focus on the identified problems; it should be appropriate for the survivor's level of functioning and state of dependence; it should be consistent with the survivor's culture and lifestyle; and it should be realistic, time limited, concrete, and renegotiable. ***Intervention*** involves helping the individual to express feelings and to develop a personal understanding of the crisis that fosters the acceptance of reality. It may also be necessary to develop new ways of coping with immediate problems and to interact with supportive others. ***Follow-up*** procedures should be defined in the overall plan developed with the survivor. The purpose of follow-up is to assess the plan's effectiveness and to reinforce new coping skills. It is also a much-needed opportunity for the individual and the practitioner to come to closure following their experiences together.

Disaster Survivors

Disasters are extreme or violent acts of nature, such as floods, earthquakes, and tornadoes, or catastrophes, such as an explosion or a plane, train, or automobile accident. Epidemics of life-threatening diseases, famines, war, and other armed conflicts are also disasters. For the individuals involved, disasters are sudden, uncontrollable, traumatic events that subject large numbers of people to high levels of stress. Disaster survivors may develop acute stress disorder and some may eventually develop PTSD, but the actual variation in individual responses to the same disaster will be great. Individuals who were particularly vulnerable at the time of the disaster may develop dissociative symptoms of acute stress disorder, appearing dazed and confused. More often, survivors are emotionally distraught. Some survivors may appear to be completely calm and in control at the time of the disaster and may seem to have no immediate emotional response. The concern with such individuals is that they may have a significant but delayed acute stress response, which may not occur for hours or even days after the disaster, as though they had not yet absorbed the reality of the event or are psychologically paralyzed for a while. All survivors should be assessed at the time of the disaster and within the following week.

Treatment of Disaster Survivors

Once the immediate physical safety and health of disaster survivors have been addressed, crisis intervention and psychological first aid should be offered. Psychological first aid means listening to the individual verbalize the experience, providing direction and information, helping the individual to find coping mechanisms, providing structure, and focusing on the individual's need to increase feelings of self-control (Rose and Richards, 1991). Talking about the disaster is important for survivors; it helps them begin to define the personal meaning of the disaster, to undergo emotional catharsis to drain their stress arousal, and to grieve and mourn as necessary. Disaster survivors should be reassured that their responses are normal and that they are not going crazy. Appropriate reassurances and information regarding the survivor's physical well-being and the well-being of friends and relatives should also be given. Structure makes it possible for survivors to begin to actively cope with the disaster, it marks the beginning of the end of the disaster and the beginning of recovery. Structure can take the form of specific directions about what to do and where to go, as well as attending to basics such as shelter, clean clothing, food, and water.

To establish a sense of self-control and enhance coping, disaster survivors should be encouraged to perform self-care tasks. These include using their normal coping skills. For example, if prayer is a normal coping method, the individual should be encouraged to pray. Those who are dazed may need to be told to use their normal coping methods. Disaster survivors should be given information about typical responses to disaster, especially the range of thoughts and feelings they are likely to experience in the coming days, weeks, and months. Knowing what to expect gives the individual a feeling of control and can improve one's immediate coping ability. It can also help the person to trust that the experience is understood by others. The majority of individuals will recover from the psychological stress of a disaster, but a portion of survivors will go on to develop stress-related disorders. Follow-up after a disaster is critical. All survivors must be assessed a few weeks and a few months after the disaster.

Treatment for Children Who Are Disaster Survivors

Disasters are extremely traumatic for children. A child's response to a disaster is influenced by several factors, including age, cognitive development, family proximity and reactions to the disaster, and the amount of direct exposure to the disaster (Sugar, 1989). If possible, children should be with their parents or relatives. Children who are alone or separated from their family during a disaster suffer more psychological stress. A child who cannot be with the family will need to talk about being without them and, if the family is safe, to be informed of their well-being and location. Children need the same psychological support as adults, including many opportunities to talk about their experiences. They may communicate verbally or through repetitive playing or drawings. Young children will need specialized care. Children require honest and helpful information, including facts about the nature of the disaster. They require this information because without it they may develop highly distorted perceptions, thoughts, and feelings about the experience, which can increase their risk of long-term psychosocial problems and immediate behavior problems. Anticipatory guidance should be provided to the child's family or caretakers. This guidance includes information about the child's possible stress reactions (e.g., regression) in the days and weeks following the disaster. The adults who will be providing the most psychological support, but have not themselves experienced the disaster, will also benefit from being listened to, supported, given information, and possibly referred to specialized care.

Professionals' Responses to Disaster

Rescue workers and practitioners who work with disaster survivors may experience significant psychological stress during and after a disaster. This can be especially true for front-line workers such as search-and-rescue teams, fire fighters, police officers, emergency care providers, and body handlers. Although these professionals might respond effectively *during* a disaster, they can develop psychological stress in the days, weeks, or months *after* the disaster. Professionals are expected to maintain an awareness of the signs of stress that they and their co-workers experience, without viewing stress as anything more than a normal reaction to disaster and the human suffering that is involved. Professionals must take care of themselves during and after a disaster as the best way to recover and prepare for future disaster work. Researchers have shown that the cause of greatest stress for professionals during a disaster is concern for the safety of their own families, so professionals may need to have contact with their own loved ones at this time (Laube-Morgan, 1992). Debriefing has become a standard element of disaster-worker support, but these professionals also need to talk about their experiences with trusted individuals.

Sexual Assault Survivors

Sexual assault (SA) is a highly traumatic event that can lead to PTSD. Like all forms of assault, SA can be life-threatening, but it may also include torture, humiliation, and degradation. Unlike other assault victims, the SA survivor can expect that others may hold him or her responsible for some element of the attack; this inevitably leads to survivor feelings of anger, confusion, guilt, and shame. Although the use of the PTSD diagnosis for SA survivors is a recent development, these survivors make up the largest single group of PTSD sufferers (Goodman et al, 1993). The PTSD diagnosis for SA survivors offers an important advantage: the psychological symptoms of SA survivors are defined as a normal responses to an abnormal event rather than as the psychopathology of the individual who was assaulted. Prior to the use of the PTSD diagnosis for SA survivors, those who developed a stress-related mental disorder were commonly diagnosed with rape-trauma syndrome. In what has become the classic description of rape trauma, Burgess and Holmstrom (1974) have identified the immediate and long-term effects of SA. Rape-trauma syndrome is similar to PTSD, but unlike PTSD rape-trauma syndrome includes specific SA symptomatology.

The original concept of rape-trauma syndrome views SA survivor symptoms as normal responses to SA. Survivor symptoms are treated as effects of SA, which is defined as an assault in which sex is used as a weapon. There are two phases of survivor response. The initial or acute phase is characterized by a period of disorganization, and the long-term phase is characterized by reorganization. During the ***initial phase*** physical symptoms, fear, shock, and disbelief are prominent. Survivors tend to have one of two emotional response: patterns; expressed or controlled. The ***expressed style*** is expression of fear, anger, and anxiety through behaviors such as crying, sobbing, smiling, restlessness, and tenseness. The ***controlled style*** is a psychological mask used to cover distress with a layer of calm, composed, subdued affect. Physical reactions are categorized into four major groups: (1) physical trauma, (2) skeletal muscle tension, (3) gastrointestinal irritability, and (4) genitourinary disturbance. Physical trauma symptoms are soreness and bruising from the physical attack, in the hands, throat, neck, breasts, thighs, legs, arms, back, buttocks, head, and face. Skeletal muscle tension includes tension headaches, fatigue, and sleep disturbances. Gastrointestinal symptoms include stomach pains, nausea, and a decreased appetite. Genitourinary symptoms are vaginal, anal, bladder, and rectal bleeding and infection.

The ***long-term phase*** of survivor response is a period of biopsychosocial reorganization. Psychological symptoms such as depression, anxiety, and fear are prominent. This long-term phase has three components: activity, nightmares, and trauma phobia. SA survivors may engage in a range of activities, including a change of residence and telephone number as well as a variety of other personal safety and security measures. They may turn to family and friends for assistance with these activities. Survivors may make special plans to return home or to some location that symbolizes safety and social acceptance. Nightmares following SA are upsetting, violent dreams that occur for months. These nightmares may contain images that are clearly connected to the SA, but nightmare content may also fail to be obviously related to the SA.

Trauma phobia, as the term implies, is a phobic reaction to trauma in which the phobia develops as a psychological defense against the SA experience. The more common phobias are fear of being indoors, fear of being outdoors, fear of being alone, fear of being in crowds, fear of having people behind oneself, and sexual fears. Burgess and Holmstrom's (1974) concept of rape-trauma syndrome includes the concept of ***silent rape reaction***, which is experienced by SA survivors who have not reported or disclosed the assault. These individuals carry the heavy psychological burden of the SA without resolving the experience of trauma or the SA. Practitioners have only recently started to consider unreported SA as a basis for atypical psychological symptoms, such as atypical anxiety, sexual relationship problems, significant changes in sexual behavior patterns, unexplained sudden onset of phobias, and chronic low self-esteem. Fear of sexually transmitted disease (STD), including HIV, is also a powerful source of psychological trauma. It has been estimated that 4% to 30% of SA survivors are diagnosed with an STD as a result of the SA (Koss, 1993). Suicide attempts, premenstrual distress, and revictimization also have been observed among survivors (Davidson et al, 1996; Golding, 1996; Messman and Long, 1996)

Treatment of Sexual Assault Survivors

Advanced-practice SA nurse examiners specialize in acute and immediate follow-up care for SA survivors. These practitioners are immediately notified by emergency-room staff when an SA survivor arrives for treatment. By working with a specialist immediately, the survivor may be able to complete the SA exam with fewer practitioners and in less time. The specialist is also better able to meet the survivor's immediate needs for nonjudgmental practitioner attitudes and high levels of practice skills and experience. Equally important, the SA nurse examiner will be skilled in the collection of forensic evidence.

Initial treatment of SA survivors consists of the SA interview, a physical exam for assessment and forensic evidence collection, and crisis intervention. The ***SA interview*** is performed before the physical examination and usually with a police officer present. The interview should be done in a room away from the waiting areas and exam rooms and while the survivor is still fully clothed. The SA interview begins with general health information, including drug allergies, current medications, recent surgeries, major health problems, date of last menses, history of STD's, use of contraception, and most recent consensual sexual contact. The SA interview follows the general health information interview. The SA survivor is asked to give the date and time of the SA and all events surrounding the SA. Accurate collection of forensic evidence requires that the examiner locate all points of physical contact and penetration and determine the survivor's activity immediately following the SA, such as bathing, douching, urinating, brushing teeth, and combing hair.

The ***physical exam*** is the final phase of the process. The SA survivor should be informed in advance of all physical-exam and forensic-evidence collection procedures. If the physical examination is traumatic for the survivor, he or she is allowed to stop or limit it. SA survivors should be encouraged to have a support person with them during the exam who is not directly involved in the exam process. When staff, family, and friends are unavailable or would not be helpful, community rape crisis centers may be able to provide support advocates for SA survivors during an SA exam. Although SA survivors may decline such support, they should be encouraged to accept it. Having an individual present tends to be more important to the survivor after the exam than before or during it.

The ***physical exam*** begins with the removal of all items of clothing. If the clothing was worn at the time of the SA, each item is placed in a separate bag, and then signed over to the police as forensic evidence. Physical forensic evidence that can be found on clothing include hair, blood, semen, and saliva. If the clothing has not been washed, these items can be found up to a year later. A brief physical exam is performed to determine the presence of injuries (e.g., bruises, lacerations, teeth marks, swelling). Blood samples for pregnancy and an STD test are obtained. The SA kit should contain all the necessary materials. Survivor forensic evidence includes samples of the individual's hair (head and pubic) and saliva; oral, vaginal, and rectal swabs; and fingernail scrapings. Information obtained during the interview will determine the forensic evidence to be collected. Pelvic, vaginal, and rectal exams are completed at the end of the exam. Semen can be found and collected within 72 hours after the SA. Although forensic evidence should be collected as soon as possible, exams performed several days after the SA can still produce findings.

The final stage of SA treatment is to initiate ***crisis intervention***. The principles of crisis intervention discussed earlier also apply, but SA survivors have additional concerns specific to the nature of the assault. These concerns include prevention of pregnancy and/or STDs, physical safety, and the need for specialized SA psychotherapy and community support groups. Physical safety becomes a focus of concern for anyone who has just been assaulted. SA survivors can become preoccupied with the fear that their attacker will try to hurt them again. This is especially true when the survivor knows the identity of the attacker or when the SA occurred in the survivor's home. Practitioners can help survivors start to solve their long-range safety concerns and help them meet their immediate needs for safety. Some individuals may elect to live with friends or family until they begin to feel safe again, but others may insist on not living their lives in fear.

In addition to these concerns, SA survivors benefit from the same psychological support as survivors of disasters and other traumatic events. The one area of difference may be in the survivor's ability to hold the attacker, rather than oneself, fully responsible for the SA. Practitioners and specialists should inform all SA survivors that they do not deserve to be assaulted, no matter what. Finally SA survivors should be encouraged to participate in the support services available from community rape crisis centers. Each person should at least be given a 24-hour crisis hotline phone number. Many individuals may not feel they need this support because their families and friends are there for them, but survivors continue to be at risk for long-term problems and may have grief and mourning needs long after the immediate crisis has passed and significant others have come to believe that the crisis is over.

Some rape crisis centers are also able to furnish legal or court advocates. Rape crisis centers may offer these services free of charge or at greatly reduced rates.

There are a great deal of services and supports that are available and helpful to SA survivors, but these may be of less value when the survivor cannot identify the attacker, when there is more than one attacker, when the assault was so violent that the survivor was close to death, or when the survivor has been assaulted before. These individuals may experience the same extreme responses as soldiers who barely survived heavy combat and who continue to live with that experience.

Two additional points must be made regarding basic treatment for SA survivors. Practitioners must know interview and exam procedures, and also be prepared to testify in court about what they have observed. Practitioners who are not prepared, skilled and accurate make it possible for the forensic evidence to be rejected as inadmissible due to improper collection or handling.

Second, children who are sexually assaulted should be referred to practitioners who specialize in child sexual assault. The interview and exam of child SA survivors is difficult, complex, and has been successfully challenged by defendants.

Adult Survivors of Childhood Sexual Abuse

The long-term effects of childhood sexual abuse (CSA) vary. Some individuals can appear to have little or no ill effects, just as others may experience severe psychopathology, including PTSD, depression, anxiety, isolation, low self-esteem, self-injury behaviors, sexual dysfunctions, substance abuse, revictimization, and parenting and relationship problems (Browne and Finkelhor, 1986). Briere (1992) defines five types of long-term effects of CSA: post-traumatic effects, cognitive distortions, altered emotionality, dissociation, and impaired self-reference. ***Post-traumatic effects*** include symptoms similar to PTSD symptoms. Adult survivors of CSA report intrusive, avoidant, and arousal symptoms, but the most prominent PTSD symptoms in adult survivors are flashbacks and intrusive CSA thoughts and memories. As with combat veterans who have flashbacks, adult survivors may relive the experience of CSA. Their flashbacks can include all of the images, smells, sounds, and bodily sensations that they experienced at the time of the sexual abuse. ***Cognitive distortions*** cause the adult survivor to hold strong negative views of oneself, the world, and the future. As adults, these survivors may chronically overestimate the amount of danger in the world and underestimate their abilities and their worth. Cognitive distortions such as these are extremely high risk factors for chronic severe depression and anxiety disorders.

Altered emotionality in adult survivors almost always takes the form of depression and anxiety, with depression being the most commonly reported disorder (Browne and Finkelhor, 1986; Messman and Long, 1996). Severe cases include significant suicide risk (Davidson et al, 1996). Anxiety in adult CSA survivors may occur as somatization, with CSA-related symptoms such as headaches, stomach pain, nausea, sleep disturbance, anorexia, asthma, shortness of breath, and muscle spasms. ***Dissociation*** related to CSA is the same as dissociation with PTSD. The individual experiences a disconnection between his or her feelings, thoughts, behavior, and memories that, during times of stress, may take the form of disengagement or a cognitive separation of the individual from the environment. Survivors sometimes describe this experience as "spacing out," during which time they are not cognitively aware of what is going on around them. Dissociation also occurs as detachment or numbing, in which the survivor is cognitively aware of the environment but emotionally detached from it. Amnesia and multiple personality disorder are the most extreme forms of dissociation experienced by adult survivors of CSA.

The final symptom category is ***impaired self-reference***. Adult survivors of CSA can have a poor relationship with themselves or a poor self-awareness (Briere, 1992). Severe CSA can literally interfere with the individual's ability to be aware of who one is and what one feels, thinks, cares about, or believes. What little sense of self the individual has may not be stable; as life situations change, the individuals's sense of self may change. A stable sense of self allows one to feel that one knows who one is and is not. An unstable sense of self may be experienced as identity confusion or as an identity that is defined by external events rather than internally determined. Without a stable, internal sense of self, adult survivors are vulnerable to severe identity problems, interpersonal boundary problems, and chronic feelings of emptiness. The distress and confusion associated with these experiences explains why adult survivors are so often diagnosed with borderline personality disorder rather than PTSD.

Treatment of Adult Survivors of CSA

Treatment of adult survivors of CSA can be in the context of individual, couples, family, or group therapy. Due to the nature of their needs, adult survivors usually require more than one form of therapy. Specialists must tailor the treatment to meet a range of patient needs. Whatever the form of therapy, the focus of treatment includes working through CSA memories. Therapy that focuses only on the obvious symptoms of a disorder that is associated with CSA (e.g., depression) is usually not effective. A treatment balance between past experience and present symptomatology is necessary. For example, if an adult survivor abuses alcohol, treatment should focus on alcohol abuse *and* on CSA as the basis of the alcohol abuse.. Working through or coming to terms with traumatic memories requires specialized training, partly because when adult survivors engage in this work, CSA memories may increase and intensify self-destructive behavior, such as cutting and burning one's arms and legs, substance abuse, and sexual acting out. Regardless of how self-destructive or impulsive the behavior is, the individuals who engage in it almost always state they do so because it relieves their psychological pain. Talking about CSA memories can increase the pain of those memories. Specialists should try to work with the adult survivor to decrease the need to engage in self-destructive behavior.

Adult Survivors of CSA in the Primary Care Setting

Repressed CSA memories and somatization often lead adult survivors to seek primary care with vague complaints of depression, anxiety, headaches, stomach aches, or sexual dysfunctions. When sexual history is included in the routine health history, CSA may be reported. Disclosure of a history of CSA to the practitioner may not necessarily be traumatic for the individual. Patients may answer "yes" to the question of CSA and then say they don't remember much of what happened other than, for example, that the offender was arrested. In the middle years of life, remembering a little about CSA can lead to remembering a lot. After years of silence some individuals develop greater recall. Should this occur, practitioners can provide emotional support and avoid judgment of the individual's recalled memories. Practitioner belief or disbelief in CSA memories is not likely to be relevant to the individual's treatment needs, and adult survivors rightly resent having to second-guess whether a practitioner believes what they have said. Should the patient become upset or blank out when recalling or disclosing CSA, the practitioner should focus on helping the individual to regain self-control by stopping the disclosure and reassuring the individual. These measures can be sufficient but in some cases disclosure of CSA can lead to increased self-destructive behavior.

False Memories

The validity of repressed CSA memories has been a topic of heated debate. On one side of the debate are researchers and clinicians who work with adult survivors and state that CSA is prevalent and significant, and that its memories can be repressed. On the other side are members of the False Memory Syndrome Foundation, an advocacy group of parents and other family members who have been accused of sexually abusing a child. The False Memory Syndrome Foundation states that many, perhaps most, memories of CSA are false and have been implanted by unethical therapists, who use hypnosis and age regression to produce such memories.

At this point, there is very little empirical evidence to support either side of the debate. There is no documented empirical evidence to support the existence of false memories of CSA. There is clinical evidence to suggest that false memories of CSA do sometimes occur and that CSA memories can be repressed. The ramifications of the false memory debate are mostly legal and political, with the following clinical ramifications. Specialists should be cautious when using techniques such as hypnosis and age regression for the recall of CSA. There is no evidence to suggest that asking an individual without using hypnosis or regression if he or she has been sexually abused will implant a false memory of CSA.

References

Aquilera D: *Crisis intervention: theory and methodology* (7th ed.), St.Louis, 1994, Mosby.

Briere J: *Child abuse trauma: theory and treatment of the lasting effects*, Newbury Park, 1992, Sage Publications.

Browne A, Finkelhor D: Impact of child sexual abuse: a review of the research, *Psychological Bull* 99(1):66, 1986.

Burgess AW, Holmstrom LL: Rape trauma syndrome, *Am J Psychiatry* 131(9):981, 1974.

Davidson JR, Hughes DC, George LK, Blazer DG: The association of sexual assault and attempted suicide within the community, *Arch Gen Psychiatry* 53(6):550, 1996.

Eth S, Pynoos R: *Post-traumatic stress disorder in children*, Washington DC, 1985, American Psychiatric Press.

Golding JM, Taylor DL: Sexual assault history and premenstrual distress in two general population samples, *J of Women's Health* 5(2):143, 1996.

Goodman LA, et al.: Male violence against women, *Am Psychologist* 48(10):1054, 1993.

Hoff LA: *People in crisis: understanding and helping*, Redwood City, CA, 1989, Addison-Wesley Publishing.

Koss MP: Rape: scope, impact, interventions, and public policy responses, *Am Psychologist* 48(10):1062, 1993.

Laube-Morgan J: The professional's psychological response in disaster: implications for practice, *J of Psychosocial Nursing* 30(2):17, 1992.

Lundin T: The treatment of acute trauma, *Psychiatric Clin of N Am* 17(2):385, 1994.

McFarlane AC: Individual psychotherapy for post-traumatic stress disorder, *Psychiatric Clin N Am* 17(2):393, 1994.

Messman TL, Long PJ: Child sexual abuse and its relationship to revictimization in adult women: a review, *Clin Psychology Review* 16(5):397, 1996.

Rose J, Richards D: Post-traumatic stress: healing the mind, *Nursing Times* 87(14):40, 1991.

Southwick S, Bremner D, Krystal J, Charney D: Psychobiologic research in post-traumatic stress disorder, *Psychiatric Clin of N Am* 17(2):251, 1994.

Sugar M: Children in disaster: an overview, *Child Psychiatry and Human Development* 19:163, 1989.

Sutherland SM, Davidson JT: Pharmacotherapy for post-traumatic stress disorder, *Psychiatric Clin N Am* 17(2):409, 1994.

Tomb DA: The phenomenology of post-traumatic stress disorder, *Psychiatric Clin N Am* 17(2):237, 1994.

van der Kolk BA, Pelcovitz D, Roth S, Mandel FS, McFarlane A, Herman JL: Dissociation, somatization and affect dysregulation: the complexity of adaptation to trauma, *Am J Psychiatry* 153(7):83, 1996.

Weinrich S, Hardin S, Johnson M: Nurses respond to hurricane Hugh victims' disaster stress, *Archives of Psychiatric Nursing* 4(3):195, 1990.

Suicide 18

Suicide is actualized hopelessness. In the absence of a thought disorder, psychosis, or intoxication, an individual is suicidal when one has thoughts and feelings of wanting to cause one's own death. Suicidal thoughts and feelings may or may not lead to suicidal behavior. When individuals engage in suicidal behavior, regardless of the nature of that behavior, the full intentionality of their suicidal behavior can never be completely known to others. Therefore the goal for practitioners is to strive to identify the patient with current or recent suicidal thoughts, feelings, or behaviors and to take actions aimed at reducing the immediate risk of suicide. This chapter reviews basic suicide risk factors and the counseling needs of potentially suicidal patients. Practitioners should follow their practice standards regarding specific interventions with suicidal patients.

➲ Who Is at Risk

Suicide risk assessment is the determination of the probability that suicidal behavior will occur within a specified time period. Retrospective and prospective studies of completed suicides have revealed numerous factors that are helpful in assessing an individual's suicidal risk (Roy, 1986). The general suicide risk factors reviewed here must be considered within the context of each individual's unique personal circumstances. This section is a review of basic personal, social, and psychological suicide risk factors.

Personal risk factors

- Gender
- Age
- Ethnicity
- Income and employment
- Education
- Health

Social risk factors

- Relationship conflict

Psychological risk factors

- Problems, trauma, or loss
- Mental disorder
- Ineffective coping skills
- Substance disorders
- Suicide plans or previous attempt
- Family or significant-other suicide
- Impaired impulse control
- Hopelessness
- Depersonalization, derealization, or detachment
- Suffering

Risk Factors

Gender

Women and men grow up learning different coping skills and different standards regarding the amount of personal control they can expect to have over events in their lives. Traditionally, males are socialized to exact solutions to problems and thus they are more likely to expect their coping efforts to directly influence events. As little boys they are more likely to learn to play to win, to disdain defeat, and to place high value on aggressive actions. When distressed, males are therefore more likely to engage in aggressive behavior and, when suicidal, to use violent means such as firearms or hanging. Distressed females may also behave aggressively, but females are more likely to use nonviolent suicidal methods, such as overdosing. Therefore, males complete suicide at twice the rate of females, but females are more likely to attempt suicide. These gender distinctions are beginning to fade as more females grow up with fewer social restrictions on their aggressive feelings and behaviors.

Age

The normal ups and downs of life are emotionally and psychologically upsetting regardless of age, but adolescents tend to interpret their upset feelings differently from adults and elders. In youth, common life events are new experiences, and personal coping skills and social resources are usually few and untested. Maturity allows one to adopt the helpful viewpoint that single life events are small pieces of the big picture of life. It can be difficult for adolescents to adopt this perspective when events in their lives seem bigger than life itself. Individuals who have yet to live through enough life events to have learned how to protect themselves are more likely to experience the full psychological impact of those events. Disappointments in the fourth decade of life hurt no less than disappointments in the second, but experience can make them easier to understand and cope with. Adolescents may not be more likely to become suicidal, but they are more likely to have events in their lives that are extremely distressing to them. Adolescent suicidal behavior is troubling and difficult to predict, but factors (e.g., substance abuse) that help identify suicidal adults can also identify suicidal adolescents (Buzan and Weissberg, 1992; Conwell et al, 1996).

Children can have suicidal thoughts and feelings and may engage in suicidal behavior. They are diagnosed and treated for mental disorders (e.g., depression) and distressing psychosocial problems (e.g., sexual abuse) known to be related to suicidal behavior. These disorders and problems cause pain and suffering in children just as they do in adults, but unlike adults, children are less able to understand, express, or cope with such experiences. Children who have been diagnosed with a mental disorder, who have been the victims of abuse or neglect, or who have been diagnosed and treated for serious physical illness can begin to think about death in general and, from there, begin to wish for their own deaths. Children who exhibit severe anger, aggression, apathy, withdrawal, or intense feelings with which they are unable to cope can also be at risk for self-harm (Pfeffer, 1986).

Adult suicide risk factors are presented throughout this chapter, but a few additional factors should be noted. Suicide is no longer the absolute taboo it once was. Living wills, death with dignity, and assisted suicide are just a few of the new social definitions of death as a personal right. Second, increasing numbers of adults are socially isolated, living in disconnected communities. For many, work has taken the place of family, friends, and community. For this population, stressful life events, personal crisis, or chronic problems can quickly exceed personal coping skills and coping resources thereby increasing the risk of extreme feelings of hopelessness.

Elders can use their larger frame of reference for life events to reduce some of the day-to-day hassles. A superior frame of reference, however, does not diminish the experience of loss, and elders have to deal with many painful losses. Regardless of age, loss is a powerful depression risk factor, and elders face the loss of meaningful work, income, loved ones, health, and independence as well as the losses that take the form of regrets and unfulfilled dreams. Elders must also deal with a culture that has not been able to construct valued social roles for people over 65. Elder women in particular undergo numerous social losses, including social identity, whereas elder men continue to have powerful loss of social roles in American politics, corporations, religion, finance, and entertainment (Alarcon, 1995). Untreated depression is a major suicide risk factor for both male and female elders (Fogel, 1993).

Ethnicity

More completed suicides are Caucasian, and the incidence rate of suicide among ethnic/minority groups is relatively lower, but for some individuals the stress of minority social status rather than ethnicity can become a suicide risk factor. Minority social status is a stable characteristic of all ethnic/minority groups. In relation to the majority social group, minority social groups have less power, less control, fewer resources, more stress, and higher social visibility. For some individuals these social group characteristics can be extremely stressful, difficult to cope with, and a significant source of hopelessness (Seivewright et al, 1991).

Income and employment

The most predictive income-related suicide risk factor is unemployment or the serious threat of it (Westreich, 1991). Unemployment and the subsequent crushing experience of poverty can easily exceed the coping skills of most people. Poverty, with or without employment, is an endless source of disabling, stressful life events that can lead to depersonalization and hopelessness. When individuals are overwhelmed by the stress and hardship of poverty, they can feel as though their life is without meaning or value. Similar experiences of depersonalization and hopelessness can develop in response to work environments that are hypercompetitive, hostile, or unpredictable. This risk is particular salient for individuals who make work the center of their lives.

Education

Less education is a potential suicide risk factor because higher levels of education support more effective appraisal styles and coping skills that in turn are better protection against stress. Less education can also mean less income for those who are employed and fewer chances of employment for the unemployed. However, academic education itself can be a highly stressful life experience. It is a performance-evaluation process in which individual achievement is the single measure of success. Students who are unable to learn under these conditions or who are unable to cope with the inherent stress may find the process dehumanizing or experience feelings of worthlessness. Students who feel they must excel at all cost may also be vulnerable.

Health

Health is related to suicidal behavior in the following ways. Illness can lead to depression and subsequent thoughts of suicide. Individuals with illnesses that cause pain, suffering, fear, humiliation, or disability may feel suicide is a means of escape (Westreich, 1991). Any health condition that produces lingering illness before death is a suicide risk factor for individuals who are unwilling or unable to endure such suffering. However, regardless of the actual diagnosis, illness has different meanings to different people. The nature, magnitude, and duration of a specific illness does not in itself predict an individual's response to it (Fogel, 1993). For example, an ill person may become despondent based on the belief that the illness is unfair and that he or she should have been spared. Research findings show a significant correlation between a recent visit to a family physician and completed suicide. In a study of 100 completed suicides, 59 patients had seen a family care physician and 18 had seen a psychiatrist within a month before the suicide (Westreich, 1991). It is important to be aware of this relationship, but it cannot be viewed as explanatory because few patients volunteer information about their suicidal thoughts or feelings. Practitioners can, at the time of the visit, remain unaware of the patient's psychological distress (Roy, 1986).

Relationship conflict

Many psychosocial problems increase the risk of suicidal behavior. Legal, financial, and employment problems, for example, can be extremely difficult to cope with. But in terms of dangerous behavior in general and suicidal behavior in particular, relationship conflict is a significant risk factor. Conflict within important relationships can quickly exceed the individual's ability to resolve the conflict, thus allowing it to escalate (Janicah et al, 1993). Conflict within important relationships can have many patterns, from sudden and unexpected to predictable and chronic. Important relationships are susceptible to intense conflict because, by definition, participants enter the conflict standing to lose or gain significantly. For this reason partner relationships can be particularly volatile, especially when the relationship is the only source of satisfaction for strong emotional, psychological, physical, and social needs. Uncontrolled conflict within partner relationships can be threatening to individuals involved because it can end the relationship or expose unspoken needs, a process that for some causes feelings of worthlessness and abandonment. If either partner has a substance disorder, conflict becomes even more dangerous (Murphy, 1967) (See Chapter 19).

Problems, trauma, or loss

Problems that are upsetting and cannot be ignored, avoided, or resolved produce stress that can lead to anxiety and depression. When patients describe problems, they usually describe their appraisal of them and their ability to cope with them. In patients with suicidal thoughts and feelings, suicide feels like a solution to the problem.

Trauma refers to any event or experience that "shocks and stops." A traumatic event is emotionally bewildering (shocks) and interferes with (stops) functioning. Two types of traumatic events are strongly related to immediate, intense, and sometimes impulsive suicidal behaviors: natural disasters (e.g., flood) and victimization (e.g., assault). Both experiences rewrite reality. The experience itself can lead to suicidal thoughts and feelings, but in some cases individuals are able to withstand the traumatic event yet cannot face the work that will be needed to put their lives back together again.

Loss events can be perceived losses, potential losses, or actual losses. The psychological experience of loss occurs even when the loss is by choice, such as choosing to leave a job or a marriage. Loss related to a traumatic event can produce the same struggle for psychological survival that is generated by disasters and victimization (See Chapter 17).

Mental disorder

Severe depression, psychosis, substance disorders, post-traumatic stress disorder (PTSD), and personality disorders are mental disorders that are associated with increased risk of suicide (Westreich, 1991). An individual who is diagnosed with any of these disorders can suffer acute and chronic suicidal thoughts and feelings as a symptom of the disorder or as a reaction to having a disorder. Recurrent suicidal behavior is particularly common with alcohol disorders, PTSD, borderline personality disorder and antisocial personality disorder (Isometsa et al, 1996). With these disorders, recurrent suicidal thoughts and feelings can be related to the individual's recurrent experiences of disinhibition, rage, and crisis. Suicidal thoughts and feelings are symptoms of depression, and therefore a diagnosis of depression directly increases the risk of suicidal behavior. Suicidal behavior related to psychosis can occur as a result of delusions and/or hallucinations. The chronic stress of living with severe mental disorders, such as bipolar disorder or schizophrenia, can generate intense suffering and hopelessness that may increase the risk of suicide (Strakowski et al, 1996).

Ineffective coping skills

This refers to the inability to decrease stress or to cope with problems effectively. Without effective coping skills, an individual will experience high levels of stress or chronic stress leading to feelings of despair, worthlessness, and hopelessness. Ineffective coping can also imply the presence of ineffective coping skills (e.g., alcohol) as well the absence of effective skills. Coping skills can be ineffective for many reasons, but in terms of suicide risk one of the most troubling consequences of ineffective coping skills is that problems are made worse.

Substance disorder

Individuals with substance disorders, especially alcohol disorder, frequently have suicidal thoughts and feelings and, when intoxicated or hung over, are likely to engage in impulsive suicidal behaviors (Murphy and Wetzel, 1990). Suicidal behavior may be related to feelings of self-hate that develop with substance disorders, unpleasant consequences of the disorder (e.g., arrest), or the chemical effects of the substance (e.g., paranoia). Substance disorders also subject the individual to multiple losses (e.g., divorce) that are, in turn, difficult to cope with and can increase feelings of self-hate. Substance-induced disinhibition, as well as a desire for substance-induced disinhibition, are related to impulsive suicidal behavior. A large percentage of individuals who attempt suicide get drunk or high first. The hope is usually that intoxication will decrease the feelings of fear and ambivalence that always precede suicidal behavior. Individuals may assume that intoxication will prevent the physical pain associated with violent suicide attempts. Finally, intoxication can increase suicidal thoughts and feelings, and the individual may interpret it as meaningful despite feeling suicidal only when intoxicated and not when sober. Evidence of active substance abuse, long-term substance abuse, severe psychosocial problems caused by substance abuse, or relationship conflict due to substance abuse indicates a potential for suicidal thoughts and feelings.

Suicide plans or previous attempt

Having thought out a suicide plan or having previously attempted suicide are both high risk factors. A suicide plan has three components: means and methods, access and availability, and emotional attachment. Individuals may not be willing to tell a practitioner if they have a suicide plan, let alone disclose information about it. Those who are willing to disclose may give information that is misleading or false, or they may withhold critical details. But there are also individuals who are quite willing to disclose completely and accurately; they may even have written journal accounts of their suicidal thoughts and feelings that they are willing to show to a practitioner. They may have prepared suicide notes that contain a great deal of information about their plans and wishes. Learning the means and method of an individual's suicide plan is very difficult, and even with cooperative patients it will require 30 to 45 minutes (Westreich, 1991).

An individual's suicide plan may not sound lethal or realistic to a practitioner, but all plans should be given serious consideration. Common ***means*** of suicide are overdose, gunshot wound (GSW), jumping from a bridge or a building, motor vehicle accidents (MVA), wrist cutting, and hanging. ***Method*** refers to the time, place, and arrangements that may be planned. Experimental suicidal behaviors are not uncommon. Experimental suicidal behavior refers to any and all behavior that could have resulted in death or serious injury, such as near miss or actual MVAs, falls, cuts, burns, and ingesting "too much" of something that causes sickness. Individuals may experiment with their suicide plans by not showing up at school, work, or home for days at a time, causing others to become concerned, or they may engage in symbolic experiments by dramatically changing their appearance and behavior so that they are no longer themselves. Sudden increases in substance abuse, preoccupation with death-related symbols, self-mutilation, regression to childlike behaviors, and rejection of previously valued relationships, possessions, or hopes may also be indicative of an undisclosed suicide plan.

A plan may be presented without evidence that the individual has access to a means or method; access might only be achieved with great effort, or the means and method may be immediately available to the individual. The practitioner should make every effort to avoid giving the impression that he or she is trying to second-guess the patient. The fact that an individual may not know how to obtain lethal poison, for example, is not relevant. Too often trial and error proves a good teacher. In all cases it is important to ask if the individual has access to or could obtain access to firearms. When access to a weapon is disclosed, the immediate goal is to remove the access. The weapon should be given to a responsible person who will confirm possession of the weapon. If there are no relatives or friends for this purpose, the local police department can assist.

Individuals can develop emotional attachment to their suicide plans. A strong emotional attachment can mean that the plan itself is meeting an important emotional need. When this is true the suicide plan may have great value to the individual, who may seem to cling to the idea of suicide or take comfort in having a plan. Practitioners can take note of the individual's attachment but should not assume that a highly valued plan signals less risk of acting on it.

Family or significant-other suicide

Being a survivor of someone close who committed suicide is a high risk factor. Individuals with family/significant others who have died as a result of suicide have an immediate as well as a long-term risk for suicide. When a loved one takes his or her life, significant others experience shock, loss, betrayal, anger, anxiety, and depression. It can require a great deal of time, energy, and effort to come to terms with the death. Some people may worry that they did or said anything that led to the suicide, if the suicide was a message to them, and if they could have prevented it. Feelings of guilt and thoughts of real and imagined wrongdoings are common. The suicide of a significant other also delivers the subtle message that suicide is a real choice. This message can be disquieting for the vulnerable survivor. The suicide death of a significant other within the previous 2 months should be viewed as a trauma and a loss.

Impaired impulse control

Impulse control is the weak link between suicidal thoughts and suicidal behavior. People routinely experience momentary impulses to act, and once in a while an impulse occurs so quickly or with such impact that people act without thinking. Without fail, they will wonder about their actions after the fact. Normal impulse control develops with maturity. Children, adolescents, and individuals with severe mental disorders (such as schizophrenia, bipolar disorder, personality disorders, and substance dependence) often have poor impulse control. They are very likely to act first and think later. The individual with suicidal thoughts, a suicide plan, and impaired impulse control may act on a suicidal thought impulsively. The impulsive suicidal patient is likely to have a range of impulsive behavior patterns that can alert practitioners to the fact that he or she may act with little or no warning. Common examples of poor impulse control are impulsive sex, stealing, lying, and spending. Individuals who are not normally impulsive can become so if their suicidal thoughts become intrusive or too strong to resist. A range of conditions can impair normal impulse control. Physical exhaustion and emotional despair can significantly decrease an individual's ability to resist strong impulses. Circumstances can also increase or decrease individual impulse control. For example, isolation can simultaneously increase impulse intensity while decreasing impulse control.

Hopelessness

Hopelessness is directly related to suicidal behavior (Beck, Brown, Berchick, Stewart, and Steer, 1990). Beck and associates view hopelessness as an indicator of the belief that suicide is the only strategy for coping with problems or events perceived as unsolvable. Hopelessness can also represent the conviction that a hoped-for positive experience will not be realized or that a negative experience cannot be avoided (Kisis, Kosier, and Robinson, 1996). Psychologically, hope operates as a semiconscious open window between today and tomorrow. The individual who is hopeful has a personal vision of the future and moves toward it. Hopelessness is, in effect, a closed window on the future. The individual who is hopeless cannot envision things being better or different, only the same or worse. Beck and associates (1990) provide an expansive clinical definition of the experience of hopelessness as a temporary mood state, a character trait, a symptom of disorder (e.g., depression), a personal pattern or style, or a stable belief. Suicidal thoughts with hopelessness increase the risk of suicidal behavior. Individuals may not be fully aware of their experience of hopelessness. Those who are aware typically describe their lives as purposeless, with flat statements such as, "My life has no meaning." Whether the individual's hopelessness is acute or chronic, in most cases appropriate intervention can decrease the intensity of the hopelessness enough to decrease the risk of suicidal behavior.

Depersonalization, derealization, or detachment

Depersonalization is the experience of not being oneself, derealization is to experience something real as unreal, and detachment refers to cutting off one's connections to people, places, and possessions. Depersonalization is clearly a significant suicide risk factor because it allows the individual to act against the self without feeling that this is indeed the case (Seivewright et al, 1991). Derealization and detachment are significant risk factors because they can enable suicidal behavior. These conditions are experienced as being outside of oneself or outside of one's circumstances. These robotic feelings of being removed or at a distance from reality can numb the individual and so have a disinhibiting effect on suicidal behavior. Others may react when an individual detaches from them by giving away prized possessions or ending a relationship, but the concurrent depersonalization and derealization may not be recognized. Depersonalization, derealization, and detachment can develop under any number of circumstances, but people are particularly vulnerable to them after trauma, disaster, or crisis.

Suffering

As the term is used here in relation to suicide, suffering is a vague yet unendurable mental pain that may be acute, recurrent, constant, or unpredictable, and it is caused by emotional, physical, psychological, or spiritual changes (Peck, Farberow and Litman, 1985; Roy, 1986). Suicidal behavior is related to an individuals ability to endure suffering, whatever the source. Suffering is an all encompassing experience that feels limitless and endless. When an individual is unable to endure the suffering associated with physical illness or the death of a child, for example, the risk of suicide occurs as a means to end the suffering. Practitioners should note that the experience of suffering is subject to each individuals faith in the teachings of their culture, spirituality, and religion. Most people are only able to suffer so much and for so long without relief. For some individuals, particularly those with a serious illness (e.g., cancer, schizophrenia), the risk of suicide is directly related to suffering (Lish et al, 1996; Conwell et al, 1996; Kisis, Kosier and Robinson, 1996).

Suicide Assessment

In summary, the risk factors presented in this chapter can be assessed with the following suicide risk interview questions. The assessment goal is to determine if the patient who discloses suicidal thoughts and feelings can be said to have a low, high, or unpredictable risk of suicidal behavior within the next 24 to 72 hours. Patients with low immediate risk of suicidal behavior will have suicidal thoughts and feelings, but will find such thoughts and feelings unacceptable or upsetting and deny any intention of acting on them (Olfson et al, 1996).

Interview Questions

1. Are there severe or chronic problems, trauma, or loss?
2. Is there a mental disorder?
3. Are coping skills and resources active and effective?
4. Is there a history of family or significant-other suicide?
5. Is there substance abuse or dependence?
6. Is there a suicide plan?
7. Have there been previous attempts?
8. Is impulse control impaired or intact?
9. Is there hopelessness, depersonalization, derealization, detachment, or suffering?

* Common Symptom Onset Patterns

Suicidal behaviors can be categorized as having chronic, acute, impulsive, or unpredictable onset patterns, but an individual may have more than one pattern. ***Chronic suicidal behavior*** is associated with personality disorders, chronic depression, anxiety, or substance abuse disorders. Some individuals with these disorders are never completely free from suicidal thoughts and feelings. Chronic suicidal behavior may have a recurrent pattern; that is, the suicidal behavior tends to occur in episodes with periods of remission. Chronic suicidal thoughts and feelings are the most common basis for recurrent episodes of suicidal behavior, but impulsive suicidal behavior may also be recurrent (Barraclough et al, 1974; Fogel, 1993).

Acute suicidal behavior refers to the sudden onset of suicidal behavior. Often acute suicidal behavior is related to an identifiable causal event or an experience that has generated sudden and intense suicidal thoughts and feelings. An acute episode of suicidal behavior can also occur as a result of the gradual intensification of chronic suicidal thoughts and feelings. ***Impulse*** refers to suicidal behavior onset with little or no warning (Murphy and Wetzel, 1990). When individuals experience suicidal behavioral as an impulse, the impulse may be perceived as intrusive, demanding, and frightening, or the individual may be semiaware of the impulse. The more intense and sudden the impulse is, the more difficult it may be to resist.

Unpredictable suicidal behavior refers to behavior that is literally unpredictable because the individual's response to suicidal thoughts and feelings is unpredictable (Barraclough et al, 1974).

❑ Common Assessment Problems

The most important problem in assessing suicide risk is getting the information needed to make a meaningful assessment (Badger, 1995). To be meaningful, information about suicidal thoughts, feelings, and behaviors must be accurate. Numerous individual and interpersonal obstacles interfere with the process of obtaining this information. Time is the primary obstacle. Except in emergency cases, suicide assessment takes time. Practitioner reluctance and patient resistance are the second and third major obstacles (Fogel, 1993). Why are practitioners sometimes reluctant and patients sometimes resistant? The list of possible explanations is too long to present here, but practitioners can feel ambivalent towards learning about a patient's suicidal thoughts and feelings for the reason that this knowledge obligates them to intervene. Intervening with a suicidal patient may not be easy, fast, effective, or welcomed by the patient. Practitioners can also be reluctant to assess a patient who is suicidal because such human suffering can be painful to behold. Finally, for personal reasons some practitioners may feel that suicide assessment is not appropriate.

Patients can be extremely resistant to talking about their suicidal thoughts, feelings, or behaviors, even when they do not appear to be resistant. Resistance may have to do with the patient's tolerance, ability, and willingness to confront suicidal thoughts, feelings, and behaviors (Goldman, 1995; Roy, 1986). Patient resistance can take many forms, the most common of which are superficial explanations or complete denial. Practitioners should note that patient resistance can also occur as a result of fear: fear of what to expect from the practitioner and fear of one's own thoughts and feelings. The most troubling forms of patient resistance are misleading information and withheld information. When a practitioner encounters patient resistance, rather than automatically assuming the worst—that the patient is planning to attempt suicide in the next 24 hours—it may be helpful to start out by acknowledging the obvious, that the practitioner is willing and able to help. Power struggles with patients over their disclosure of information routinely fail.

The most difficult assessment problem is that of immediate risk. Is the patient going to attempt suicide today or within the next 72 hours? The rationale for limiting the time frame for immediate risk to the next 24 to 72 hours is that even though it is not possible to predict the behavior of others, in most cases a reliable assessment of immediate risk is possible (Badger, 1995). If immediate risk cannot be assessed, the patient should be referred to a specialist. ***High immediate risk*** implies that, based on the information disclosed, the patient is likely to engage in suicidal behavior within the next 24 to 72 hours. ***Low immediate risk*** implies that the patient is not likely to engage in suicidal behavior within the next 24 to 72 hours. ***Unpredictable immediate risk*** implies that the patient has suicidal thoughts and feelings, but the probability of the patient engaging in suicidal behavior within the next 24 to 72 hours cannot be determined.

In theory, the lethality of the suicide plan should be considered when determining immediate risk. However, this criteria should only be used when practitioners have access to a great deal (3 to 6 months) of reliable patient behavior information. Without this information the focus of risk assessment should be on whether suicidal behavior will occur rather than on the nature of suicidal behavior most likely to occur. Unless the patient's behavior patterns are well-documented, there is always the possibility that a patient may have more than one suicide plan or may become impulsive. Disclosure of a non-lethal over-the-counter overdose can, on impulse, be replaced with a high-speed motor vehicle accident. Suicide risk assessment only refers to the ***immediate*** probability of suicidal behavior (Goldberg, 1995).

Management of Suicidal Behavior

➢ Counseling

The psychiatric primary care counseling goals for low-risk suicidal patients are to decrease the risk of suicidal behavior, support effective coping, and promote well being (Lazare, 1979). These primary care goals are most appropriate when a patient is willing and able to disclose suicidal thoughts and feelings and able to participate in counseling. Basic mental health care skills of cognitive-behavioral therapy, emotional support, teaching, family counseling, and developing a plan of action are applicable. High risk and unpredictable risk patients should be referred to a specialist. Assessment and treatment referrals for suicidal patients should be same-day appointments if there is evidence of recent or impulsive suicidal behavior. In counseling low-risk suicidal patients, a friendly but professional approach is recommended. Appearing rushed or indifferent is nonproductive. Practitioners should strive for an interaction style that allows for patients to talk about sensitive information comfortably and respond to professional recommendations. The suicide assessment presented in this chapter can be used for the initial risk assessment and for routine reassessment of risk at follow-up visits until the patient is relatively free of suicidal thoughts and feelings.

Patients with low suicide risk who are found to have an undiagnosed depression, anxiety, or stress disorder should also receive treatment for the disorder, but the first focus of counseling should be to decrease the risk of suicidal behavior. These disorders, however, can produce low-intensity or background suicidal thoughts and feelings that may not completely resolve. Acute suicidal thoughts and feelings usually subside within 3 to 10 days. If this is not the case and acute suicidal thoughts or feelings continue, the patient should be referred to a specialist. Some patients who improve with psychiatric primary care counseling may wish to participate in counseling with a specialist for longer periods of time than are feasible in primary care.

Decrease the risk of suicidal behavior

The process of helping patients decrease the risk of suicidal behavior can begin with the deconstruction of suicidality from a single phenomenon into personal thoughts, feelings, and behaviors. Suicidal thoughts and suicidal feelings should be viewed as different from, but connected to, suicidal behavior, which is the ultimate concern. Patients should be asked to make every effort to talk about, rather than act on, their suicidal thoughts and feelings.

Patients can be encouraged to use cognitive and emotional self-care techniques to decrease their suicidal thoughts and feelings. The self-care goal is to decrease the risk of suicidal behavior and increase personal feelings of comfort and control. A self-care plan increases the probability that the patient can immediately act when troubling thoughts and feelings occur. A self-care plan should identify the exact steps to be taken by the patient. Practitioners can help patients think of positive steps to take. Positive steps must be varied, portable, and suitable for any of the patient's routine settings such as work, school, and home. One of the most portable and positive self-care skills is ***thought-stopping***. Thought stopping is the use of a thought to stop a thought. Thought stopping can be used to reduce the duration, intensity, or content of suicidal thoughts. Take, for example, the following suicidal thought: "I wish I would just kill myself and be done with it." A thought stop might be, "Not true." Every time the suicidal thought is experienced, the patient's immediate self-care response is, "Not true." It is important for patients to use self-care and avoid constantly relying on others to decrease their suicidal thoughts for them.

Patients should identify meaningful, daily self-care behavior goals. These behaviors should have personal value or importance to the patient and provide positive moments, for example, walking 20 minutes in a nature setting, writing a letter to a close friend or relative, or working on a relaxing project. The patient's plan should include scheduled time to be with significant others, but the purpose of such interactions should not be limited to emotional support. Interactions should include some sort of activity, such as preparing a meal, visiting an art center, or participating in a community program, but any plan will be helpful if used. If suicidal thoughts or feelings are so severe and troubling that it is extremely difficult for the patient to engage in self-care, or if the patient needs a great deal of emotional support from others, specialized care may be needed.

Support effective coping

When patients attribute their suicidal thoughts and feelings to specific events or problems, they may become focused on those events or problems rather than on their coping. Just the opposite should be true. Focusing on problems rather than on their solutions can lead to feelings of hopelessness. This is not to imply that all problems have solutions or that individuals should be able to solve all their problems. What is important is that individuals try. Taking actions aimed at resolving a problem has two benefits. First, the problem may be reduced or resolved, but second, the mental effort of problem solving *in itself* protects the individual from becoming psychologically overwhelmed.

Effective problem solving does not require individuals to have no emotional response to their problems. Such an expectation would be unrealistic and unnecessary. Individuals should strive for progress rather than perfection. ***Effective*** refers to the fact that the individual is focused, whereas ***ineffective*** coping refers to unfocused mood-alterating activities and avoidance. Effective problem solving can also protect against excessive ineffective coping (e.g., isolation, overeating, denial), thereby protecting long-term functioning.

Promote well-being

As suicidal thoughts and feelings decrease and functioning is stabilized, the promotion of well being becomes important. In order to promote well being, the patient must clarify his or her definition of it. A personal definition of well being makes it possible to engage in actions that promote well being. For example, if well being is defined as feeling healthy, actions related to feeling healthy should be identified and performed. Specific steps, such as designating time every day for sleep, relaxation, exercise, and conversation, can serve as an active promotion of well being.

℞ Prescribing

When suicidal thoughts, feelings, and behaviors are symptoms of a mental disorder, medications can be prescribed to reduce these symptoms. Low-risk suicidal patients who do not have a mental disorder may benefit from a short course of antianxiety or sedating antidepressant medications, prescribed for relief from tension and distress and to promote rest and sleep. Chronic suicidal thoughts, feelings, and behaviors as symptoms of severe mental disorders such as schizophrenia or bipolar disorder require long-term medication management with antipsychotic medications or mood stabilization medications. Patients with a personality disorder, a substance disorder, acute symptoms of a mental disorder, and those who are severely suicidal or impulsive may require brief hospitalization for their immediate safety needs and before medication can safely be prescribed for treatment or relief. Brief hospitalization can provide structure as well as respite, allowing the acute patient to reorganize as quickly as possible.

☎ Consultation and Referral

Practitioners should consult with a specialist when the following conditions exist: (1) The immediate risk for suicidal behavior cannot be assessed, (2) the immediate risk for suicidal behavior is high or unpredictable, (3) the suicidal patient has a chronic or long-term history of suicidal behavior, (4) the suicidal patient requires treatment for a severe mental disorder, or (5) there are recurrent unexpected changes in the patient's behavior. Consultation with a specialist is also indicated when patients are not willing or able to fully disclose information about their suicidal thoughts, feelings, or behaviors. Consultation with and referral to a specialist is recommended for these serious clinical situations with the assumption that practitioners have immediate access to a specialist by phone or in person. The need for emergency consultation or referral may be rare, but when it is needed any delay will prove unacceptable. Consultation and referral options, including emergency treatment options, should be standard practice. If a patient is found to be highly suicidal with direct access to a violent plan, all efforts should be made to protect the patient, but physical restraint should be avoided unless it is absolutely vital. If a patient requires involuntarily treatment as a danger to self (and/or others), practitioners should follow state and practice rules and, if necessary, consult with police or EMT services.

References

Alarcon RD: Cultural psychiatry, *Psychiatric Clin N Am* 18(3), 1995.

Badger J: Reaching out to the suicidal patient, *The Am J of Nursing* 3:24, 1995.

Buzan R, Weissberg M: Suicide: risk factors and prevention in medical practice, *Ann Review Med* 43:36, 1992.

Barraclough B, Bunch J, Nelson B, Sainsbury P: A hundred cases of suicide: clinical aspects, *Br J Psychiatry* 125:355, 1974.

Conwell Y, Duberstein PR, Cox C, Herrmann JH, Forbes NT, Caine ED: Relationship of age and Axis I diagnoses in victims of completed suicide: a psychological autopsy study, *Am J Psychiatry* 153(8):1001, 1996.

Fogel BS (editor): *The Psychiatric Care of the Medically Ill*, New York, 1993, Oxford University Press.

Goldman H: *Review of General Psychiatry,* 4th Edition, East Norwalk, 1995, Appleton & Lange.

Isometsa ET, Henriksson MM, Heikkinen ME, Aro HM, Marttunen MJ, Kuoppasalmi KI, Lonnqvist JK: Suicide among subjects with personality disorders, *Am J Psychiatry* 153(5):667, 1996.

Janicah PG, Davis JM, Preskorn SH, Ayd FJ: *Principles and practice of psychopharmacotherapy*, Baltimore, 1993, Williams & Wilkins.

Kisis Y, Kosier JT, Robinson RG: Suicidal plans in patients with acute stroke, *The J of Nervous and Mental Disease* 184(5):274, 1996.

Lazare A (editor): *Outpatient psychiatry diagnosis and treatment*, Baltimore, 1979, Williams & Wilkins.

Lish JD, Zimmerman M, Farber NJ, Lush DT, Kuzma MA, Plescia G: Suicide screening in a primary care setting at a Veterans Affairs medical center, *Psychosomatics* 37(5):413, 1996.

Murphy GE, Robins E: Social factors in suicide, *JAMA* 199:303, 1967.

Murphy MD, Wetzel RD: The lifetime risk of suicide in alcoholism, *Arch Gen Psychiatry* 47(5):383, 1990.

Olfson M, Weissman MM, Leon AC, Sheehan DV, Farber L: Suicidal ideation in primary care, *J of Gen Internal Med* 11(8):447, 1996.

Peck ML, Farberow NL, Litman RE: *Youth suicide*, New York, 1985, Springer Publishing Company.

Pfeffer C: *The suicidal child*, New York, 1986, Guilford Press.

Roy A: *Suicide*, Baltimore, 1986, Williams & Wilkins.

Seivewright H, Tyrer P, Casey P, Seivewright N: A three-year follow-up of psychiatric morbidity in urban and rural primary care, *Psychological Med* 21:495, 1991.

Strakowski SM, McElroy SL, Keck PE, West SA: Suicidality among patients with mixed and manic bipolar disorder, *Am J Psychiatry* 153(5):674, 1996.

Westreich L: Assessing an adult patient's suicide risk: what primary care physicians need to know, *Postgrad Med* 90(4):59, 1991.

Partner Violence 19

Out of every 10 cases of partner violence, 9 are committed by men against women. Only a fraction of a percent of cases involves female violence against men. Regardless of who is the violent individual, violence is unacceptable, but given the high incidence of male violence, practitioners have a critical role to play in the social movement to offer women more protection. This chapter reviews male violence toward female partners.

At the start of the 1900s wife abuse was socially acceptable and legal. Old English Common Law held that a man could beat his wife in order to "correct" her behavior if it was objectionable to him. Wife beating was restricted by the Rule of Thumb, which stated that a man could not beat a woman with a stick larger in circumference than his thumb. The concept of ***battering*** as a social problem did not become widely accepted until the mid-1960s (Kashani et al,1992). Currently in the United States, 16.5% of all murders occur within families. Three out of four American women who are murdered are killed by their male partners. And 75% of lethal male violence against female partners occurs when the woman acts on her intentions to end the relationship (Jordon and Walker, 1994)

Because 95% of the victims of partner violence are women (Abbott et al, 1995; Kashani et al, 1992; Gazmararian et al, 1996), the focus here is on women who currently or recently have had an intimate relationship with a violent man, with the understanding that the partners involved are not the only people affected. Partner violence affects everyone in the household, especially children. Children suffer when they must live with violence, but the true magnitude of the effect of partner violence on children is made clear by the fact that when these children reach adulthood, many will become involved in partner violence, either as victims or as perpetrators (Devlin, 1994; Malinosky-Rummel, and Hansen, 1993).

The relationship between child abuse and partner violence as an adult is also very strong; the experience of child abuse can, in fact, be viewed as a forecast for partner violence (Friedlander,

1993). In a study of battered women and their children, children were significantly more likely to be targets of violence when their mother was a target of violence (McCloskey, Figueredo, and Koss, 1995). This particular study found that in some cases children who were beaten were not sexually abused, and those who were sexually abused were not beaten. The researchers found that some men rationalize their abuse of children (sexual, physical, or both) as a means of hurting the child's mother (McCloskey et al, 1995).

A satisfactory comprehensive explanation for male violence toward their female partners has yet to be developed, but numerous personal (e.g., disregard for consequences) and situational (e.g., opportunity) factors have been found to be important (Friedlander, 1993; Kashani et al, 1992). Understanding partner violence begins with understanding the violence. Partner violence is not an abstract concept or a faceless statistic. Male violence toward female partners consists of punching, slapping, kicking, burning, pushing, dragging, choking, restraining, and rape. Fists, feet, teeth, objects, weapons, and vehicles are used intentionally to cause fear and inflict pain, injury, harm, and, suffering. Some women become victims of violence without warning; others are able to predict when their male partners will become violent with a high level of accuracy. An episode of violence may last for hours, causing a woman to fear for her life, or may occur so quickly that she feels uncertain of what just happened to her. In most cases the pattern of violence will include a combination of these extremes. Whatever form or pattern the violence takes, the scars will be physical, psychological, social, emotional, and behavioral. Every cut, bruise, burn, and broken bone causes seen and unseen damage.

Violent men must rely on powerful psychological defenses to rationalize their behavior. These defenses include justification, comparison, displacement, generalization, depersonalization, blame, and minimization (Ordona, 1995). ***Justification*** is a claim of personal privilege or right, expressed with statements such as, "I pay all the bills around here; I can do whatever I want." ***Comparison*** alters the context of the violent behavior for the purpose of redefining it; for example, comparing himself to someone whom he believes is worse with statements such as, "My mother had something to complain about; you don't." ***Displace-***

ment is the attribution of violent behavior to specific external forces, then disowning his own behavior; for example, attributing his violent behavior to a football game in which "his" team was defeated. ***Generalization*** is taking the position that being male means being violent, or that violence is normal behavior for the male. ***Depersonalization*** is viewing the woman as subhuman and therefore an appropriate target for male violence; for example, instead of using her name, always referring to her as "that hag." ***Blaming*** is making the woman responsible by claiming that if only she were different (e.g., thinner, younger, more fun) he would not be violent towards her. ***Minimizing*** is the insistence that no matter how severe or dangerous his behavior is, "it's not that bad." A classic example of minimizing is the statement, "I didn't hit her, I slapped her." The man's primary defense objective is to make sense of his violent behavior in a way that is acceptable to him. He may not make the same defense of his behavior to the woman he has harmed, the children who have witnessed, or the authorities. Because of the immediate danger and long-term consequences of partner violence, practitioners must be prepared to fully assess and act on reports of violence.

➲ Who Is at Risk

Partner violence occurs in all social groups and cannot be predicted by the ethnicity, education, income, or employment level of the individuals involved (Centerwall and Race, 1995). The high-risk models of partner violence reviewed here apply to all social groups. Risk related to partner violence refers to both the probability and the severity of violence. On both counts, male-female intimate relationships are the highest-risk type of relationship. Reports of male violence toward female partners, excluding homicide, indicate that as many as 1 in 8 males in a 1-year period are physically violent toward their female partners. When homicide is included, up to 25% of all homicides in the United States are committed by a husband or a wife (Holtzworth-Monroe, 1995). Physical violence in partner relationships occurs in same-sex as well as heterosexual relationships. In a study of married or dating heterosexual, homosexual, and lesbian couples; the combined rate for partner violence for the total sample was 16% (Bitler, Linnoila, and George, 1994) These statistics are disturbing, but they also show that the majority of adult intimate relationships are free of physical violence.

Numerous violence risk factors have been identified, but two specific factors, alcohol abuse and having been beaten as a child, have been shown to be critical in affecting the risk and severity of partner violence. Alcohol abuse is an important correlate of partner violence, but alcohol consumption does not cause or explain violence. Individuals who abuse alcohol are more likely to also have chronic, complex, and severe psychological, social, emotional, and behavioral problems, including difficulty with intimate relationships. There also appears to be a strong interactive effect between violent behavior and the biochemical changes that occur as a result of alcohol abuse.

For example, Virkkunen and Linnoila (1993) studied early-age onset alcoholism (Type II) and violent behavior in a sample of 27 adult male volunteers and 58 alcoholic violent male offenders. Predictably, 62% of the offenders reported that they had been drinking at the time of their criminal behavior (murder, physical assault, sexual assault, family violence). Measures of alcohol abuse as a risk factor for partner violence produced an interesting finding when the lumbar, cerebrospinal fluid serotonin levels of the volunteers and offenders were compared. Lower serotonin levels, associated with negative mood states, were found in offenders with a pattern of impulsive violence and in volunteers with close relatives who were diagnosed with alcoholism or depression. The researchers observed that in Type II alcoholic violent offenders, lower serotonin levels were significantly correlated with several negative states, such as irritability, impulsiveness, and sleep disturbances. This study does not show if changes in serotonin levels are a cause or an effect of violent behavior, but they highlight the complex biopsychosocial interactions of alcohol abuse, negative mood state, and violent behavior. The observation of lower serotonin levels in volunteers with a family history of alcoholism and depression is consistent with the family transmission models of alcoholism and depression. The significant finding of the study in terms of alcohol abuse and partner violence is that in men who are violent, alcohol abuse can increase the risk (probability and severity) of violence by increasing the risk of impulsive behavior. Alcohol abuse is an important risk factor, but the relationship between alcohol abuse and violent behavior is largely mediated by individual characteristics (e.g., self-concept). Alcohol intoxication, on the other hand, is a more universal risk factor in that most people become disinhibited when intoxicated. For the violent individual, disinhibition can directly increase the risk of violent behavior.

Being beaten as a child has been shown to be significantly related to adult partner violence. When children observe adult violence or are the victims of violence, they experience strong, typically unexpressed, physical and emotional reactions to that violence, such as rapid heart rate, tremors, hyperventilation and anxious feelings of entrapment, threat, and interpersonal rejection. These physical and psychological hurts can remain buried until adulthood, when new hurts revive them and make hurt feelings an emotional flashpoint capable of igniting violent behavior (Bitler, Linnoila, and George 1995). As with alcohol abuse, the connection between a history of having been beaten as a child and adult violence is well documented, but the exact nature of this connection has yet to be defined. What is certain is that violence begets violence. In a study of hospitalized battered women and incarcerated male batterers, 76% of the women and 78% of the men grew up with both parents in the home; half of both women and men had fathers who were alcoholic; most had mothers who were not alcoholic (76% of the women, 78% of the men); but the majority of men (83%) and women (78%) had been beaten as a child (Bergman and Brismar, 1992). Many explanations for the correlation between adult violence (offender or victim) and having been beaten as a child have been developed, but the most obvious conclusion is that children who are forced to learn to accept violence are less likely to become adults who reject violence.

Biological, psychological, social learning, stimulated aggression, and systems theories are among the most well-developed formal theories of violent behavior. Hypothesized ***biological risk factors*** for violent behavior include the potential of chromosomal abnormalities, hormonal imbalance (testosterone and estrogen), and neurotransmitter (GABA, serotonin) and brain tissue abnormalities. ***Psychological theories*** view the mental disorders that are commonly diagnosed in offenders and victims (depression, substance abuse, antisocial personality disorder, borderline personality disorder) as risk factors for violence. ***Social learning***

theory points out the intergenerational or family transmission of violence from generation to generation. ***Aggression theory*** proposes that certain individuals develop or somehow establish a pattern of responding to painful internal (e.g., low self-esteem) and external (e.g., interpersonal conflict) experiences by inflicting pain or suffering upon others. ***Systems theory*** attributes individual violence to membership within a family or a household that is characterized by a give-and-take system of violent interpersonal interactions (Kashani et al, 1992). The clinical usefulness of any single theory is limited by the fact that in most cases, a combination of risk factors will apply.

The risk of violence within male-female intimate relationships is increased when: the woman is physically, emotionally, or socially isolated; weapons are kept in the home; there is severe or chronic conflict about money or parenting; the female partner has significantly less social status, power, and control than the male partner (e.g., an accomplished middle-age man with a teenage girl). These and similar circumstances can generate high levels of relationship stress and conflict that can suddenly and chronically exceed the couple's ability to cope. Violations of role and relationship expectations can trigger intense emotions and old hurts that in turn increase the risk of violence. America's transition from fixed to negotiated roles and expectations in relationships has effectively deregulated what had previously been standardized. Partners may define their roles and their relationships, delineating what each person is "supposed" to do. Agreement on these issues supports the development of the positive emotional attachments that are needed to sustain a healthy intimate relationship. Without such agreement, individuals may silently assume roles that they perceive as theirs and relationship expectations that they perceive as correct. Although fragile, an intimate relationship can work under such circumstances as long as neither partner violates, intentionally or unintentionally, the other's silent assumptions. Even minor violations would put a great deal of stress on an intimate relationship based on unspoken role assumptions. As a risk factor for partner violence, all violations may be significant, but sex-role violations can pose a major threat. The physical, emotional, and psychological needs that define a sexual relationship also expose personal needs. Believing that these personal needs will be satisfied is a way of coping with the vulnerability of being in an intimate relationship. Dysfunctional, maladaptive, or irrational personal needs can create a great deal of stress for the relationship, such as a man who has a psychological need to feel in control of a woman if he has a sexual relationship with her.

In conclusion, multiple individual and relationship factors can increase the risk of partner violence. Of these many factors, the most critical are alcohol abuse, having been beaten as a child, and intimate relationship stress.

☐ Common Assessment Problems

Complex assessment problems can add to what may already be a difficult and time-consuming process. Violence, including male violence against female partners, cannot be predicted, but accurate and early assessment may decrease the risk of violence. The first goal of assessment is to determine whether or not a woman is a target of violence, and the second is to evaluate the level of danger. Professional assessment of risk and danger can create an opportunity to protect the woman and prevent violence. The most critical assessment problems related to partner violence can be summarized as fear, denial, danger, and negative attitudes of health care providers.

Being a target of violence triggers feelings of ***fear*** that can range, in a clinical setting, from sarcasm to terror to silence. For two very different reasons, fear can prevent women from reporting actual, threatened, or potential violence against them. First of all, the woman's state of fear is the violent man's goal: he actively generates or strives to maintain her fear without relief. Second, reporting violence may not gain a woman protection but may only increase the man's violence against her, lead him to rationalize his previous violence, or give him an excuse to expand the targets of his violence to include her children, her job, her supportive relationships, her personal possessions, her income, or her home. Creating and maintaining fear is a basic element of partner violence. During the assessment a woman who has been a target of violence may silently ask herself, "What am I most afraid of?" Her answer will determine her level of participation in the assessment. To fully participate in the assessment, a woman will have to manage her fears, including the fear that is relived in telling her story. Her response to each assessment question may be the result of careful decision making.

Above all, assessment of partner violence is personal. Intimate information must be disclosed. Women who struggle with disclosing intimate information can seem to practitioners to be calculating, perhaps dishonest, or in some way suspect, and practitioners may react negatively to this. This negative reaction tells the woman that the practitioner is reacting to *her* rather than to her report of violence, causing her to wonder why she should bother to tell her story. It is unrealistic to expect a woman who has been, or currently is, the target of violence to strive to be pleasant when reporting that violence. Practitioners can expect disclosure to trigger a run of intense and conflicting emotions. If a woman is describing having been hit, kicked, bitten, pushed, shoved, slapped, dragged across the floor, or raped, the fear attached to those experiences, however it is expressed, should be anticipated and assessed without judgment.

Denial at some point during the assessment can practically be assumed. Both partners may totally or partially deny the violence. Practitioners are understandably baffled by the denial of violence when, for example, there is obvious physical evidence or an arrest has been made. In a study of 59 husbands who were convicted of wife abuse, placed on probation, and court-ordered to participate in treatment, 6 of the men denied that they had ever assaulted their wives (Palmer, Brown, and Barrear, 1992). The researchers reported that a sizable number of these men simply ignored the court order to participate in treatment. As this study indicates, no matter how severe the violence or its consequences, there are men who will not admit to their violence. This is not surprising, since a man who uses violence to establish control over a woman is not likely to want to "trade places" with her by submitting to the will of authorities.

Just as men deny their violence, women may deny that they have been, or currently are, the victims of violence, or they may simply fail to volunteer this information. The basis for a woman's denial may be less obvious than a man's. Both may deny the violence in order to "protect" themselves, but women may deny the violence out of the need to protect themselves from more violence. Denial is such a common assessment problem that some experts recommend that practitioners ask all women direct and specific questions about violence (Golden and Frank, 1994). As explained by these researchers, violence functions as a means of establishing rules and expectations that govern the woman's actions whether or not the violent male is present. Her denial may result from intimidation and thus simply be a matter of "obeying his rules." When this is the case, making the assessment safe becomes an important issue (Hyman, Schillinger, and Bernard, 1995).

Finally, women's denial may be used as a strategy. For example, a woman could inform her partner that the injuries inflicted by him were noticed, but when she was asked about violence she denied it. It is not unusual for a battered woman to believe that she can change the man's behavior. Telling him that her injuries were observed but she did not report him can be a bargaining chip with which she gambles. The folly of this strategy is apparent to others, but most battered women go through a period when they need to believe that they can find a way to have some level of control or power within the relationship.

A woman may also deny her partner's violence because she loves him and believes that the violence can be ended without ending the relationship. The most extreme assessment problem related to denial is that a threat of consequences for the man's violence (e.g., arrest, unemployment) can rejoin the couple in what becomes their shared effort to defeat a common enemy. A woman may go to extreme lengths to defend a man who has been violent with her. The woman's denial and her subsequent defense of the violent man usually brings the assessment to an end.

The absolute ***dangers*** of male violence are injury and death. Therefore danger, though variable and difficult to assess, must be considered in every case of partner violence. The basic problems related to the assessment of danger consist of whether the violent man has a mental disorder, including alcohol abuse, the level of violence at the time of the assessment; and the woman's readiness to leave the relationship. The mental disorders commonly diagnosed in violent men are alcoholism, depression, post-traumatic stress disorder (PTSD), panic disorder, impulse control disorder, and personality disorder (Bitler et al, 1994; Holtzworth-Munroe, 1995). Dysthymia and subclinical symptoms of depression have also been shown to be correlated with male violence (Collins and Bailey, 1990). It is tempting to assume that when a violent man has an undiagnosed or untreated mental disorder, successful treatment of the disorder would also end his violent behavior. However, the majority of men who are diagnosed and treated for mental disorders (except antisocial personality disorder) are not violent. Other individual factors mediate the effects of the disorder on violence and psychosocial functioning, including functioning as an intimate partner. That is, a mental disorder alone may not explain violent behavior, but a disorder can generate relationship stress and interfere with the individual's ability to cope effectively.

The level of violence at the time of the assessment directly impacts the assessment. The typical cycle of violence includes five recurring stages: tension, conflict, violence, withdrawal, and calm, followed by a return of tension. Violence is only the middle stage of the relationship cycle; the events and behavior that routinely precede and follow the violence are also important. In terms of the assessment, violence should not be equated with a relationship dysfunction. Even the most severely dysfunctional relationships can avoid violence when individuals are able to identify a line of aggression that they choose not to cross. That line protects the individuals and the relationship from reaching a stage of conflict that leads to violence. In relationships where there is violence, the amount of time it takes to complete a cycle may be days, weeks, or months, and this time frame may wax and wane. Whatever stage is occurring at the time of assessment impacts the assessment. A woman whose batterer is withdrawn or calm will appear differently to the practitioner than if she is seen just prior to or in the midst of a violent episode (Kashani et al, 1992).

If a woman has decided to end the relationship, how close is she to actually leaving? Women leave violent men gradually; that is, they may leave and return several times (Maher-Sharp, 1995). There are many reasons for doing so: women leave when they believe it is safe, when they have somewhere to go, and when they believe they can avoid the male's response. Women who have small children or who are unemployed may feel that leaving is impossible. A successful escape requires that the woman be able to navigate considerable barriers (financial, legal, physical, social, or religious) that have been constructed by the violent man for the express purpose of stopping her. Therefore some women deal with each problem, each barrier, and each response of the man until they are out of the relationship. Physically leaving the relationship is only the first stage. After that the woman must leave the relationship financially, emotionally, sexually, and socially and, if the couple is married, she must also leave the relationship legally.

At any point the violent man may decide that she has gone too far and may take action to stop her. From his point of view (once supported by common law), he is stopping the woman from behaving in an objectionable manner. If he has already used barriers, intimidation, threats, and violence and she has not conformed, he may view her defiance as *his* failure or inability to control her and may then use these feelings to rationalize killing her. Women who are leaving a violent man should be viewed as being in a potentially life-threatening situation. Women who realize this danger may express intense emotions such as suicidal thoughts, aggressive self-destructive behavior, or may be demanding of and impatient with practitioners who do not seem to understand their danger. Women who do not realize the danger may appear to be confused, ambivalent, or unrealistic. Leaving may also be complicated by intense feelings of grief over the loss of her partner and the relationship. The entire issue of leaving a violent man is all the more complicated when the woman's current relationship is not her first with a violent man. It is not uncommon for women to report that they have had a series of relationships with violent men. What may appear to be self-defeating patterns might, in fact, have to do with the realities of getting out of such relationships. Whether the problem is one violent man or a series of violent men, getting out once and for all requires resolve and resources. For this reason practitioners must focus on the violence, rather than each individual man.

Negative attitudes of practitioners toward women who are in relationships with violent men are not unusual, but they pose important assessment problems (Gremillion and Evins, 1994). Those of us who are not victims of violence feel certain that we would leave a violent partner immediately; this is a common reaction. With or without resources, many women do leave. But others, such as women who have been beaten as children, may be less able to find the resolve needed to take an absolute position against violence. Experience may have schooled them to believe that they cannot avoid or escape violence but must live with it.

For personal or professional reasons, practitioners may stereotype a woman who is with a violent man, sometimes even letting her know that they find her situation repulsive or something not tolerated by decent people. This negative attitude is all the more troubling when, because of this attitude, practitioners fail to assess violence (Gremillion and Evins, 1994). Some practitioners may hold negative attitudes toward women in relationships with violent men because they believe that anything they could say or do would be futile, or that any help they offered would be rejected. There may also be concern about taking on excessive professional liability by trying to address partner violence. Perhaps the most difficult negative practitioner attitude is the belief that partner violence is only a social-legal problem, and not a health problem. There are no easy answers to these negative attitudes, but they do not alter the fact that partner violence is a social-legal problem with serious health and well-being consequences. Primary care should be a safe point of access to help (Feldman, 1992.

Assessment Guidelines

The Nursing Research Consortium on Violence and Abuse has developed a five-item abuse assessment screen for pregnant women (McFarlane and Parker, 1994). A *yes* answer to one or more of the assessment questions indicates that the woman is a target of violence and an assessment of danger should be performed, such as the Danger Assessment screen developed by Campbell (1986). Both the assessment and the danger screens are short and take only a few minutes to complete; they can then serve as the basis of a more comprehensive interview. When should a woman be asked to complete an assessment about partner violence? Without a policy of assessing all female patients, practitioners will have to decide on a case-by-case basis. The hazard is that a woman may be the victim of violence but not say so; she may wait for the practitioner to ask, but the practitioner may not ask unless the woman makes some reference to violence. There is no ideal method for knowing when to assess for violence. Women who are ready to report having been a victim of violence may view the assessment process as an important validation of their needs for assistance. Women who are not ready to report could still view the assessment as a valuable opportunity to talk about violence, but may refuse to disclose personal information. With all assessments, women should be informed of what to expect, what actions will and will not be taken, and how the information she has provided will be recorded. The process of assessment should not cause a woman to feel that she has no choice over what will or will not happen. Because a battered woman has already had little say over events in her life, being forced to submit to well-meaning protocols can feel abusive.

Abuse Assessment*

1. Have you ever been emotionally or physically abused by your partner or someone close to you? Yes/No
2. Within the last year have you been hit, slapped, kicked, or otherwise physically hurt by someone? Yes/No. If yes, by whom? Total number of times:
3. Since you have been pregnant, have you been hit, slapped, kicked, or otherwise physically hurt by someone? Yes/No. If yes, by whom? Total number of times: (Optional)
4. Within the last year, has anyone forced you to have sexual contact? Yes/No. If yes, who? Total number of times:
5. Are you afraid of your partner or anyone else?

Danger Assessment**

Answer each question yes or no.

1. Has the physical violence increased in frequency over the past year?

* *From McFarlane, J, Parker, B: Preventing abuse during pregnancy: an assessment and intervention protocol, Maternal Child Nurse, 19(Nov/Dec): 321, 1994.*

** *From Campbell, J: Nursing assessment for risk of homicide in battered women, Ans Adv Nurs Sci, 6:36, 1986.*

2. Has the physical violence increased in severity over the past year? Has a weapon or a threat with a weapon been used?
3. Does he ever try to choke you?
4. Is there a gun in the house?
5. Has he ever forced you to have sex when you did not wish to do so?
6. Does he use drugs ("uppers" or amphetamines, speed, angel dust, cocaine, "crack," street drugs, heroin, or mixtures)?
7. Does he ever threaten to kill you and/or do you believe he is capable of killing you?
8. Is he drunk every day or almost every day (in terms of quantity of alcohol)?
9. Does he control most of your daily activities? For instance, does he tell you whom you can be friends with, how much money you can take with you to shop, or when you can take the car? (If he tries, but you do not let him, check here_____.)
10. Have you ever been beaten by him while you were pregnant? (If never pregnant by him check here_____.)
11. Is he violently and constantly jealous of you? (For instance, does he say, "If I can't have you, no one can"?)

Management of Partner Violence

➢ Counseling

The aim of primary care counseling with battered women is to provide access to the support and resources that they need to make choices and take action (Yam, 1995). Without blaming her, practitioners can point out that from the start the woman has been making choices. She can feel responsible for her choices but not for the choices made by her partner. This empowerment is emotionally meaningful, but it is also necessary. Once a woman has reported violence, her subsequent actions should be measured in terms of whether they move her toward or away from regaining control of her life. The partner and the relationship should not be the focus. Staying in or leaving the relationship should be a separate topic. Practitioners should address the violence, not the relationship. This is no small task, since the relationship has most likely defined her life for a long time. But without question the focus must be on acting to protect the woman and her children from harm and danger and on preventing the man from acting violently against her and her children with impunity.

When women report violence to practitioners, they may also report current symptoms of a mental disorder, such as depression, anxiety, chronic stress, substance abuse, or PTSD. When a mental disorder is diagnosed, symptom relief and treatment are required, but protection and prevention must still be priorities. Depending on the nature of the disorder, a woman may feel unable or unwilling to make choices and take action regarding the violence. She may insist that she cannot do anything until she feels better. Whenever possible, battered women with mental disorders should immediately be referred to a psychiatric specialist who is experienced in working with this complex patient profile. Outpatient crisis counseling can be a good resource. Crisis counseling is intense but brief, with usually two to three appointments per week for not longer than 4 weeks. A good guideline for practitioners would be that if a woman's symptoms of mental disorder are related to the violence, then symptom relief is required: if the violence is causing or sustaining symptoms, especially self-harm symptoms such as sexual acting out and substance abuse, these behaviors should also be addressed as such. When there is no clinical evidence of an acute or severe mental disorder or self harm behavior, the following primary care counseling strategies are recommended.

By the time professionals become involved, a woman's situation may be grim (McCauley et al, 1995; Roberts et al, 1996). To provide effective psychiatric primary care counseling for battered women, practitioners must be knowledgeable of local and state laws that apply to partner violence and familiar with services and resources for battered women, such as consultation/education/prevention services, crisis services, specialized psychiatric counseling, and community resources and shelters (Jordan and Walker, 1994). When helping a woman to access these services and resources, it should be pointed out to her early on that she may have to deal with several different agencies. Emotional support, teaching, and coaching are effective counseling skills to help the woman begin to adopt a new view of herself and of the violence that she may have lived with for years.

Although their immediate needs may be for health care, safety and shelter, women who are victims of violence will also have temporary (e.g., money) and long-term (e.g., lawyer) needs. Psychiatric primary care counseling can begin the process of addressing these needs by discussing the most recent episode of violence. The goal here is to use that episode as a point at which to begin to rethink the violence in ways that she may not have considered. This process can help to clarify her current needs. Counseling should stress the importance of adopting the view that violence is socially and personally unacceptable. This may sound like an all-too-obvious point, but, depending on how the man has rationalized his violence and the extent to which he may have abused her children as a way of hurting her, some women will try to understand or "explain" the violence. Women who are struggling to make sense of the violence against them have not yet adopted the perspective that any violence is unacceptable. Practitioners may need to restate this point often and explain that since there is no acceptable explanation for violent behavior, there is no reason to try to "figure it out."

If possible, it is helpful to discuss any counseling the woman may have already received from professionals, family members, and friends. If that counseling seems to have been negative or nonproductive, it can be helpful to try to learn from the woman why it was not helpful and what would have made it more useful. For example, she may have received more than one unwelcome lecture accusing her of making a mistake that other women would not have made. Others may have told her repeatedly that there is nothing she can do to improve her situation. Practioners who understand this negative counseling can avoid making similar mistakes.

A female practitioner may encounter the rather difficult experience of being told that, unless she herself has been the victim of violence, she can't understand or be of help. Since the practitioner's goals are to help the woman to protect herself, prevent the violence, and gain access to resources, this is not true. This negative patient reaction can occur when a battered woman compares herself unfavorably to the practitioner, such as viewing the practitioner as someone who would never tolerate being abused or degraded. The female practitioner may become a mirror in which the woman sees an extremely negative image of herself. Patience and a professional manner can ease this negative reaction and help the woman to resist giving in to feelings of self-hate.

For many women, counseling means getting an answer to the question, "What should I do?" The counseling response to this question is to help the woman reduce this generic question into smaller personal questions that have answers. Practitioners should avoid spending much time on generic questions. Advice should be specific and offered with the expectation that the woman will choose what advice to accept and follow. Despite their hope of obtaining useful assistance, women who report having been victims of violence may make excessive requests and demands of practitioners, few of which can be satisfied, and then imply that the practitioner is of no use or not willing to help. This is almost always an expression of hopelessness that is best dealt with by focusing on what can be done rather than on lifelong wants and needs that have never been fulfilled. Effective psychiatric primary care counseling does not require that a woman do more than be willing to begin the process of ending the violence in her life. Unless there is evidence of danger, each woman should be allowed to make her own choices in her own time.

Psychiatric primary care counseling is not couples therapy. Severe relationship problems will be reported, but these problems are best handled by referring the woman to specialized care. Practitioners can point out that regardless of what happens to the relationship, the violence must stop. Many women may assume that if certain details of their relationships were different, there would be no violence. In rare cases this may be true, but the problem with this logic is that violence is not caused by a bad relationship, just as a bad relationship is not necessarily violent. Psychiatric primary care counseling cannot focus on the nature or pattern of a relationship. A woman may sincerely wish to talk about her relationship and believe that the violence can be understood by trying to understand the relationship, but practitioners should point out that the best way to improve the relationship is to stop the violence, and then return the focus to the violence and refer to specialized care.

Finally some women need to warm up to the idea of talking about violence. This is one of the many reasons why written assessments are so helpful, but even after reporting violence some women may seem intent on testing the practitioner's interest and skill, hinting at problems, then refusing to describe them. Patience is still the best strategy. If the assessment cannot be completed or the woman somehow rejects or resents the practitioner's efforts, a practitioner who has patience may still be remembered and might be called on in the future when the woman is prepared to take one more step toward safety.

Consultation and Referral

Two types of consultation and referral should be made, regardless of whether or not the woman is prepared to act. Each woman who reports having been a victim of violence should be provided with direct access to legal, professional (e.g., a psychiatric specialist) and community programs that help victims of domestic violence. Whether the current relationship is the first one in which a woman has experienced violence, or just one of a series, practitioners should focus on helping her to regain control of her life. Unless there is a clear reason not to, each woman should be given an appointment to consult with a psychiatric specialist for the purpose of obtaining a psychological evaluation of her mental health and psychosocial functioning. If this evaluation indicates a mental disorder, severely impaired psychosocial functioning, or behavior that is dangerous to oneself or others (e.g., sexual acting out, alcohol abuse, child abuse), individual psychotherapy should be arranged.

Consultation and referral with community programs is also necessary. Effective community programs have a range of staff, including women who have successfully stopped the violence in their own lives. Preferably, the community program can respond immediately to a call for help at any hour of the day and has an established record of being helpful. Community programs can be effective in many ways, but they should offer comfort, respite, support, safety, and expertise. For primary care practitioners, the bottom line in arranging for consultation and referral for a battered women has to be the following: if the woman makes the call, will she benefit? The answer to this bottom-line question largely rests with the woman herself, in her ability to effectively utilize professional and community resources. When practitioners have the luxury of making consultation and referral choices, they should strive for a good match between the woman and the resources. Handing a woman who has reported violence a list of generic resources is unacceptable. Despite the practitioner's best efforts, some women who are victims of violence may not make use of the resources they need, but these resources should still be made available. Finally, violent male partners may be prepared to respond to any noticeable change in the woman's attitude or behavior, viewing them as cues to re-establish his control. Flyers, phone numbers, unaccounted-for time away from home, or phone calls and visits from strangers can be perceived by a violent man as a personal threat against him. Every effort should be made to decrease the risk that a woman's request for help will become another opportunity for violence.

References

Abbott J, Johnson R, Koziol-McLain J, Lowenstein SR: Domestic violence against women: incidence and prevalence in an emergency department population, *JAMA* 273(22):1763, 1995.

Alpert EJ: Violence in intimate relationships and the practicing internist: new disease or new agenda? *Ann Intern Med* 123(10):774, 1995.

Bergman BK, Brismar BG. Can family violence be prevented? A psychosocial study of male batterers and battered wives, *Public Health* 106(1):45, 1992.

Bitler DA, Linnoila M, George DT: Psychosocial and diagnostic characteristics of individuals initiating domestic violence, *The J of Nervous and Mental Disease* 182(10):583, 1994.

Campbell J: Nursing assessment for risk of homicide in battered women, *Ads Nurs Sci*, 8:36, 1986.

Centerwall BS: Race, socioeconomic status, and domestic homicide, *JAMA* 273(22):1755, 1995.

Collins JJ, Bailey SL: Relationship of mood disorders to violence, *The J of Nervous and Mental Disease* 178(1):44, 1990.

Devlin BK: Child abuse, *Am J of Nursing* March:26, 1994.

Feldman MK: Family violence interventions, physicians find it's more than treating injuries, *Minnesota Med* 75:19, 1992.

Friedlander BZ: Community violence, children's development, and mass media: in pursuit of new insights, new goals, and new strategies, *Psychiatry* 56(1):66, 1993.

Gazmararian JA, Lazorick S, Spitz AM, Ballard TJ, Saltman LE, Marks JS: Prevalence of violence against pregnant women, *JAMA* 275(24):1915, 1996.

Golden GK, Frank PB: When 50-50 isn't fair: the case against couple counseling in domestic abuse, *Social Work* 39(6):636, 1994.

Gremillion DH, Evins G: Why don't doctors identify and refer victims of domestic violence? *North Carolina Med J* 55(9):482, 1994.

Holtzworth-Munroe A: Marital violence, *The Harvard Mental Health Letter* 12(2):4, 1995.

Hyman A, Schillinger D, Bernard L: Laws mandating reporting of domestic violence, do they promote patient well-being? *JAMA* 273(22):1781, 1995.

Jordon CE, Walker R: Guidelines for handling domestic violence cases in community mental health centers, *Hosp and Comm Psychiatry* 45(2):147, 1994.

Kashani JH, Dandoy AE, Holcomb WR: Family violence: impact on children, *J of Am Acad Child Adolescent Psychiatry* 31(2):181, 1992.

Maher-Sharp K: Why do they stay? *Iowa Med* 85(1):24, 1995.

Malinosky-Rummell R, Hansen DJ: Long term consequences of childhood physical abuse, *Psychological Bull* 114(1):68, 1993.

McCauley J, Kern DE, Kolodner K, Dill L, Schroeder AF, DeChant HK, Ryden J, Bass EB, Derogatis LR: The battering syndrome: prevalence and clinical characteristics of domestic violence in primary care internal medicine practices, *Ann Inter Med* 123(10):737, 1995.

McCloskey LA, Figueredo AJ, Koss MP: The effects of systemic family violence on children's mental health, *Child Development* 66(5):1239, 1995.

McFarlane J, Parker B: Preventing abuse during pregnancy: an assessment and intervention protocol, *Maternal Child Nursing* 19(Nov/Dec):321, 1994.

Ordona T, Understanding domestic violence, *Iowa Med* 85(1):35, 1995.

Palmer SE, Brown RA, Barrear ME: Group treatment program for abusive husbands: long term evaluation, *Am J of Orthopsychiatry* 62(2):276, 1992.

Roberts GL, O'Toole BI, Raphael B, Lawrence JM, Ashby R: Prevalence study of domestic violence victims in an emergency department, *Ann of Emergency Med* 27(6):747, 1996.

Virkkunen M, Linnoila M: Brain serotonin, Type II alcoholism and impulsive violence, *J of Studies of Alcohol* Suppl 11:163, 1993.

Yam M: Wife abuse: strategies for a therapeutic response, *Scholarly Inquiry for Nursing Practice: An International Journal* 9(2):147, 1995.

Part V

Practice Notes

Mental Health Care Laws and Patient Rights 20

This chapter presents information related to legal issues in mental health care. Five areas will be discussed:

1. Mental health care patient rights
2. Involuntary mental health care treatment criteria
3. The *Tarasoff v. Regents of the University of California* case
4. The Americans with Disabilities Act
5. Patient treatment needs versus patient treatment rights

Each state defines the specific scope and range of mental health care patient rights and involuntary treatment criteria that will govern practice in that state. Practitioners should obtain this information and become familiar with the patient rights laws and the involuntary treatment process for their state. Most state laws specifically apply to mental health care professionals who, by education, training, and license, are obligated to comply. Practitioners of psychiatric primary care could also be subject to these laws as standards of practice and should therefore understand their intent and application.

Mental Health Care Patient Rights

By law, patients have numerous mental health care treatment rights. The two most fundamental are the right to receive appropriate mental health treatment and the right to refuse mental health treatment. Mental health care patient rights have been defined by law because prior to the enactment of these laws, individuals who were admitted to mental hospitals had few if any civil rights. Individuals could be sent to a mental institution for years or even for life without recourse, and never receive any mental health treatment. To end the abuse of individuals with mental disorders, patients and their families used the courts to win the legal right to demand appropriate treatment for a diagnosed mental disorder and, under certain conditions, to refuse mental health care. As they currently exist, patient rights include personal rights, treatment rights, communication and privacy rights, record access and privacy rights, and grievance of patient rights violations. A partial listing of Wisconsin patient rights is presented later in this chapter to demonstrate the potential scope of patient rights laws. The scope of mental health patient rights is so broad that it is possible for a patient's treatment needs to conflict with that patient's treatment rights.

For example, a mental health care professional may be aware that a patient will have a profoundly negative reaction to reading his or her mental health treatment records, but the patient's reaction cannot be taken into consideration should that patient request a complete copy of his or her mental health treatment records. Many states allow for limitations to be placed on patient access to mental health treatment records, but in Wisconsin and California patient access to treatment records following treatment discharge is not restricted. While there are no calls to repeal patient treatment rights, there is a growing interest in taking steps to decrease the risk that patient treatment rights will directly conflict with patient treatment needs or the practice of mental health care professionals.

Patients, their families, mental health care professionals, and lawyers regularly dispute the positive and negative impact of patient treatment rights laws on patient care, but all agree that the current problems are preferable to the days of no patient rights. Practitioners should be aware that patients who have been diagnosed and treated for mental disorders or psychosocial problems may elect to obtain their treatment records. Mental health treatment records are now routinely requested by patients for reasons that may not be directly related to their mental health care treatment, such as pending legal actions regarding social security-disability income, employment disputes, divorce, or child custody.

The right to refuse mental health treatment becomes a clinical problem when, as is often the case, the refusal of mental health treatment is the result of mental disorder symptoms that treatment is intended to relieve (Urrutia, 1994). The most dramatic example of patient treatment rights potentially conflicting with patient treatment needs is the preventable winter deaths of homeless, mentally ill individuals who exercise their legal right to refuse mental health treatment. Unless it can be shown to a court of law that an individual is gravely disabled due to a mental disorder or is a potential risk of dangerous behavior toward oneself or others, the individual may be able to refuse treatment from which he or she could reasonably be expected to benefit.

In most states the right to refuse mental health treatment is contingent on whether the individual's treatment refusal can be considered valid. An individual's refusal of recommended mental health treatment may be deemed invalid if it can be shown to be the result of delusional thinking, mental incompetence, or severe mental illness (SMI), if there is a significant history of mental health improvement with medication treatment; or if there is significant potential for violent behavior (Urrutia, 1994). Although the term ***treatment*** is used in the discussion of patient rights, it almost always refers to medication and hospitalization.

Forcing an individual to take medication or be hospitalized is difficult for all concerned. In addition, many of the most advanced medications can have a very long onset time or a half-life duration, and therefore they cannot easily be prescribed for a short period of hospitalization. The newer medications for SMI tend to have significantly fewer side effects and health risks, but disturbing and disabling side effects can occur. Despite improvement in efficacy, medication treatment of mental disorders continues to be far from 100% effective. In other words, it is possible that an individual may receive only limited benefits from involuntary treatment.

Nevertheless, potential patient rights problems must continue to be weighed against actual patient treatment needs and a reasonable potential for treatment benefits. In the final analysis, the pain and suffering of untreated mental illness is the first concern of the practitioner.

Wisconsin Patient Treatment Rights*

1. You must be provided prompt and adequate treatment, rehabilitation and education services appropriate for you.
2. You must be allowed to participate in the planning of your treatment and care.
3. You must be informed of your treatment and care, including alternatives and possible side effects of medications.
4. No treatment or medication may be given to you without your consent, unless it is needed in an emergency to prevent serious physical harm to you or others, or a court orders it. If you have a guardian, however, your guardian can consent to treatment and medication on your behalf.
5. You must not be given unnecessary or excessive medication.
6. You cannot be subject to electro-convulsive therapy or any drastic treatment measures such as psychosurgery or experimental research without your written informed consent.
7. You must be informed of any costs of your care and treatment that you or your relatives may have to pay.
8. You must be treated in the least restrictive manner and setting necessary to safely and appropriately meet your needs.
9. You may not be restrained or placed in a locked room (seclusion) unless in an emergency when it is necessary to prevent physical harm to you or to others.

Wisconsin Patient Privacy Rights**

1. Your treatment information must be kept private (confidential).

* *Wisconsin Department of Health and Human Services, 1995.*

** *Wisconsin Department of Health and Human Services, 1995.*

2. Your records cannot be released without your consent, unless the law specifically allows for it.
3. You can ask to see your records. You must be shown any records about your physical health or medications. Staff may limit how much you can see of the rest of your records while you are receiving services. You must be informed of the reasons for any such limits. You can challenge those reasons in the grievance process. After discharge, you can see your entire record if you ask to do so.
4. If you believe something in your records is wrong, you can challenge its accuracy. If staff will not change the part of your record that you have challenged, you can put your own version in your record.

Wisconsin Patient Grievance Rights***

1. You may sue someone for damages or other court relief if they violate any of your rights.
2. Involuntary patients can ask a court to review the order to place them in a facility.
3. If you feel your rights have been violated, you may file a grievance.
4. The service provider or facility must inform you of your rights and how to use the grievance process.
5. You may, at the end of the grievance process, or any time during it, choose to take the matter to court.

Involuntary Mental Health Care Treatment Criteria

States have similar involuntary treatment criteria, but these can vary a great deal in terms of the process of admitting an individual to involuntary treatment. Practitioners should understand their state's criteria and involuntary treatment process and how to initiate the process from their practice setting. Most important,

*** *Wisconsin Department of Health and Human Services, 1995.*

practitioners should know what authorization is needed to start the process. The primary intent of involuntary mental health treatment is to provide mental health care to individuals who need treatment but who are unwilling or unable to consent to it. The process itself is designed to address the issues of treatment need and consent but the driving forces behind involuntary treatment are potential or actual dangerous patient behaviors, appropriate patient responsibility, and appropriate provider authority (Beahrs and Rogers, 1993).

The process of involuntary treatment is mostly the product of involuntary treatment criteria, clinical and legal checks and balances, and patient rights versus public rights checks and balances. Clinically, the first step of involuntary treatment should be the determination of whether voluntary treatment with informed consent is more appropriate. Informed consent is the individual's voluntary agreement to treatment after receiving full information about it. The individual must be able to make a knowing and willful decision, without constraint or coercion, to volunteer to participate in treatment (Miller, 1994). To volunteer for mental health treatment, the individual must be mentally competent to sign a legal treatment agreement.

Although the question of an individual's mental competence to consent to mental health treatment would appear to be the major criterion for involuntary treatment, the most important consideration to date has been potential or actual dangerous behaviors (Lindenthal and Thomas, 1992). Involuntary treatment criteria for most states are grave disability due to mental disorder, danger to oneself, or danger to others. ***Grave disability*** is commonly defined in terms of basic functioning, or the ability to meet one's immediate food, clothing, shelter, and safety needs. Some states have expanded the concept of grave disability to include the individual's immediate and long-term needs for mental health care. In those states, severe psychiatric symptomatology and impaired independent functioning are additional criteria for involuntary treatment (Kapp, 1994).

Danger to oneself or others refers to any dangerous or injurious behaviors, actual or potential, including suicide and homicide. Without exception, risk of danger is the most complicated, criterion clinically and legally, for involuntary treatment. Clinical evidence of immediate or severe risk of dangerous behavior must be presented to the court. The aim of the court's review of a petition for involuntary treatment due to dangerous behavior is to protect the individual's civil rights and the public's right to safety. The range of behaviors that satisfy or fail to satisfy this involuntary treatment criterion is so great that absolute standards cannot be defined. Verbal threats, harmful acts, and lethal plans may all be considered.

Assuming that the individual is competent to agree to treatment and there is clinical evidence of a need for mental health care treatment, the danger to oneself and others becomes the primary consideration of clinicians and the court. Many states require that police officers, on the advice of clinical staff as well as by direct observation, initiate all petitions for involuntary treatment. This arrangement partly reflects a belief that danger to oneself or others may not be directly related to mental illness and that, in the eyes of the court, the individual is being taken into custody. Therefore the individual has the right to be represented by a lawyer and to request immediate release.

Society fully expects that individuals who are found to be a potential or an actual threat of harm or injury to others will be prevented from doing so. Families and friends equally expect that, if their loved one is set on a course of self-harm, the authorities will act to prevent the self-harm and provide the necessary treatment. In some states, acute substance intoxication is included in the scope of dangerous behaviors. At the same time, patient rights laws instruct the courts to deny excessive restrictions on personal liberty. At each step of the involuntary treatment process the state, via the courts, must provide the individual with a real opportunity for clinical reassessment and release from custody (Monahan et al, 1995).

Regardless of the individual's actual conduct before appearing in court, should the individual appear to be competent and not an immediate danger to oneself or others, the court must place a great deal of weight on this evidence. Clinicians, family members, and police officers must be able to present overwhelming evidence to refute this. The court must apply every possible means of safeguarding the individual's freedom. State and community standards vary in terms of the actual behavior that constitutes the level of risk of danger that is required for involuntary treatment. The individual's age, race, gender, education, and income can have a negative or positive effect on the process and on the ruling.

Individuals who are taken into custody involuntarily are entitled to immediate court review of their admission, usually within 24 hours. At this time the court may support or revoke the involuntary admission. The initial duration of involuntary commitment is 72 hours. This time is intended to be used more for assessment and psychiatric evaluation than for actual treatment. Based on the findings of the first 72 hours, the clinical staff may recommend to the court that an additional 14 or 21 days of involuntary assessment and treatment are necessary. This recommendation is based on the same involuntary treatment criteria but may include more evidence of the individual's need for treatment. At any point in the process the individual can agree to treatment, if his or her agreement meets the test of informed consent and if the individual is not seeking voluntary patient status for the purpose of circumventing the involuntary treatment process.

Efficacy is one of the most important questions regarding involuntary treatment. Does involuntary treatment produce improvement? Are the outcomes of involuntary treatment the equivalent of outcomes normally associated with voluntary treatment? Along with these questions, there is a concern that the individual's treatment needs can become secondary if the individual's efforts to resist involuntary treatment, and the clinical staff's efforts to document the need for involuntary treatment, become excessive (Monahan et al, 1995). The dilemmas inherent in involuntary treatment make it apparent that despite the efforts of many people, involuntary treatment is far from an ideal solution to an extremely difficult social and mental health problem.

Some communities have tried to split the difference by establishing outpatient involuntary treatment as a condition for the release of involuntarily hospitalized patients, as an alternative to hospitalization for patients who meet involuntary treatment criteria, or as an alternative for patients who may not currently meet involuntary treatment criteria but, unless preventive measures are taken, soon will (Kapp, 1994; Swartz et al, 1995; Sanguineti et al, 1996; Smith, 1995).

The *Tarasoff v. Regents of the University of California* Case

Tarasoff v. Regents of the University of California (1974, 1976) refers to the case of a California male who told his therapist of his plans to murder Tarasoff, a woman he had dated, and then carried out his plan. The original 1974 *Tarasoff* ruling held that mental health professionals have a duty to warn known potential victims of potential dangerous patient behavior. This ruling was expanded in 1976 to state that mental health professionals have the duty to protect the public against the dangerous actions of their patients (Pettis, 1992).

The *Tarasoff* ruling is unique because according to this law, mental health professionals have a duty to both their patients and the public (Rudegeair and Appelbaum, 1992). Practitioners may be required to act to protect the patient's rights and the public's rights by recognizing potentially dangerous patient behaviors and taking action to protect the public (Kagle and Kopels, 1994). Health care professionals are not expected to be able to predict patient behavior, however. The aims of *Tarasoff* are to ensure that practitioners will take action when it is called for, since they may be the first to detect any sign of potentially dangerous behavior.

According to *Tarasoff*, neither patient rights nor patient-provider confidentiality exceeds the public's right to protection. States define the specific actions that mental health professionals are expected to take in order to fulfill their duty to protect the public. The clinical as well as social drawbacks of this requirement, which in effect makes practitioners into officers of the court under the threat of malpractice litigation, may sometimes exceed the hoped-for benefits of *Tarasoff*. Patients who understand the *Tarasoff* ruling can argue that the mental health professional represents a threat to them or has not made their treatment needs the priority (Cartensen, 1994). The duty to third parties continues to be a complex practice problem (Applebaum and Zoltek-Jick, 1996; Pettis, 1992).

The Americans with Disabilities Act (ADA)

The 1990 Americans with Disabilities Act (ADA) protects the civil rights of individuals with a physical or mental disability (Parmet, Daynard, and Gottlieb, 1996; Ravid and Menon, 1993). Under the protection of the ADA, individuals with a mental disability (a mental disorder) cannot be subject to discrimination. Qualified individuals with a mental disability who are able to perform the essential functions of a job, with or without reasonable accommodation, may not be disqualified due to the mental disability. The ADA does not protect sexual behavior disorders, compulsive gambling, kleptomania, or substance disorders. Individuals who no longer have a mental disability diagnosis, but have in the past received treatment for a mental disability, are also protected (Ravid and Menon, 1993).

The overall effect of the ADA is that individuals with mental disorders cannot be discredited by their disorder alone; employers with 15 or more employees may take steps to determine if an individual is able to meet job performance standards, but they cannot simply assume that an individual who was treated for a mental disorder is unable to perform the work. Individuals who have been diagnosed with or treated for a mental disorder need not disclose this information to potential employers. As with all civil rights legislation, ADA laws protect individuals against discrimination (actions) but can provide little or no protection from prejudice (attitudes). However, the ADA gives individuals the right to decide whether to disclose a mental disorder diagnosis without fear of discrimination.

Patient Treatment Needs versus Patient Treatment Rights

The patient rights and treatment laws reviewed in this chapter can create complex practice concerns for mental health professionals who must address patient needs, patient rights, public rights, and immediate and long-term treatment outcomes. Take, for example, a single young woman with SMI who frequently suffers episodes of psychosis that have been difficult to treat. She is sexually active but is unwilling, and sometimes unable, to use contraception to prevent pregnancy, but she would be at significant risk of losing custody of a child should she become pregnant

As a mental health patient she needs health care that can help build her self-esteem, support effective coping, help her to retain personal autonomy, and manage her SMI. But her family insists on being fully informed of the woman's sexual behavior and, as her caretaker, they want to insure that the woman uses contraception (Petrila and Sadoff, 1992). The family does not want the woman to become pregnant because they feel she would not be able to care for a child at this time in her life, and they worry that the woman might unintentionally harm an infant. The mental health professional is concerned about possible pregnancy, because it is a contraindication for the woman's treatment medication, but is also hesitant to prescribe a long-acting IM contraceptive to someone who cannot give her consent.

At odds here are the young woman's physical and mental health care needs, her treatment rights and reproductive rights, the safety rights of the child should she become pregnant, and the family's right to obtain and participate in the best possible health care for their loved one, including medication for her SMI and contraception. This example further illustrates the potential conflicts between patient health care needs and rights that health care professionals must face. There are no easy solutions to the problems presented here, but practitioners are an important voice in advocating for full consideration of patient health and well-being needs as well as patient treatment rights.

References

Appelbaum PS, Zoltek-Jick R: Psychotherapists' duties to third parties: Ramona and beyond, *Am J Psychiatry* 153(4):457, 1996.

Beahrs JO, Rogers JL: Appropriate short-term risk in psychiatry and the law, *Bull Am Acad Psychiatry Law* 21(1):53, 1993.

Carstensen PC: The evolving duty of mental health professionals to third parties: a doctrinal and institutional examination, *Inter J of Law and Psychiatry* 12(1):1, 1994.

Kagle JD, Kopels S: Confidentiality after *Tarasoff*, *Health and Social Work* 19(3):217, 1994.

Kapp MB: Treatment and refusal rights in mental health: therapeutic justice and clinical accommodation, *Am J Orthopsychiatry* 64(2):223, 1994.

Lindenthal JJ, Thomas CS: Confidentiality in clinical psychiatry, *Medicine and Law* 11:119, 1992.

Miller RD: The U.S. Supreme Court looks at voluntariness and consent, *Int J of Law and Psychiatry* 17(3):239, 1994.

Monahan J, Hoge SK, Lidz C, Roth LH, Bennett N, Gardner W, Mulvey E: Coercion and commitment: understanding involuntary mental hospital admission, *Inter J of Law and Psychiatry* 18(3):249, 1995.

Parmet WE, Daynard RA, Gottlieb MA: The physician's role in helping smoke-sensitive patients to use the Americans with Disabilities Act to secure smoke-free workplaces and public spaces, *JAMA* 276(11):909, 1996.

Pettis RW: *Tarasoff* and the dangerous driver: a look at the driving cases, *Bull Am Acad Psychiatry Law* 20(4):427, 1992.

Petrila JP, Sadoff RL: Confidentiality and the family caregiver, *Hosp and Comm Psychiatry* 43(2):136, 1992.

Ravid R, Menon S: Guidelines for disclosure of patient information under the Americans with Disabilities Act, *Hosp and Comm Psychiatry* 44(3):280, 1993.

Rudegeair TJ, Appelbaum PS: On the duty to protect: an evolutionary perspective, *Bull Am Acad Psychiatry Law* 20(4):419, 1992.

Sanguineti VR, Samuel SE, Schwartz SL, Robeson MR: Retrospective study of 2,200 involuntary psychiatry admissions and readmissions, *Am J Psychiatry* 153(3):392, 1996.

Smith CA: Use of involuntary outpatient commitment in community care of the seriously and persistently mentally ill patient, *Issues in Mental Health Nursing* 16(3):275, 1995.

Swartz MS, Burns BJ, Hiday VA, George LK, Swanson J, Wagner HR: New directions in research on involuntary outpatient commitment, *Psychiatric Services* 46(4):381, 1995.

Tarasoff v Regents of the University of California, 118 Cal Rpt 129, 1974.

Tarasoff v Regents of the University of California, 17 Cal 3d 425, 1976.

Urrutiu G: Medication refusal, clinical picture, and outcome after use of administrative review, *Bull Am Acad Psychiatry Law* 22(4): 595, 1994.

Practice Problems 21

This chapter discusses potential problems that practitioners hope never to encounter but that may be unavoidable. Reviewed here are three of the most serious of these problems:

1. The practitioner misses important assessment information
2. The patient becomes physically threatening toward the practitioner
3. The patient is potentially dangerous to one's self or others.

These issues and specific problem-solving steps that can be taken immediately are presented here with the intent of helping practitioners to think through the problem quickly and respond effectively.

The Practitioner Misses Important Assessment Information

The practice of psychiatric primary care requires that practitioners strive to assess the patient's psychiatric symptoms, psychosocial problems, and personal and social coping resources; provide counseling, treatment, and referrals as needed; consult other practitioners and specialists as needed; and plan for follow-up. Along with these demanding expectations, practitioners may have additional concerns about their ability to recognize the importance of specific assessment information or to obtain patient assessment information that should not be overlooked (Lieberman, 1996)

If practitioners saw patients weekly for one-hour appointments, their concerns might decrease somewhat but would not disappear completely due to mental health assessment. In the absence of laboratory tests and high-technology scans, patient assessment information in psychiatric primary care practice is the product of the patient interview. Practitioners must rely in part on the information that patients choose to disclose. In addition, even if it were possible to assess every psychosocial characteristic of the individual's life, important aspects of this information would be outdated within 24 hours. The essential building blocks of the patient assessment are the patient's thoughts, feelings, and behaviors, each of which is dynamic, undergoing constant changes in content, process, and meaning.

Therefore, rather than trying to generate large amounts of assessment information, it is more effective to establish a level of assessment that supports the effective practice of psychiatric primary care, given the practice setting and patient population, and to consistently maintain that level with each patient. This standardized approach reduces the risk of missing basic assessment information or overemphasizing the individual's interpersonal style. The difficulty of recognizing and obtaining important assessment information is, in large part, a matter of experience, but specific assessment questions can be used to decrease the probability of missing important assessment information.

Take, for example, a man who describes his recent experience of fatigue as a symptom of depression and offers a great deal of specific and useful information. The practitioner completes a depression assessment and finds that the man's symptoms are consistent with a diagnosis of major depression. The practitioner also realizes that major depression affects all areas of psychosocial functioning and therefore continues to assess the effects that the depression has had on the man's life by asking more questions about functioning. Any diagnosis or problem that affect the individual's ability to function is important information and should not be overlooked. If the same man makes a casual remark during the assessment such as, "I would rather be dead than feel like this," and because of his casual manner the practitioner does not ask him about this statement, the practitioner is in the position of overlooking potentially important assessment information. Most casual remarks by patients are exactly what they appear to be, but if a patient makes a statement that does not fit in with the rest of the assessment or with the individual's general presentation, or if it appears to suggest a totally different view of the patient, that information should be evaluated as potentially important.

As with physical health conditions, it is helpful to ask patients to describe unusual experiences, such as out-of-the-ordinary thoughts, feelings, and behaviors. This open-ended questioning can take a little more time, but it can be effective when there is an increased risk of failing to recognize important information. Important information may not be recognized or obtained if the patient is highly focused on one or two concerns to the exclusion of all other concerns that are presented by the practitioner. Therefore, the following short list of assessment questions should always be considered: (1) Has the patient experienced significant changes or alterations in mental status? (2) What substances does the patient use? (3) Is the patient involved in important interpersonal conflicts that are aggressive or that involve hitting of any kind? (4) Is there any indication that the patient has been, currently is, or potentially is impulsive?

Changes in mental status, from psychosis to impaired concentration, should be noted as potential symptoms of severe mental illness (SMI) but they can also reveal potential problems that might not have otherwise been considered. All patients should be asked about their substance use, all substance use should be discussed, and all such information should be viewed as important. Individuals who are involved in aggressive or violent interpersonal conflicts should be assessed for counseling and referral needs that could lead to conflict resolution, and additional diagnostic assessment should be considered to ascertain if the conflict is related to a mental disorder. Impulsivity is always important assessment information, but it is particularly important as a risk of dangerous behavior or as a symptom related to substance abuse or personality disorder.

If despite these measures the practitioner becomes concerned that important information was not recognized or obtained, the practitioner should telephone the patient and, if necessary, arrange to complete the assessment. In cases in which some element of the assessment takes on new meaning and importance some time after the patient appointment, the same immediate response of telephoning the patient is recommended. If the individual can be reached by phone and is willing to complete the assessment, this approach is effective. When this is not the case and additional assessment is not possible, the practitioner can document the assessment areas of concern and the measures that have been taken to address that concern. Individuals who are intent on misleading the practitioner or who give information in an ambiguous way may cause concern about the possibility of missing information, but reassessment is not likely to solve the problem.

Who can help?It is almost a given that a patient will present a slightly different profile to different practitioners. When missing assessment information is a concern, it may be helpful to have the patient speak to another practitioner. When this option is not practical and the patient is available and cooperative, a friend or family member may be able to assist with the assessment.

The Patient Becomes Physically Threatening Toward the Practitioner

One of the last experiences that practitioners expect to have is to be physically threatened by a patient. Whether the threat is personal or professional, implicit or explicit, planned or impulsive, to be threatened by a patient violates the unspoken agreement of goodwill between practitioner and patient (Cembrowicz and Ritter, 1994; Whittington, Shuttleworth, and Hill, 1996). Along with this rather intellectual response to a physical threat by a patient, practitioners may also have a strong emotional response, with the moral indignation that comes from being made aware of one's vulnerability. Practitioners today may be more likely to have the experience of being threatened by a patient because society as a whole is more aggressive than it used to be.

Individuals who are delusional, paranoid, or antisocial can have a dramatically threatening presentation without becoming an actual physical threat to the practitioner. They may sit silently and stare at the practitioner as though searching for the right moment to attack. They may have a confrontive manner or an aggressive street style that is physically threatening, and practitioners may find it difficult to distinguish the patient's style from substance. Patients may also adopt a physically threatening stance toward a practitioner because they feel threatened by the practitioner. The individual may, for example, expect an experience of discrimination and act aggressively in anticipation of being treated poorly. Individuals who are fearful of receiving a diagnosis of serious illness may develop acute anticipatory anxiety that is expressed as hostility until they learn their actual diagnosis. The individual who is confused or intoxicated can strike out unpredictably.

These types of situations are not difficult for practitioners to recognize or handle effectively; the more serious problem is the patient who launches a verbal or physical assault without warning. The patient may even have a weapon or may turn one of several suitable items in the treatment room into a weapon. In this situation, practitioners have to deal immediately with three distinct elements of the physically threatening patient: the patient, the threat, and the practitioner's response to both (Cembrowicz and Ritter, 1994). ***The only unacceptable practitioner response to a physically threatening patient is no response.*** Aside from this rule, most practitioners can immediately execute an effective plan of action before a physical assault occurs. By focusing on the three elements, practitioners may be better able to assess which element of the physical threat is most important. If the patient has a weapon or is employing an object as a weapon, the practitioner should immediately move to safety.

Experienced health care providers plan in advance how they could leave a patient care area should the patient become physically threatening, and they ensure that their access to this exit is not blocked. Primary care settings should have a policy for ensuring the safety of staff that includes a system for verbally calling for help and for notifying security staff or the police. These policies should include a planned response to a patient who carries out an assault or who holds a practitioner hostage. This may sound like high drama and appear improbable, but with a physically threatening patient such measures are common sense.

If a patient who has become physically threatening does not have a weapon, the practitioner should immediately focus on the three elements noted above. Is the patient impaired (e.g., intoxicated) in any-way? What is the nature of the threat? Is the patient talking or silent? Is the patient responsive to the practitioner or unaware of what is said to him or her? Is the first response of the threatened practitioner a perception of immediate danger?

If the patient is not impaired, is still talking (albeit in a threatening way), and continues to be responsive, practitioners may consider an immediate limit-setting response to try to defuse the situation. There can be no "wiggle room" in this limit setting: the patient must stop all threats immediately. Practitioners should not negotiate this limit or allow continued threats. The patient's first threat marks the end of the health care visit, and the practitioner should take the position that he or she is now assessing whether the appointment remains ended. Should the patient appear to be manipulative, such as laughing and insisting that no harm was done or intended, the practitioner who decides to continue should have a second practitioner in the room for the remainder of the appointment.

Individuals who become frightened in a small treatment room may engage in threatening talk, but few practitioners feel threatened in this situation. This is perhaps the only situation in which it may be reasonable to say or do something that might reassure the patient or make the appointment less stressful for the patient. Practitioners should not second-guess their first response to a physically threatening patient. Instinct is not perfect, but it should not be ignored. If the practitioner's gut response is that the situation is out of control, there must be objective evidence to the contrary before this response can be invalidated. No one wants to overreact and end up feeling foolish, but health care professionals can learn to live with such feelings.

What can be done? If no assault has occurred and the threatening patient is responsive, not impaired, and not acting manipulative, the practitioner should prepare to exit the area and then offer the patient the opportunity to stop all threats. If the patient continues to threaten, the practitioner should leave the area, maintain eye contact with it, and call for assistance according to the practice protocol. If the patient stops threatening and agrees to continue with two practitioners rather than one, the appointment can be completed, but others practitioners in the area should be notified of the potential problem. An assessment of the risk of dangerous behavior to oneself or others should be made.

Who can help? Just about anyone can join the practitioner who decides to continue or who evaluates the threatening patient as potentially dangerous to oneself or others. An emergency request for mental health services should be made if there is reason to believe that the patient's conduct is related to SMI or substance abuse. Practitioners should be prepared to notify police or request their assistance.

The Patient is Potentially Dangerous to Oneself or Others

A delusional woman points to tiny red pin marks on the arms of her infant daughter and says that they are the mark of Satan and the child must be saved. A middle-age man about to be released from a prison halfway house complains of headaches, then rages about his much younger wife, who has filed for divorce and is living with another man. A high school senior asking for antidepressant medication discloses a history of attempted suicide. A college freshman, complaining of severe gastric upset, describes binge drinking beer for the last three months and almost hitting an oncoming car when driving home last Saturday night.

All these individuals are potentially dangerous to themselves or others. The mother could harm her infant. The husband could act out his rage toward his wife. The adolescent could once again attempt suicide. The college student could cause a fatal motor vehicle accident. In each case, in assessing the mental disorder or psychosocial problem, determination of the immediate risk of potentially dangerous behavior is most important.

Practitioners should act to protect patients and others from the immediate risk of potentially dangerous patient behaviors. A wide range of county and state services are available to help practitioners meet this obligation, but each practice setting should have well-defined protocols. In cases where there is a potential for dangerous behavior but there is no evidence of immediate risk, where the patient shows concern or insight into the problem behavior and appears to be open to making positive changes, an immediate referral to specialized care may be appropriate. If there will be a delay of more than 48 hours before the patient can see a specialist, temporary arrangements should be made.

Although the actual steps required to protect the patients and the public are relatively clear-cut, for some practitioners the severe ramifications of potentially dangerous patient behavior can create nagging self-doubts. Practitioners may find themselves struggling with the endless implications of failing to act on their assessment of immediate risk but being greatly concerned about unnecessary safety measures. Potentially dangerous behavior toward oneself or others are two of the three criteria for involuntary psychiatric treatment. But unlike the third criteria, being gravely disabled, the assessment of risk of potentially dangerous behavior can require a great deal of clinical judgment. Small variations in the patient's disclosed thoughts, feelings, and behaviors can significantly alter the findings of the assessment.

Using the risk-assessment criteria of access, means, motivation, and controls, what is the immediate risk of dangerous behavior in the examples presented? ***Access*** refers to the individual's ability to get hold of the ***means*** of injury and or the potential target. In the examples presented, the mother has ample means of injury and unlimited access to her infant. Her ***motivation***, fearful delusions, are powerful and not easily subject to change. ***Controls*** refer to internal and external influences on the individual's behavior. In this example, there are very few internal or external controls over the mother's actions. Based on these assessments, the immediate risk of harm to the infant is considered to be high. However, if there is evidence of additional injuries (old or new) to the infant, if the mother appears to be psychotic, if there is evidence of acute substance abuse, or if the mother has harmed other children in the past, the immediate risk in this case would be severe.

But say that the mother is aware of and alarmed by her delusional thoughts, that her infant is well cared for, that there is no evidence of a history of child abuse or neglect, and that the pin marks are uncomplicated, very superficial, and recent. Immediate specialized care and social services for the mother and the infant might significantly lower both the immediate and the long-term risk of harm to the infant. This example also demonstrates the psychological impact of dealing with potentially dangerous patient behaviors. The practitioner may find his or her thoughts persistently returning to images of this helpless infant and the possible harm the infant might suffer. As disturbing as these images may be, they cannot take the place of accurate assessment as the basis for intervention.

The other three examples are more typical of the ambiguity that can make an assessment of danger difficult. Living in a prison halfway house and being angry at his wife does not make the husband an immediate risk of potentially dangerous behavior toward his wife. Just as a history of attempted suicide or disclosed reckless driving are not in themselves predictive risk factors. The same criteria of access, means, motivation, and controls should be applied, but in all cases easy access to the means of dangerous behavior or to a vulnerable target is included as a risk factor.

The most deadly means of dangerous behavior is always assumed to be firearms, but every household has suitable alternatives: knives, automobiles, over-the-counter medications, matches, and household products. The presence of a clear motivation for dangerous behavior should be considered, but dangerous behavior can be motivated by numerous factors (e.g., love, hate). The most common is motivation based on anticipated results of the behavior, especially when the anticipated result is the satisfactory solution to a problem the individual has not been able to resolve.

For example, the prior suicide attempt of the high school senior was an aspirin overdose following an argument with a peer. The student vomited immediately and never told anyone about the overdose. Two weeks later the student became depressed and disclosed the aspirin overdose to a trusted teacher at school, who subsequently arranged for the student to see a practitioner for assessment of depression. In this case the high school senior has adequate access and means, uncertain motivation, and external controls. But what if the student's motivation was to escape the pain of a lost peer relationship, and, by refusing to attend school or speak to family members, the student is not subject to external controls? Under these circumstances the risk might be higher.

The college student also has full access to the means of his or her dangerous behavior (alcohol and an automobile), and binge drinking requires little motivation. But the risk would be low if, for example, having seen the same self destructive behavior in family members, the student is willing to do whatever is necessary to prevent following the same path and agrees to give his or her car keys to a responsible person until entering a substance abuse treatment program.

Each example of potentially dangerous behavior can and should be assessed based on clinical criteria rather than practitioner alarm, but few practitioners will encounter such cases without being emotionally impacted by them.

Finally, potentially dangerous behaviors must be assessed in terms of immediate risk, which in most practice settings is defined as the next 24 to 72 hours. For example, what is the risk that the high school senior will attempt suicide in the next 48 hours? By defining the risk period, the assessment of risk becomes more meaningful, and the indicators for necessary intervention to protect the individual or the public are brought into focus. The high school senior may struggle with suicidal thoughts and feelings for the remainder of this development period, but the immediate risk, and thus the need for protection from oneself, can be said to be low.

Whether an individual is assessed to be at low, high, or severe risk for dangerous behavior, human behavior is unpredictable, and events and circumstances can change an individual's immediate risk with little or no warning.

What can be done? Accurate assessment of risk and, when indicated by the assessment, action to protect the patient or the public. When the assessment indicates potential dangerous behavior but not immediate risk, internal or external controls can be developed to help the individual remain in control of his or her behavior. Evaluation by a specialist is a recommended policy for individuals with high or severe risk of dangerous behavior.

Who can help? Most health professionals can offer an immediate second opinion on the assessment of risk of dangerous behavior. In all cases practitioners should be able to employ procedures for involuntary admission to a hospital should this be necessary. Practitioners should also know how to access immediate child-protection services, crisis services, and acute substance abuse treatment.

References

Cembrowicz S, Ritter S: Attacks on doctors and nurses. In Shepherd J (editor): *Violence in Health Care a practical guide to coping with violence and caring for victims*, New York, 1994, Oxford University Press.

Lieberman JA: Compliance issues in primary care, *J Clin Psychiatry* 57(suppl 7):76, 1996.

Whittington R, Shuttleworth S, Hill L: Violence to staff in a general hospital setting, *J Advanced Nursing* 24(2):326, 1996.

Clinical Examples 22

This chapter is a selected presentation of clinical examples. Each example contains the approximate amount of clinical information that might be available to practitioners and includes an assessment and management statement. The intention is to provide additional information about the some of the mental disorders described in this book. The examples are brief and are not intended to be used as treatment guidelines. Patients in each example are identified by age, marital status, and gender only. However, race, ethnicity, religion, culture, education, family, and income are also important personal characteristics that can significantly affect the experience and expression of mental disorder symptomatology.

Personal characteristics also interact in ways that greatly influence the nature of the stressors to which an individual is exposed and the coping skills upon which he or she has learned to rely, including the ability to cope with having a mental disorder. In actual clinical practice these characteristics are important patient information and are not excluded from the assessment or management process.

For space consideration purposes, the examples presented are intended to reflect important, defining characteristics of the mental disorder rather than to highlight potential or actual individual differences.

Paranoid Schizophrenia

A. is a 44-year-old single woman who is being seen for a large cut on her right leg that looks dirty and possibly infected. Although the wound looks painful, A. seemed to be uninterested or unaware of her injury. Her neighbor, a 28-year-old woman who lives in A.'s apartment building, brought A. in because she was concerned about A.'s leg injury and because A. seemed to be upset or scared. The friend states that A. lives alone and seems to have troubles now and then but had always appeared to be "basically okay." During the drive to the clinic she said A. seemed to be confused and once looked at her as though she were a total stranger.

The practitioner asks A. if her leg hurts, and A. smiles and stares at the practitioner but says nothing. Then she asks A. if she can touch her leg and get a better look at her cut. Again A. smiles, stares, and says nothing. As the practitioner moves to examine A.'s leg, she asks if A. has ever had a cut like this before. At that moment A. claps her hands and screams "Bingo!" Then she beams at the practitioner, hugging her arms across her chest and rocking back and forth. The practitioner smiles at A. and repeats the word "bingo" with a puzzled look on her face.

At that point A. begins to talk. She informs the practitioner that by asking three questions in a row, the practitioner qualified for a bingo, which means A. can talk to her. A. tells the practitioner that she hurt her leg three days ago. While running outside she fell over something, but she is not sure what. She is pretty sure it was three days ago. Yes, her leg hurts a lot, all the time, but she is not suppose to say anything or she will have to fall again. In one breath, A. tells the practitioner that she is very happy to see her, the clinic is a very nice place, and her neighbor is a very nice person, but sometimes she changes into a person that A. has not met.

The practitioner then asks A. to tell her a little more about "bingo." A. says that actually it's not much fun, not as much fun as the other kind of bingo, anyhow. But the radio told her she was going to have a bingo today and that she should wait. A. explains that she can hear the radio playing pretty much all the time, but it has been playing really loud lately, and this makes it hard for her to think. At this point A. laughs and smiles and tells the practitioner that she is a nice person, the clinic is a nice place, and she thinks it is nice to have her leg fixed because it was awfully sore. A. then tells the practitioner, "You can call John, my social worker; he'll tell you."

Assessment and Management

According to the social worker, A. has been treated for paranoid schizophrenia for 10 years. When A. does not take antipsychotic medication she experiences auditory hallucinations that give her commands and frighten her. Her social worker usually takes A.

to the mental health center for intramuscular injections of antipsychotic medication every 2 weeks and psychotherapy appointments with a clinical specialist, but 3 days ago A. refused her medication and has been in hiding ever since. The social worker agreed to come to the clinic and take A. to the mental health center to receive antipsychotic medication and to be seen by her therapist. After bandaging her leg and informing A. that her social worker is on his way to the clinic, A. smiles at the practitioner and softly whispers "Bingo."

Bipolar Disorder

B. is a 25-year-old married man who has been treated for bipolar disorder for 1 year. B. is very dissatisfied with this diagnosis and wants to have a complete physical exam and treatment for hypertension. B. has made a complete study of hypertension on the Internet, and it is clear to him that this is his actual diagnosis. B. informs the practitioner that he does not have much time today, and so he needs to have his exam and treatment completed within the hour in order to attend an important meeting. The practitioner asks B. to talk about his Internet research. B. congratulates the practitioner, commenting that he is smarter then he looks, since obviously he can see that B. is a very intelligent and busy man.

B. explains to the practitioner that it took him a while to complete his research, but he did not mind because it was important work. He estimates that it took him 4 days to obtain what he is certain is the most accurate and current research on hypertension. B. states that the total value of his research is about 20 million dollars in federal funding, but he admits that he had to estimate this amount. The practitioner asks B. to talk about what he did during the 4 days he was doing his research. B. flies into a rage, informing the practitioner that he obviously spent the four days doing research, and that if this is too complicated for the practitioner to understand, he should say so in which case A. wants to see his supervisor, or someone who is more intelligent. The practitioner asks if B. has ever worked for 4 days and 4 nights in the past, and B. assures him that he has, and in fact he has worked for much longer periods of time.

At this point B. becomes impatient again and demands to see the practitioner's supervisor. The practitioner asks B. if his research had bothered anyone at home, and B. informs the practitioner that he is able to conduct research correctly and therefore did not bother anyone; besides, his wife was away visiting her parents and would be returning tomorrow, so he needs to have his hypertension taken care of now or else she will become worried and the practitioner could be liable for "causing my wife to have a mental illness," just like that other "so-called health professional" who told his wife that he has to take lithium. B. gladly gives the practitioner his therapist's name and instructs the practitioner to inform his therapist of his research findings.

Before calling B.'s therapist, the practitioner asks B. to talk a little more about his hypertension. B. informs the practitioner that he should know what hypertension is if he is going to work in a clinic, but that he will be happy to teach him about this condition. B. explains that when he has hypertension he feels a lot of pressure, and that when the pressure is really high it is important to keep busy and to do important work, but the work must be truly important. He says that sometimes he has a headache but most of the time he is able to handle a great deal of work exceptionally well—an experience, B. states, the practitioner has probably never had. B. states he stopped taking lithium 2 weeks ago since, this medication is a "leading cause" of hypertension.

Assessment and Management

According to B.'s therapist, B. was diagnosed with bipolar disorder after a severe episode of mania, but neither he nor his wife have been able to accept his diagnosis. B.'s current symptoms of irritability, rapid speech, grandiose thinking, insomnia, and feelings of pressure are symptoms of hypomania. B. agrees to have his lithium plasma level checked and reluctantly agrees to speak with his therapist on the phone. The practitioner arranges with B. to have his older brother come to the clinic and take B. to see his therapist. In speaking to B.'s brother, the practitioner learns that B. has been very worried about an ongoing conflict between himself and his wife. B. seems to feel that if he had a different diagnosis, there would be less conflict with his wife.

Antisocial Personality Disorder

C. is a 50-year-old single man who has recently been diagnosed with noninsulin-dependent diabetes. His diabetes can be managed with diet, exercise, and weight loss, but although he has worked with a practitioner for 2 months, he still has not made important changes in his life-style and has not brought his diabetic symptoms under control. C. has a significant family history of diabetes. He knows that his father was diagnosed with the condition, but C. has very little information beyond this because his father died in prison when C. was 19 years old. C. describes his father as "a mean old man that was always in trouble."

C. had been employed as a shop manager in a paint factory but lost his job 1 month ago. He talks about having been the "boss man" at work and that all of the employees in his department "knew what would happen if they crossed me." He says no one ever crossed him twice; he always made sure of that. C. was fired last month after he chased, then physically assaulted, an employee in his shop. The employee found out that C. had been stealing cases of paint and selling the stolen paint around town from the back of his truck. The employee threatened to report C. for stealing, and C. immediately hit him. The man ran, but C. chased him and continue to assault him. C. is satisfied with this behavior and is pleased with the fact that, although he was fired, he was not reported for stealing paint.

After reviewing C.'s diet and exercise goals with him, the practitioner tries to engage C. in a discussion of his life-style and the changes he should make to protect his health. C. listens to the diet and exercise recommendations—limiting his intake of fast-food meals to one a week and walking 45 minutes everyday—but he makes it clear that he is not interested. In response to C.'s show of uninterest, the practitioner invites C. to talk about his goals and the changes that he would like to make. C.'s response is "Now that you've wasted 10 minutes of my time I'll be glad to tell you what you need to know." He shows her a large stack of forms and explains to her that she must sign the forms so that he can get a disability paycheck.

The practitioner asks C. to say more about his plan, since she is not certain what he has in mind. He explains that this is how the system works: you either get them or they get you. C. says he knows how this whole thing works and all the practitioner has to do is sign the forms and he'll take care of the rest. The practitioner explains to C. that what he is proposing is fraud, and she will be happy to work with him in learning to manage his diabetes, but she cannot sign the forms. C. immediately becomes enraged and tells the practitioner that he is going to get her for malpractice. The practitioner does not respond to this statement. C. then stands up and informs the practitioner that she has crossed him, and "she knows what that means for her." Then he says that if she won't sign, he knows a guy who will, and he walks out of the treatment room laughing.

Assessment and Management

C. does not submit to rules of any kind. In his mind he makes the rules, and everybody follows his rules or else. He is pleased with his ability to get what he wants and has no interest or concern in how he affects other people. What is most important to him is that at all times and in all situations he is the victor. C. tries to manipulate others in order to get them to do what he wants; when this does not work he uses threats of violence or actual violence. He seems to have some insight into his father as a man who was "mean" and a "troublemaker," but he has no insight into his own antisocial characteristics. His plan to demand the practitioner's cooperation in his efforts to obtain disability income for noninsulin-dependent diabetes was acceptable to him, so he sees no need to try to disguise his request by claiming to be more ill than he actually is. He threatens the practitioner just before leaving, but this seems perfunctory. He thinks he has alternatives and sees no reason to waste his time with someone for whom he has no use.

Major Depression I

D. is a 30-year-old single woman who is concerned that she may be anemic or "something," and is seeking "lab tests" to find out what is wrong with her. She states that she is always tired, but no matter how tired she feels she is unable to sleep more than 2 to 3 hours at a time. She wakes up at least once during the night and seems to always be awake hours before her alarm rings. D. moved to the city 4 months ago to attend graduate school at the university and states that she is just barely able to keep up with the course reading assignments. She is starting to worry about her grades, but when she tries to study she has a really hard time keeping her mind on her work.

When asked, she tells the practitioner that when she was little her mother and grandmother used to complain about being tired all the time. The practitioner asks D. if she has had any major changes in important relationships or if anything has happened recently that has been more upsetting than usual. D. explains that before applying to graduate school she had been dating a man that she cared for deeply and, although she had never spoken to him about it, she states that "I kind of thought we might get married." The relationship ended when D. realized that her boyfriend liked her and they had fun together, but "that was about it." She wrote to him a few times since starting graduate school, but he has never written to her or called her.

The practitioner asks D. to talk a little more about how she has been feeling over the last 2 weeks. Her response is that she feels "half dead," then she attempts a little smile and says, "I seem to be doing a lot of things halfway now." D. states that she thinks she would feel better if she could lose some weight and maybe go out on the weekend instead of sitting alone in her apartment, but she is unable to get herself to do the things she would like to do, such as study or read a novel that she started 1 month ago. When asked if she has had any changes in her weight she replies no. When asked if anyone has commented on her appearance or weight, she says her advisor asked her if she had lost weight.

At this point the practitioner asks D. what she feels is happening to her and D. replies, "I guess I got a little depressed, I was so mad at my boyfriend, and now I just feel drained." D. has not found new friends or places to go that are relaxing for her. She feels out of place at the university and has started to seriously question her decision to go to graduate school. Her family assumes that she is doing well unless they hear differently from her. When asked how she normally handles difficult times in her life, she states that she always feels better after talking to her older sister, but she admits that she has not talked to her sister recently. D. states that her sister is very proud of her and wants to drive into the city to visit, but D. told her sister that she would not be much fun right now.

Assessment and Management

D. realizes that she has been very depressed for some time and has been falling behind in school and isolating herself. She also realizes that her anger and disappointment over her relationship with her boyfriend has been overwhelming for her, but she did not use her normal coping method of talking with her sister. She seems to have a family history of depression, with her mother and possibly grandmother having had recurrent untreated depression. D.'s symptoms can be relieved with a selective serotonin reuptake inhibitor (SSRI) antidepressant, and the practitioner helps D. to make the decision to allow her sister to visit and to speak to her advisor to make some arrangements to protect her academic standing.

Major Depression II

E. is a 40 year-old-married man who has been having severe headaches nearly every day for more than 2 weeks. On the advice of a co-worker, he is requesting a CAT scan to find out what is wrong with him. The practitioner asks E. to talk about his headaches; in particular, when the headaches first started, when do they usually occur, what makes them worse, and what makes them better. E. states that he has never had headaches like this before. "The headaches just started, and once they start they just keep 'eating at me'." Nothing makes them better. I've taken every single one of those pills they advertise on TV and not a single one of them saved me, and after your head has been pounding for hours you just get sick of it. I try not to think about it, since I just seem to feel worse when I do, like right now. So if you don't mind, let's get on with the CAT scan."

The practitioner assures E. that he will have whatever "tests" are necessary, but he would like to find out a little bit more about how things have been going for E. and about events in his life over the last 2 to 4 weeks. E. responds that nothing bad has happened "if that's what you're getting at. Do you think I have some kind of mental problem?" The practitioner's response is,

"What kind of mental problem would that be?" E. stands up and moves toward the door to leave and the practitioner states, "I think there is something on your mind, and since I really would like to help you I have to ask you questions. For example, what did you mean when you said nothing "saved" you?" E. says to the practitioner, "I know what your thinking; you think this is about my wife's breast biopsy." Exactly 3 weeks ago E.'s wife had a positive mammograph finding, followed by a needle biopsy that was negative. E. and his wife have been married for 2 years, and this is his first marriage. E. admits that his headaches started a few days after he and his wife got her biopsy results. They were both relieved that she did not have cancer, but they never sat down and talked about their anxiety or relief; they just returned to their normal daily routines.

The practitioner says to E. that it seems he had been badly shaken by his wife's "test" for cancer.

E. says nothing in response to the practitioner's observation.

At this point the practitioner invites E. to talk a little more about his headaches and any other bothersome "aches" that he may have. After thinking about it a minute or two, E. says that sometimes he doesn't feel hungry, and mostly all he wants to do is sleep. The practitioner asks if he is having any problems being around people, at work for example. E. says that everything at work is fine, or at least it would be if people would do their job and leave him alone. Some of his co-workers were complaining about him to his supervisor, and E. says that when his supervisor spoke to him he told her that everything would be okay if people would just mind their own business. At this point the practitioner asks E. if he thinks that all of the stress in his life recently might have affected him, since he has not really been able to talk about his feelings. E.'s response is "I guess that's possible."

Assessment and Management

E.'s primary depression symptoms are negative thinking, irritable mood, hypersomnia, withdrawal, and headaches. Although he has supportive people around him, he seems to be too on-edge to interact with anyone in a meaningful way or to express his needs directly. He is clearly very upset about his wife's "tests" and seems to have been alarmed both by the possibility of his wife being diagnosed with cancer as well as with the idea of cancer. This experience seems to have caused him to become preoccupied with his health and his wife's health. Like many people, E. experiences psychological distress as somatic symptoms, which in this case added to his distress. Antidepressant medication can relieve his irritable sadness and the negative changes in his social functioning, sleep, and appetite. It will be important for E. and his wife to talk about their feelings and provide each other with needed emotional support, so the practitioner refers E. to a specialist for couples therapy.

Major Depression III

F. is a 15-year-old girl who currently lives with her grandmother. F. does not know where her father is. Her mother has a long history of substance abuse and unemployment, and her 14 year-old-sister is pregnant. Because F. has skipped nearly every day of school this term, she has just learned that she will have to repeat this school year. Last month F.'s mother sent her to live with her grandmother because, according to F., her mother says she is "trouble looking for a place to happen." E. is seeing a practitioner because she wants to start taking "shots for birth control," adding, "I don't want to end up like my sister." The practitioner assures F. that she will be happy to help her, and that she is interested in hearing more about some of the things with which F. is trying to cope right now.

F. says she is doing fine right now; it's just that her mother "gets on my nerves, so I get mad." She says that when she gets mad she does things she shouldn't, like shoplifting and getting drunk or high. She got into a fist fight at school with a boy who was making fun of her, and she got suspended but "nothing happened to him, and he started it." F. says she doesn't know why she got into a fist fight, just that sometimes she feels like fighting. She describes things at home as "the same" and that it is not a big deal being sent to live with her grandmother. "She tries to tell me what to do and I just ignore her. One time she was yelling at me, and I got mad and threw a full can of soda at the wall, and it went everywhere. Grandma just ran to her room. She didn't do anything; what can she do? Nobody can make me do anything. I do whatever I feel like doing."

The practitioner asks F. what she feels like doing. F.'s response is "That's just it, I never know how I'm going to feel. Sometimes I cry for hours, listen to music, and smoke cigarettes. Then I usually go somewhere and get high. Sometimes I get mad and yell at people and throw things, and then everybody gets all upset and everything, but I don't care...I mean, I care, but most of the time I don't care."

The practitioner then asks her what she thinks about most of the time. F. says she thinks about her mom. F.'s plan is to stay out all night this weekend, and this will make her grandmother "nuts," and "then she'll send me home to my mom."

The practitioner asks her what she'll do all night, and F. says "I know some guys that will let me hang out with them. They like to party."

The practitioner asks F. to describe the single most important thing she is worried about right now. F. thinks about this for a little while and asks if it has to be just one thing. When informed that it does she says, "I'm not sure, maybe school—maybe my sister and her baby. I don't know. Nobody just has *one* problem to worry about; at least I don't. I can't say one problem; that's a dumb question. So are you going to give me a birth control shot?"

The practitioner explains to F. that she has to have a negative pregnancy test and then take the medication after she starts her menstrual period. F. seems surprised to hear of the delay and is not happy about it, asking, "What am I supposed to do in the meantime?" F. refuses to discuss her sexual activities or the possibility that she is pregnant.

Assessment and Management

F. is sad, angry, and bewildered by the chaos that seems to define her young life. She does not have a stable adult in her life; she has an established pattern of acting out when she feels emotionally distressed, a pattern which includes substance abuse and possibly high-risk sexual activity. She may feel abandoned by her mother, and she uses negative behavior to try to gain support from her. At the same time (as is often true with adolescents), she may believe that she can and should rescue her mother from drugs and alcohol.

Although F. is somewhat ambivalent about trusting the practitioner, the practitioner represents a potentially reliable adult resource for F., and if a relationship can be established, it may then be possible to make additional referrals for F., such as an adolescent girls' support group. To avoid putting F. into the position where she might on impulse reject an offer of support, the practitioner avoids offering F. too much too soon.

Acute Stress Disorder

G. is a 28-year-old woman with a large superficial burn that covers most of the surface of her right arm. A week ago she came home from work to find her neighbors' house on fire. The neighbors are a couple in their late 60s. G. called the fire department and then went to see if her neighbors were in the house. G. apparently tried to open the back door because she thought the fire had not reached this part of the house, but when she opened the door the intense heat of the fire on her arm caused her to move away from the house. Just as she turned away she thought she saw the neighbor's cat on the floor, not moving. She later learned that the neighbors were okay and had not been home, but that their cat died in the fire.

G. describes these events each time she comes in to have her burns assessed and cleaned. She seems to be numb and dazed by the experience and is unable to talk about it. She says she has mental images all the time of "the little cat" lying on the floor and can't seem to make them go away. She has not been able to sleep through the night since the fire and has not gone to work for three days. She states that she doesn't really remember the fire, calling the fire department, or returning home. All she can "recall" is the cat lying on the floor. She tells the practitioner that sometimes she thinks none of these things really happened, but she knows that the fire occurred because she can see her neighbors' house, but sometimes she is not certain she saw the cat.

Assessment and Management

The practitioner consults with the psychiatric specialist in the clinic, and the specialist confirms that G. has the following symptoms of acute stress disorder: feeling nothing or numb, a persistent daze or mild state of confusion, and recurring thoughts that are very upsetting to her. At times she is not certain if she actually went to the house or saw the cat, despite the burns on her right arm. She has not been able to sleep through the night and has not left her house except to come in for clinic appointments. The specialist recommends 3 days of lorazepam 1 mg TID to relieve G.'s acute symptoms, and immediate crisis therapy with the goal of helping G. to return to work and to discharge the intense fear reaction she experienced when she opened the door to the neighbors' house, saw the fire, and felt the pain in her arm when she was burned. The specialist has hypothesized that the image of the cat is a psychological defense for G. against the more frightening experience of the fire itself and of her arm being burned.

Suicide I

H. is a 33-year-old man who has been employed for 3 years as a computer programmer. He is being seen for severe cold and flu symptoms, including a high temperature, vomiting, and mild dehydration. The practitioner observes that H. looks very tired and underweight, and he is wearing summer clothing although it is the middle of winter and very cold outside. H. seems to be uninterested in his symptoms and states that he only came to the clinic because he promised his younger sister that he would. The practitioner attempts to engage H. in ordinary conversation but is unable to do so. He suspects that H. may be suffering from severe depression.

A brief symptom assessment confirms that H. has recently lost about 12 lbs. H. has not slept through the night for over a week, and he is not sure when he last ate a prepared meal. He says that if he feels hungry he has a bowl of cereal or microwaves some frozen burritos. He admits to having a great deal of trouble concentrating at work and has made a few "major mistakes," one of which shut down the computer network system at his company for almost an hour. H. then volunteers some information about himself when he states, "You're right, I feel kind of down, but mostly I guess I'm angry." The practitioner makes a neutral response to this statement, saying, "I would like to understand."

H. instantly flares into a rage and seems ready to lash out, but just as suddenly his shoulders drop and he looks like a person who has been totally defeated. His eyes become red and fill with tears, but he never actually cries. He sits silently, staring at the floor.

The practitioner allows H. to sit silently because it seems as though he is using the time to regain his composure, and the practitioner is aware that H. will not continue until he is ready to do so. H. does look up again a few minutes later. At that time the practitioner again tells H. that he wants to understand, and then adds that he is willing to help. H. states, "Well, if you must know, I was supposed to get married, but 4 days before the wedding she decides she doesn't want to marry me because I'm too serious. She said I'm not much fun to be with."

The practitioner asks when and how H. found out about his fiancée's decision. H. says her father called him, told him her decision was final, and said that he expects H. to respect his daughter's decision. H. replied that he wanted to talk to her and hear her decision from her. His fiancée's father then informed H. that his daughter and her mother were out of town for a while, that H. heard her decision from him, and that that was the way it was going to be.

The practitioner then asks H. to describe his actions after hanging up the phone. H. says he got mad and threw things around for a while. Then he drank a bottle of vodka; "I cried for a couple of hours, got tired of doing that, then I took a couple of handfuls of pills." H. says he thinks the pills were over-the-counter (OTC) sleeping pills and some other pills. He vomited almost immediately, passed out, and woke up the next day sick as a dog, vomited some more, and has been sick ever since. He didn't go to work and did not tell anyone about his overdose. His sister came by, and he told her about the wedding being called off; "she got all worried" and tried to take him to a counselor. She wouldn't leave until he promised to get some help. H. did not tell his sister about his overdose, "but she keeps calling; she knows I'm totally confused by all this."

Assessment and Management

H. has experienced the painful and confusing loss of an important relationship, and the phone conversation with his ex-fiancée's father was humiliating to him. He has significant mood changes (sadness and anger), weight, sleep, and cognitive symptoms of depression. He is unable to function at work or talk to his sister, a person to whom he has always been close. His abuse of alcohol combined with his depression symptoms make him a high risk for more impulsive self-harm behaviors. The fact that he told no one about his overdose and would not have been observed if the overdose had been lethal are also important risk factors. Finally, there is a significant risk of H. being retraumatized when he learns more about his ex-fiancée's reason for calling off the marriage, or if he is able to speak to her.

The practitioner informs H. that his situation is serious, that he will need help if he is going to deal with his depression and his loss, and that help must start now. H. agrees but says he will "get help" only because of his job and "not because of her." Per clinic policy, the practitioner refers H. to a psychiatric specialist for crisis therapy and evaluation for possible voluntary hospitalization. The practitioner obtains H.'s permission to call his sister and have her come to the clinic immediately and to go to the crisis clinic with him. The practitioner confirms the sister's arrival and confirms that H. is seen by the specialist.

Suicide II

I. is a 14-year-old girl who was brought into the emergency department after telling a teacher at her school that she took a full bottle of acetaminophen while at school after having a "stupid fight" with her best friend. The teacher states that the school tried to notify I.'s mother but she was out of town.

I. is very pretty and clearly puts a great deal of time into her appearance. She is very outgoing and friendly and seems to be very comfortable in the emergency department. Her acetaminophen level is high enough that she will be hospitalized for 72 hours or until her level has dropped. In starting an IV in I.'s left arm, the practitioner observes several thick scars across I.'s left wrist. After the IV is started the practitioner sits down with I. and asks the young girl about the scars.

I. assumes a matter-of-fact attitude and informs the practitioner that the scars are from cutting her arm with a razor blade last year on New Year's Day. I. says she was in the hospital for 3 days then, too. The practitioner says to I., "You seem to understand what is going on here. Maybe you can help me, because I don't quite understand." I. pats the practitioner's hand and says "Oh that's okay, you don't have to worry about me, I'll be okay, but you're very nice to sit here and talk to me."

The practitioner then asks I. to tell her about the overdose she took today. I. responds, "Oh, I got mad and went into the store across the street from school and put a bottle of pills in my pocket and walked out, then I just started taking them. I took one every 10 minutes." The practitioner then asks I. to describe what she did after she had finished taking the bottle of pills. I. says, "I didn't do anything, I felt better then." The practitioner asks how I. got around to telling her teacher that she took the pills. She says, "I guess I must have looked funny or something, but she took me to the office, and the nurse asked me if I took anything, and I told her what I took, and then they brought me here."

At this moment I.'s father bursts into the treatment area demanding to speak to the person in charge. I. is clearly surprised to see her father, and her entire manner changes immediately. Her face turns into a mask that is impossible to read. Instead of the outgoing person she has just been, she now seems to be far away. Her father is removed from the treatment area and taken to speak with the practitioner in a separate interview room. When the practitioner returns to I., the young girl is anxious, with beads of sweat forming on her forehead. She asks if she is going to be able to stay in the hospital for 3 days and is informed that she is. This does not seem to relieve her. When asked about the change in her mood, she says, "He's never come to the hospital before."

The practitioner asks I. again about her overdose today, but this time she asks about the fight with her girlfriend. I. says it was about her father, but that is all she will say. Then I.'s father returns to the treatment area, demands to speak to I. alone, and about 2 minutes later, he leaves the hospital. When the practitioner returns this time, I. is crying without making a sound and will not say anything to the practitioner. No matter what the practitioner says to I. she will not respond. After making all of the arrangements for transfer to the inpatient unit, the practitioner is able to travel with I.. On the way to the unit, I. says to the practitioner, "You've been very nice to me, but don't ask me anything else. He thinks you might be able to make me tell."

Assessment and Management

I. seems to be fully aware of her behavior and has not acted on impulse, although she is clearly acting out. She has a history of recurrent self-harm or suicide attempts so although her immediate risk is low this behavior will recur. The cuts on her left arm appear to have been very deep, serious wounds, indicating that there are circumstances in which she is willing to do serious harm herself. I. seems relieved to be able to stay in the hospital for 3 days, which suggests that she may be trying to escape or avoid something, perhaps at home or at school. The change in her mood and behavior and her surprise when her father comes into the treatment room indicate that the argument I. had with her girlfriend this morning may have had something to do with her father. The practitioner is concerned that I. may be a target of physical or sexual abuse and makes a referral to a specialist to have I. evaluated before she leaves the hospital.

Substance Abuse I

J. is a 40-year-old married woman who moved to town a few weeks ago and wants to establish a relationship with a health care provider. She says she always makes sure that she finds a new practitioner when she moves to a new town because "you never know what will happen." During the routine physical exam the practitioner learns that J. has had several car accidents and last year fell forward onto cement steps, fracturing her arm in two places and breaking her nose. The practitioner asks her about these incidents, and J. states that she used to have a problem once in a while with alcohol, but she's finally had enough of that and has quit drinking, "this time for good." J. states that her husband is in a 90-day inpatient treatment center for alcoholism, but that his drinking was "way worse than mine, so he really needed to check himself into one of those places." According to J., her last drink was 3 weeks ago and "I never felt better in my life."

In completing the assessment of J.'s substance use, the practitioner learns that J. started abusing alcohol about 10 years ago.

Prior to that time she drank when she was out with friends but did not drink to the point of intoxication. She admits that, starting her senior year in high school and as a college student, she "partied" a lot. She states that both her parents are big wine drinkers, but they don't have a problem with it. She describes them as drinking a bottle of wine together every night, but it's with their meal and they "don't get into any trouble or anything." J. and her husband have been married for 9 years and he has had problems with alcohol "on and off" most of that time. J. met her husband when they were both in college.

J. admits that she used to drink a little in the morning "once in a while" and she has "quit" before, but this time is different. When asked how this time is different, she states that her husband will be different and that will make it different for her because she really only drank because he didn't like to drink alone. According to J., if her husband is not drinking, she won't drink. J. describes having had serious financial problems because of her and her husband's alcohol abuse. They have both lost jobs, had to pay expensive drunk driving traffic citations, and now their car insurance is extremely high.

J. and her husband moved to town to get a fresh start "because so many people were too nosy about my business, and they put your name in the paper if they say you're drunk, even when you can prove you're not drunk." J. admits that her employer asked her to resign; otherwise he would have to fire her. The main reason was that she had a lot of "colds" this past winter and had to call in sick. But when she went to work she did a good job, there were no problems, and she got along well with everyone. Her current job is going to be better because the people are easygoing and "you don't have to pretend like you're not sick when you are sick."

J. indicates that her husband will be coming home in a few days, and part of the reason that she came into the clinic was that she told him she would do so before he came home. J. says they forced her to go to a "big family meeting type of thing" and made her say she would see a practitioner. J. states, "I hope I still recognize him when he comes home. He talks different, he even looks different. But I'll be glad to see him; we always have a lot of laughs together."

Assessment and Management

J. has a history of alcohol abuse starting in high school. Her drinking increased acutely in college, but after graduation she was able to achieve a brief period of controlled drinking. At that time she married a man who had an alcohol abuse history that was similar to hers but who is now making a very serious effort to live sober. J.'s husband has been her drinking partner since they have been married, and as in her parent's relationship, a drinking couple tends to cover up each other's drinking. J. is clearly very threatened by the loss of her husband as a drinking partner and the loss of his drinking as a way of denying her own alcohol abuse. J. does not deny her past or recent alcohol abuse or the many psychosocial problems that have been caused by her alcohol abuse, but she denies her current abuse of alcohol.

If her husband comes home sober and intent on remaining so, J. will be facing an extremely difficult loss, with very few support resources. She will be alone in a new town with a new job and essentially a new husband, who may seem to be a total stranger to her. Under these circumstances she is much more likely to increase, rather than decrease, her alcohol consumption.

At this point, the practitioner's goal is to meet J.'s stated request, which is to have a "relationship" with a provider "just in case something happens." Despite her fragile denial, J.'s request suggests that she has some insight into her alcoholism and concern about her relationship with her husband. The practitioner tells J. that her request for a "relationship" with a provider is an excellent plan and that she will be happy to work with J. The practitioner schedules a series of appointments with J. and gives her an information brochure about the various available alcohol-related services. J.'s assignment is to read the material and come prepared to talk about the services and ask questions. Before J. will be able to make a serious effort toward alcohol treatment, she will have to build her motivation. The practitioner then recognizes J.'s current efforts to "quit" and defines quitting, for now, as no drinking and driving and no drinking at work.

Substance Abuse II

K. is a 31-year-old man who works in the kitchen of a large popular pizza restaurant. He does not have a car, so he travels by bus or gets rides with friends. He lives alone in a small room that he rents in a boarding house not too far from work. Although he doesn't like living in the boarding house, it is so inexpensive that he does not want to leave. K. has smoked marijuana every day since he was 14 years old. Currently he smokes 2 to 4 times a day in order to avoid withdrawal symptoms. If he has not been able to smoke within 1 to 2 hours after the day has started, he "feels lousy."

K. is seeking a prescription for antidepressant medication. He states that he has been worrying about a lot of things and this has made him feel depressed, so he has not shown up for work a few times this month. If he gets any more points at work he "technically" could be fired. He told his supervisor that he was going to the clinic today to get treatment for his depression, so the supervisor gave him time off. K. really likes the people with whom he works. He describes it as a "really laid-back place, and the people are pretty cool, and everyone gets along."

He knows he has a problem with marijuana because he can't go a day without smoking. Sometimes he drinks too much beer, but he says he can cut back on it a little. At some point, he says, he would like to stop smoking cigarettes, but he knows there is no point in trying that until he has stopped the "pot and beer." He says that he has taken antidepressants before, and "they really helped me; I cut way back on the pot and stopped drinking beer completely." He cannot remember the name of the medication he took.

K. is very vague about his depression. He says that the main thing he notices is that he has a bad attitude. He knows he could be doing more with his life, but he always seems to let things slide, saying, "There's lots of stuff I can do. There's no problem there; I'm good at a lot of things." When asked to describe his bad attitude, K. states that "maybe it's not a bad attitude so much as I get up in the morning, and I sit down at the table, and then that's as far as I get sometimes. When I do that I think about things too much." K. does not feel that he has any other symptoms of depression, but "this is bad enough." When asked, K. states that he spends most of his time alone. He watches a lot of sports on TV, especially basketball. K. used to play basketball in high school and with friends at work, but he is not sure if they are still playing. K. also requests that the practitioner give him something in writing about the fact that he will be taking medication for depression so that he can turn it in at work.

Assessment and Management

K. has a 17-year history of marijuana dependence, nicotine dependence, and alcohol abuse. His description of depression is consistent with the amotivational syndrome associated with marijuana dependence. K. works in a very popular and busy restaurant and it is difficult to imagine that work there would be "laid back" and easygoing. Just the opposite would make more sense, because in such a work environment, there will be a lot of pressure to get things done quickly and a lot of work to be done. K. is so specific about the written documentation that there is a possibility he may have more problems at work than he is willing to reveal. K. seems to be very isolated, with few relationships or activities other than drug and alcohol use.

There is also the potential of a serious developmental crisis: K.'s life-style may be very different from that of his same-age friends, or he may not be living the life he thought he would have when he reached his 30s. K. clearly would benefit from counseling and treatment for substance abuse. It is difficult to determine at this point, but he appears to have a substance related mood disorder. However, although K. does not deny his substance use behavior, he seems to use his substance abuse to rationalize his substance abuse—that is he can't quit one drug until he quits the other, and so forth.

The practitioner offers to schedule a series of brief appointments with K. to fully evaluate his treatment needs, with the knowledge that if K. is only seeking a prescription that he can present to his work supervisor, he may not return to the clinic.

Substance Abuse III

L. is a 48-year-old man who drinks a 12-pack of beer every night starting at sundown. He works as a grounds keeper for the city and has had this job for 15 years. Currently L. does not have his own apartment. He alternates between living with his parents, his ex-wife and their two children, and a male friend who drives a bus for the city. L. has never been arrested or charged with driving under the influence (DUI), and he has never been in trouble at work. L. does not become intoxicated when he drinks, and rarely does he ever drink more than one 12-pack of beer. However, neither does he drink less. He never goes to bars to drink because "those places are full of losers." He likes to drink alone in front of the television.

He says his wife never complained about his beer, but she "was always wanting to go someplace or do something, saying she was bored when she could see I was watching TV." L. says this is why they divorced. L. say he has had his current drinking pattern for "a few years," but he and his wife divorced 18 years ago. L. says he gets along okay with people "as long they mind their own business and let me mind mine." He has Sunday dinner with his parents every week, and on most Saturdays he takes his kids out for burgers. He does not have a close male friend and he is not dating. L. says that he is not interested in women and "all that fooling-around stuff anymore."

L. is concerned because "sometimes there's a little blood when I use the toilet and I don't guess that's anything good." L. admits to having first noticed blood in his stool a "few years back." Since there wasn't blood every time, he figured he had eaten something that did not agree with him. He assumed that if there was something seriously wrong he would have felt some kind of pain, but he never had pain. He has had stomach aches now and then but he "knew" that this was normal. The only reason he is asking about it now is that the last time there seemed to be a lot more blood, and he knows a little blood is okay but he wasn't sure how much was too much.

Assessment and Management

L. is completely unable to admit to his alcoholism. All references to his alcohol consumption are made as references to watching television. His parents and ex-wife frequently complain about the fact that he watches television every night and does not allow anyone to interrupt him, but no one speaks about the 12-pack of beer every night. L. goes to great lengths to disguise and deny his drinking and to maintain almost no self-awareness of his alcohol consumption. For L., the fact that he never drinks in public or in places where others are drinking, and that he looks down upon those who do drink in public as "losers" to him means that he is not a problem drinker. The television is a very important part of L.'s denial, since watching it allows him to remain relatively unaware of the amount of alcohol he consumes. The practitioner is careful to avoid direct confrontation with L., and instead keeps the focus where L. has placed it; in this case, on the changes in his stool. Given L.'s dependence on denial, the practitioner assumes that L. is much more worried about this symptom than he is willing or able to express. The practitioner's goal is to establish a trusting relationship with L. in the hope that such a relationship will make it possible to focus on L.'s nightly drinking and his fears about possible health problems.

Bulimia Nervosa

M. is a 35-year-old high school English teacher. She has two children ages 9 and 10, and has been married and divorced twice. M. is extremely upset, saying that she "can't live like this anymore." M. says she has been out of control for about 2 weeks, bingeing and vomiting at least once a day. Her children apparently are aware of her bingeing and vomiting, because she overheard them talking. Her son, the oldest child, thinks that she is dying and doesn't want to tell the others. He told his sister that when their mother dies, they will have to go live in a home for poor children.

M. says that she started bingeing and vomiting her first year in college. She was worried about gaining weight, but all of her friends went out all the time, and "there just seemed to always be lots of candy and stuff around." No one else seemed to be gaining weight, but she was, and this was very upsetting to her. She knew about bulimia and had even had classes on it, and she had a girlfriend in high school who made herself vomit. None of this stopped her. She could not make herself diet or stay away from all the junk food, but she had to do something to avoid gaining weight.

M. admits that she also is having more difficulty controlling her behavior and is beginning to binge and vomit in public places, whereas before she never binged or vomited outside her home. A large part of her anxiety stems from her fear of being discovered at work. She thinks that she might lose her job because the school would not tolerate having someone with this problem teaching in a high school. The more anxious she becomes, the stronger the compulsion to binge becomes, and she feels like she is falling down a hole, only she never stops falling. Despite everything, M. has been able to maintain her weight, which she says is the "main thing," but a few times it was very difficult to make herself vomit, and that made her very anxious.

M. admits that in the past, one way she has been able to control her bingeing and vomiting is by drinking alcohol. It seems that, for her, it is either one or the other, and she would "rather be dead than become a drunk," but she can't do that either because she has to be there for her children, who have already been "put through too much because of me." M. states that she really doesn't know what to do, but she knows that people can die from this, and she just can't take it anymore. The practitioner asks about other changes or patterns in M.'s thoughts, feelings, or behavior and the only other thing that M. is a little concerned about is that she is getting more irritable and short with her own children and at work with her students.

Assessment and Management

M. can be referred to the clinic's eating disorders program to help her regain control, but she may also have a chronic mood disorder, possibly generalized anxiety or dysthymia that becomes more severe when she is not bulimic. However, it is important to have M. enter treatment for her disorder until she is motivated and has identified clear personal benefits to entering treatment.

Anorexia Nervosa

N. is a 17-year-old girl who is 5 ft. 6 in. tall and weighs exactly 99 lbs. She has maintained this body weight for 1 year, and she stopped menstruating about 8 months ago. N. lives at home with her mother and father, both of whom are extremely angry and frightened by their daughter's condition. N.'s parents believe that she is going to die, but N. insists that by keeping her weight at exactly 99 lb she is not in any danger and in fact may be better off, because when she weighs more she becomes depressed and has many thoughts of suicide.

According to her parents, N. exercises everyday by running 5 miles in the evening and riding a stationary bike for 1 hour every morning. The only foods N. will eat are green apples, rice cakes, nonfat yogurt, canned tuna packed in water, puffed wheat cereal with nonfat milk, and whole wheat crackers. According to N. these foods can be combined in many different ways to provide the nutrition she needs. N. feels her parents are overreacting "as usual," and that she is old enough to know what she is doing. "If it were up to them," she says, "I would have to eat peanut butter sandwiches everyday."

N. does not acknowledge her parents' fear and concern, and she suggests that they need counseling for their own problems and should leave her alone. N.'s parents say they have watched their outgoing, confident daughter become rude, angry, and full of self-hate. They are not sure what may have led their daughter to try to reduce her weight in the first place. N. was never overweight, and she was always popular at school and had many friends. N. apparently agreed to see a practitioner, on the condition that the family would follow whatever recommendations the practitioner made, and they would stop arguing about N.'s "program." Therefore, throughout the entire appointment, the parents try to convince the practitioner that N.'s life is in danger, and N. tries to convince the practitioner that her parents need couples counseling for their problems.

N. denies bingeing, vomiting, or using laxatives, diuretics, or diet pills—all of which she rejects as being "unhealthy." She also denies using drugs or alcohol. N. insists that she is not depressed, that no one has abused or harmed her, and that she is not mentally ill. In her mind she has made some difficult choices that "maybe other people would not be able to do," but she is very comfortable with herself and her "program," and she wants the practitioner to get her parents off her back. At that point her parents remind her of their agreement that the family will follow whatever recommendations the practitioner makes.

Assessment and Management

N. will be referred to the clinic's eating disorders program, but the practitioner realizes that family counseling is needed before the family will accept the referral. Right now the unresolved conflict between N. and her parents, and possibly between the two parents as well, seems to effectively maintain the status quo within the family. The practitioner also realizes that if she allows the family to give up responsibility for their choices, the referral may fail. The practitioner therefore uses family counseling to accomplish two immediate goals: to give everyone a chance to speak and be heard and to arrive at their own decisions. If the practitioner can bring the family to this point, the family will have a greater investment in the eating disorders program than they would if they follow their original plan, which is to do whatever is recommended.

The practitioner explains that before the family can talk about the eating disorders program, they should talk a few minutes about some of the things that may be on their minds right now. After explaining the ground rules of listening without interrupting, the practitioner then asks who would like to start. The father speaks up first. He says, "All I have to say is that I'm sick of all this business. What is the big deal with women and food, anyhow?" N. and her mother seem taken aback by his comment. They are surprised to learn that to him this is just bickering.

N. speaks up to say, "I guess this is mostly between me and my mother. She just makes me mad, that's all I have to say." N.'s mother comments that it makes her think her daughter is insane to see her looking like this, and it makes her feel as though she did something wrong, and she is sick of feeling like she did something wrong.

With this information, the practitioner is able to help the family to find common ground. In this case each person has failed to understand the other two. By pointing this out to the family, the practitioner is then able to recommend the eating disorders program and family therapy as methods that the family can use to gain more accurate information about each other. Now that everyone's needs are going to be given equal consideration, the family is a bit more open to moving forward, and, at the same time, a little less emphasis on N.'s weight and her "program" reframes these behaviors as N's needs rather than as her misbehavior.

Index

A

B

C

D

E

F

R

S

T